# More Healthy Years

## Why a Mediterranean diet is best for you and for the planet

**Dr Richard Hoffman, RNutr**

Published by Cambridge Editions
Copyright © Richard Hoffman, 2020

A CIP catalogue record for this book is available from the British Library.

ISBN: 9798692608376

Cambridge Editions, Bath House, Cambridge, CB1 2BD, United Kingdom
Front cover photo by Lukas at Pexels

**Disclaimer**

The publisher and the author are providing this book and its contents on an "as is" basis and make no representations or warranties of any kind with respect to this book or its contents. The publisher and the author disclaim all such representations and warranties, including but not limited to warranties of healthcare for a particular purpose. In addition, the publisher and the author assume no responsibility for errors, inaccuracies, omissions, or any other inconsistencies herein. The content of this book is for informational purposes only and is not intended to diagnose, treat, cure, or prevent any condition or disease. This book is not intended as a substitute for consultation with a licensed practitioner. The use of this book implies your acceptance of this disclaimer.

## Acknowledgements

I am extremely grateful to the University of Hertfordshire, UK for all its support and resources.

And to my wife Marella Hoffman for all her help and encouragement.

"And those who were seen dancing, were thought to be crazy, by those who could not hear the music."

Friedrich Nietzsche

# 1. Preface

I was brought up in Mansfield, a mining town in the Midlands, in the 1960's. I remember the fine market selling huge amounts of fresh produce. The market is still there, but the number of stalls selling fresh fruit and veg has dramatically decreased. Fast foods shops now dominate the food scene. Their food isn't cheaper, but for many the taste of fast food has become addictive and it's oh so much easier to pop in for an instant meal rather than cook at home.

Most people want to eat healthily, particularly to lose weight. But somehow it just doesn't happen. This is especially challenging in poorer more socially deprived areas such as Mansfield. [1] Fast food companies cynically target these areas, creating obesogenic environments that can be difficult to ignore. This further exacerbates the ever-widening health inequalities between the wealthy and the less well off. [2]

People who achieve a healthy diet in a socially deprived area deserve a special mention. They are true food heroes, people who rise up beyond the norms of their environment despite their adversity. Sociologists label them positive deviants [1]. They can offer much useful advice to others who are less able to resist their unhealthy environment and deserve more attention in a society grappling with the problems of obesity.

But it's far from easy. Even the current head of the NHS Simon Stevens admitted to putting on weight when he worked in the US, a fact he attributed to the ease of eating junk food. [3] He managed to lose the excess weight when

---

1 Mansfield now has one of the worst prospects for social mobility in England
http://www.bbc.co.uk/news/education-42112436.
2 https://publichealthmatters.blog.gov.uk/2016/10/21/obesity-and-the-environment-the-impact-of-fast-food/
3 https://www.politicshome.com/news/uk/health-and-care/house/62885/simon-stevens-interview-tackling-obesity-not-just-health-issue

he returned to the UK, and he summed up his success in three words: *Eat. Less. Rubbish.*

And in a nutshell that sums up this book. It is a simple enough message and yet it does not come without controversy. Certainly, there are still areas of nutrition research where the evidence is inadequate to draw consistent conclusions. But to quote the eminent epidemiologist Sir Austin Bradford Hill "All scientific work is incomplete... That does not confer upon us a freedom to ignore the knowledge we already have, or to postpone the action it appears to demand at a given time" [2]. Although nutrition research may appear to generate conflicting conclusions and advice, there is in fact remarkable consensus amongst the real experts. It is these views that I mainly convey. Where there are still areas of disagreement even among the experts, such as an acceptable level of alcohol consumption, I have tried to give a fair account. As a Registered Nutritionist, I uphold their professional standards, and I can declare that my views have been reached with no commercial conflicts of interest.

I write this book from 20 years experience of research in nutrition as well as teaching nutrition at university level to nutritionists and dietitians.[4] I also had many years experience working in cancer research as well university training in the biochemistry of plants. So I bring a very wide perspective on the subject of nutrition, one that also includes the agricultural and medical sciences. I have been writing about the Mediterranean diet for the last 10 years - the main diet I recommend in this book - and I also published a detailed academic book on this diet in 2011 [3].

---

[4] The preferred spelling in the profession - not "dieticians".

# 2. Introduction

## A simple message

Each meal we eat makes us a little healthier or a little less healthy. It is now clear: our food choice is the single most important way we decide whether to live fewer or more healthy years. [5]

There is widespread consensus from the experts that a healthy diet consists of "minimally processed foods close to nature" [4]. Or in author Michael Pollan's famous aphorism "Eat food. Not too much. Mostly plants". [6] This consensus to eat mostly plant foods and to keep it natural has been the standard message from nutritionists, dietitians and other health professionals for many years. And yet many people are unclear what this actually means in practice and how to fit it into their daily lives. There is much confusion, much of which is generated by the many vested interests competing to influence what we eat. So how can we overcome these barriers to healthy eating in a way that is compatible with our own values and lifestyle?

A good place to start is by expanding on the definition of a healthy diet. In November 2015 in Boston, US some of the world's top nutritionists issued a statement reaffirming that a healthy diet is based on natural foods and that it should be "higher in vegetables, fruits, whole grains, low- or non-fat dairy, seafood, legumes, and nuts; moderate in alcohol (among adults); lower in red and processed meats; and low in sugar-sweetened foods and drinks and refined grains." [7] The Boston group didn't come up with a list of industrial products, nutrient supplements or even super-foods. The foundations of healthy eating have stayed constant even while ever more glorified edifices to industrialised foods are constructed.

---

[5] Poor diet has now overtaken smoking as the leading cause of premature death in England and many other western countries. Newton JN, Briggs AD, Murray CJ *et al.* (2015) Changes in health in England, with analysis by English regions and areas of deprivation, 1990-2013: a systematic analysis for the Global Burden of Disease Study 2013. *Lancet* **386**, 2257-2274.
[6] From his seminal book *In Defense of Food*
[7] Oldways Common Ground Consensus Statement on Healthy Eating 2015
https://oldwayspt.org/programs/oldways-common-ground/oldways-common-ground-consensus

Of course, simply defining a healthy diet is only a first step. It is clear that this has been insufficient to prevent the massive increase in diet-related chronic health disorders, such as obesity, heart disease and type 2 diabetes. In the UK, the official set of recommended dietary guidelines is encapsulated in the "Eatwell Guide". But overall adherence to these guidelines is very low, with one study finding that less than 0.1% of a sample of people were adhering to nine of its recommendations (such as eating five-a-day fruit and veg and oily fish once a week) [5]. If only 0.1% of patients were taking a recommended medication there would be serious concern and immediate action to remedy this. This same urgency seems lacking in removing the barriers to healthy eating.

Many people would like to be eating more healthily but do not achieve this. Because there are many reasons for this, this book takes a broad perspective on how to switch to a healthy diet. It may be taste that matters most to you, or convenience or cost or health or concerns for the environment. These are all covered in this book.

In chapter 3 I describe the current toll taken by diet-related diseases, and I argue that more public resources should be put into extending the number of years lived free from disease rather than simply extending lifespan. A healthy diet is the most important way to achieve this. Chapter 4 then delves into the sometimes murky world of the many vested interests that influence our dietary choices. Understanding how and why they are trying to influence our eating decisions can make it easier to resist them. Like fake news, these vested influences often use false or manipulated information - they are spreading "fake nutrition". To help counter this, in chapter 5 I show how nutritionists have established more trustworthy associations between poor diet and ill health. This chapter also emphasises how important its is to consider your own circumstances and not to rely on "population averages".

The next few chapters discuss what is and what isn't a healthy diet. Chapter 6 describes the building blocks of a healthy diet: its carbohydrates, fats, protein, vitamins, minerals and plant chemicals. This chapter shows why the best way to achieve an optimal balance of these nutrients is by eating a diet based on natural foods. Unfortunately, a diet of natural foods is at odds with the more typical diet in the west, which includes junk foods. These foods are described in chapter 7. They are usually high in calories and low in beneficial nutrients, and the result is that many people are "overfed and undernourished". This chapter argues that it is because we have evolved to consume natural foods that they are optimal for our health whereas we are ill adapted to handle junk foods.

Understanding nutrients is helpful, but our unit of eating is a meal and not individual nutrients. Hence we need to consider eating from the more holistic perspective of a meal, not least because it is the only way to take into account how nutrients in a meal interact. This is discussed in chapter 8. By chapter 9 we are ready to consider all the elements that make up the healthiest of all diets - and the diet of choice in this book - the Mediterranean diet. The Med diet is rich in healthy nutrients, foods and meals and minimises consumption of junk foods. A Med diet achieves an excellent balance between nutrients and calories. Although not primarily seen as a weight-reduction diet, the Med diet has been shown to be effective for preventing weight gain. By focusing on nutrient-rich foods, there is no need to count the calories when eating this diet. In other words, "Don't count the calories; make the calories count". This chapter also shows that to fully benefit from a Med diet means going well beyond just the food on the plate and to consider social aspects such as sitting down to eat together, and even the benefits of taking a siesta!

The Med diet reduces the risk of a remarkably wide range of chronic diseases, including heart disease, some types of cancer, type 2 diabetes and Alzheimer's disease. Chapters 10 and 11 argue that the underlying reason for this is that these seemingly distinct diseases have many similarities in their early stages, and it is these early stages where a Med diet intervenes. Hence a Med diet can prevent the later stages of many different diseases from developing. I have called these early common stages between chronic diseases the Core Risk States. There are three: oxidative stress, chronic inflammation and insulin resistance. I show that understanding how a Med diet suppresses these three Core Risk States provides a new framework for understanding how the Med diet works.

All this information is no good without action! And so the next few chapters show how to put eating a Med diet into practice. Chapter 12 covers the different types of foods eaten in a Med diet. I describe which foods to choose for their health benefits and how to cook foods in ways that retain their nutrients and that prevent the formation of harmful substances (particularly important for meat). Chapter 13 then shows how to create a Med diet larder and how to shop and organise meals the Med way. Shopping only once a week is entirely feasible.

The environmental crisis is highlighting that eating a healthy diet will not be sustainable without changing our farming system. The present trajectory of industrial farming is seriously harming the ecology of our planet and threatens our own survival. Chapter 14 shows how the foods for a Med diet can be produced by a highly sustainable farming system called agroecology that is good for personal health, for animal welfare and for the environment.

## Why choose the Med diet?

Every year a group of esteemed nutritionists and medical scientists scrutinise the latest scientific evidence and decide on the best diet in the world. In 2020, and for the third year in a row, this accolade was awarded to the Mediterranean diet. [8] It was not only its nutritious-ness that earned the Med diet its first place, but also because it is easy it is to follow, safe, effective for weight loss, and protective against diabetes and heart disease.

These criteria, important though they are, are not all that needs to be considered. A diet must also be socially and culturally acceptable. This broad view was incorporated in the definition of a sustainable diet by the Food and Agriculture Organisation (FAO) of the United Nations when it identified a sustainable diet as one that should also be culturally acceptable. Many diets considered healthy - such as a traditional Japanese diet, vegetarianism and veganism - are fine for their adherents, but are unlikely to be culturally acceptable to most people living in the UK and other western countries. By including a low amount of meat, the Med diet steers a middle course between high meat diets such as the paleo diet and no-meat diets. The surge in popularity of the flexitarian diet [9] - which resembles the Med diet in many ways - demonstrates the widespread support for eating less meat. According to research from Kantar Worldpanel, 41% of meat eaters currently classify themselves as flexitarian and the percentage of meat-free evening meals is on the rise in Britain. [10]

---

[8] In 2020 a team of 25 of the world's top nutritionists judged 41 diets.
https://health.usnews.com/best-diet/best-diets-overall
[9]https://www.theguardian.com/environment/2019/jan/19/could-flexitarianism-save-the-planet
[10] Cited in The Future of Food 2040. NFU

The health credentials of the Med diet have been scrutinised from all angles: epidemiologists observing and analysing the eating preferences of people living in society and in carefully controlled metabolic chambers; physiologists conducting experiments with animals and cell systems to determine how various nutrients work; and molecular biologists peering into the very DNA of cells to determine how diet switches on and off genes. It is remarkable how almost without exception these studies demonstrate that the Med diet is extremely healthy, significantly reducing the likelihood of dying prematurely from heart disease, type 2 diabetes, cancer and many others. And if the long-term benefits of eating a Med diet are not enough to incentivise you, then consider possible short-term benefits on mood. In one study, healthy young women felt more alert and content after eating a Med diet for 10 days - a benefit that was lost when they switched to their normal diet [6]. Interest in the effects of the Med diet on the brain is a growing area of research and its benefits on memory and overall cognitive function have important implications for dementia prevention [7].

So what is it about the Med diet that makes it so special? First and foremost, it is based on natural foods that have undergone minimal processing and it avoids foods that are industrially produced and highly processed. Secondly, although it is based on plant foods, the Med diet is not vegetarian. We evolved as omnivores, and animal products - meat, fish, eggs and dairy - provide essential nutrients that are more difficult to obtain or are completely absent in plants foods (such as some types of omega-3 fats and vitamin B12). Although the amount of meat eaten in the Med diet is similar to the flexitarian diet, the Med diet differs from the flexitarian diet by including two emblematic foods with well-proven health benefits, namely extra virgin olive oil and wine (drunk in moderation and with a meal). Thirdly, is the exceptional diversity of foods in the Med diet, because of its many different cuisines, such as those of Greece, Italy, Spain and Morocco. And lastly, eating a Med diet gives hope for the planet since it can arise from an agricultural system that is sustainable and respectful of biodiversity and ecosystems.

Many individuals now recognise that eating responsibly for the sake of future generations is hugely important. They are moving beyond being mere passive food consumers to becoming actively engaged food citizens prepared to make choices based on sustainability.[11] Choices based not only around dietary health and climate change, but also around issues such as animal welfare and the use of pesticides and its effects on insect and bird populations. There is a huge groundswell of voices demanding change, from lone voices through to high-level international think tanks. [12] Eating a Med diet is one of the best ways to become an active food citizen rather than a passive food consumer.

Eating healthily does not require the huge resources needed to find a cure for cancer or to create energy from nuclear fusion. Unlike these challenges, the solution to healthy eating is - more-or-less - known. Indeed, many households don't have much to learn from nutrition science since, each day, they sit down to eat a meal of traditional Mediterranean foods. They are eating foods that have been part of their culture for many generations. I hope this book will help you too make a Med diet part of your daily life.

## Using this book

This book covers an unusual breadth of topics for a book on healthy eating. Although the chapters are ordered to develop understanding, it is not necessary to read the book sequentially. If you want to go straight to the practicalities of healthy eating the Med way and how to incorporate it into daily life, a good place to start is with chapters 12 and 13. Or if you are interested in how the Med diet works, this is discussed in chapters 10 and 11. Sustainability issues are described in chapter. 14.

I give two types of references to further reading. Firstly, those designated by superscript numbers after the ends of sentences, (eg A sentence. [1]) are to mainly open-access articles in the media and are given as footnotes on each page. Secondly, those designated by superscript numbers in brackets within sentences (eg A sentence [1].) are references to scientific journal articles and reports and these are listed at the back of the book. (Some of these are not open-access.)

There are lists of abbreviations and definitions of some terms in the Appendices at the back of the book.

---

[11] Further information on how to engage as a food citizen here:
https://www.foodethicscouncil.org/our-work/food-citizenship.html
[12] See, for example, the International Panel of Experts on Sustainable Food Systems (IPES-Food) at http://www.ipes-food.org/

# 3. Putting disease prevention centre stage

## Overview

The NHS spends many millions trying to keep people alive in hospitals for a few weeks at the end of their lives. By contrast, less than 5% of the NHS budget is used to prevent or delay the chronic diseases such as cardiovascular disease, cancer and dementia that degrade people's lives for many years. And yet prevention is better than cure not only for the patient but also for society because in the long term it is far cheaper. Fortunately we have a powerful defence against the early stages of these chronic diseases. And that defence is a healthy lifestyle: not smoking, keeping a healthy weight, diet and exercise. This chapter argues that a far higher proportion of health resources should be used to promote these healthy lifestyle factors. Of these, promoting a healthy diet is the most important way of all to achieve more healthy years.

## Fewer healthy years

In 1965, when the former USSR switched spending from social services to defence, there began a period of rising insecurity, stress, and alcohol abuse. During this period there was also a significant decline in life expectancy, suggesting that when societies do not receive the support they need, lifespan can suffer.[13] Lifespan is an important social barometer.

Lifespan has now started to decline in the US too - something not seen since the American civil war [8]. The trend is similar in the UK, where life expectancy stalled in 2018, and more recently has started to decline [9]. Noting these trends, the UK pension industry in 2019 revised downwards its estimates for life expectancies for 65 year old men to 86.9 years, down from its previous figure of 87.4 years, and for 65 year old women to 89.2 years, down from 89.7 years [10]. [14] These downward trends of only a few months may seem trivial. But they are in stark contrast to the year on year increase in

---

[13] https://hbr.org/2017/06/white-americans-mortality-rates-are-rising-something-similar-happened-in-russia-from-1965-to-2005
[14] https://www.theguardian.com/society/2019/mar/07/life-expectancy-slumps-by-five-months

life expectancy experienced during the last 150 years, a period when life expectancy increased by about one year every four years.

The main reason for shorter life expectancies in industrialised countries is the rise in chronic diseases. Chronic diseases typically develop over many years, and even though symptoms can often be managed, for many of these diseases there is no cure. Chronic diseases target almost all major organs in the body. The brain, damaged from dementia, Parkinson's disease or a stroke, will kill half of women in the UK. [15] Heart disease is the number one cause of death in men and second in women in England. And lung diseases, mainly cancer and chronic obstructive pulmonary disease (COPD), rank high as causes of death - legacies of high rates of smoking. Many organs are afflicted by cancers, especially the colon and prostate in men, and breast in women, and all are significant causes of mortality. A malfunctioning pancreas results in type 2 diabetes, which, although not often a direct cause of death, will on average result in death six years sooner than someone without diabetes. This is mainly because of a diabetic's increased risk of heart disease and stroke.

Death from chronic diseases is the main reason why people from lower socio-economic groups often have lower life expectancies. It is not only in the former USSR where social factors are blamed for declining lifespans: socio-economic factors also go a long way to explaining the differences in the health of socio-economic groups in countries such as the UK. The stats are damning indeed. Life expectancy is nine years less for UK men who live in the most deprived areas compared to their counterparts in the least deprived areas (74 versus 83 years; for women the corresponding figures are 79 and 86 years). [16] In England, half of the reduced life expectancy in the most deprived fifth of society compared to the least deprived fifth is due to death from heart disease, stroke and cancers [11].

As well as overall lifespan, another important indicator of the health of a nation is the risk of dying prematurely. In the UK, the risk of dying prematurely is defined as dying before the age of 75 years. And just as overall life expectancy is decreasing, so too the risk of dying prematurely is

---

[15] https://www.theguardian.com/society/2018/oct/01/half-of-women-will-develop-dementia-or-parkinsons-or-have-a-stroke
[16] https://www.gov.uk/government/publications/health-profile-for-england/chapter-5-inequality-in-health

increasing. Chronic diseases are responsible for 80% of all deaths before the age of 75 in England. Rather than the dementias of old age, premature deaths in middle-aged women are mainly caused by lung and breast cancers and by heart disease. For men, heart disease is the top cause of death for 50 to 79 year olds.

Of course, trends in increasing life expectancy cannot carry on indefinitely - or at least not until there is some major breakthrough in our understanding of the aging process. But the life expectancies of the elderly in countries such as the UK or US have a long way to go before they catch up with life expectancies in some other industrialised countries. For instance, French and Japanese women and Swiss men live far longer than their British counterparts. This shows that far fewer people in the UK or US are living out their full biological potential.

## Healthspan

For many people, maximising the number of years lived in good health is more important than maximising lifespan. These years have been dubbed a person's "healthspan". In a memorable phrase by Professor David Katz "it is not only the years of life that matter, but also the life in those years". Improving healthspan is a huge growth area in the health care sector. Improving the number of years in good health is also more responsive than lifespan to personal lifestyle changes such as diet and exercise than overall lifespan. We now have the "wellderley" generation.

Defining "healthy years" is not straightforward. One way is by the number of years a person lives free from disability. The converse is also frequently used, namely the number of years a person lives *with* a disability (YLDs). YLD indicates the overall loss of quality of life. YLD is now increasing in some countries. In a UK government survey, adults were asked: 'How is your health in general; would you say it was... very good, good, fair, bad, or very bad?' The survey found that women on average reported living about sixty-two years in good health and men sixty-three years. [17] Comparing this with

---

[17] https://www.gov.uk/government/publications/health-profile-for-england/chapter-1-life-expectancy-and-healthy-life-expectancy

This is a subjective measure, obtained by asking a sample of people if they are in good health or not. It reports that women live in good health for 63.9 years old on average. However, recently piloted objective population-wide the NHS data shows that on average women fall out of their

previous estimates shows that as a proportion of overall lifespan the number of years lived in good health is now declining in England.[18]

As for overall lifespan, a person's socio-economic group has a major influence on their years lived with a disability. Men and women in England from the most socially deprived group live on average only 52 years in good health [12]. [19] If these men and women attained the years lived in good health of the best, they would have nineteen more healthy years. [20] This tragic deprivation of a healthy life is not only socially unjust for the individual, but it also has a huge impact on that person's family and friends and on wider society.

YLD is a metric used to compare health between countries. The largest of these studies, called the Global Burden of Disease study, has calculated the YLDs and their causes for many countries. For England, the Global Burden of Disease study found that the most common reasons for disability were musculoskeletal problems (such as lower back and neck pain), mental disorders and poor sight or hearing. Usually, these disabilities are readily noticed and diagnosed.

This is not the case, however, for many of the early pathological changes that lead to chronic disease. For instance, many people with hypertension and atherosclerosis are unaware they have these conditions - even though they are precursors to heart disease. And many people have undetected elevated blood glucose - a precursor for type 2 diabetes. For example, for every ten people with hypertension, four are undiagnosed, which equates to around 26,000 people in every local health area in England. [21] Similarly, large numbers of people with atrial fibrillation and type 2 diabetes, both conditions that dramatically increase the risk of cardiovascular disease (CVD), are undiagnosed or under-treated [13]. Hence many people at high risk of chronic

'generally healthy / well' status, by developing one of 26 serious long-term conditions, when they are only 55 years old.
See p. 6 in The Health of the Nation report 2020
[18] For EU stats see https://ec.europa.eu/eurostat/statistics-explained/index.php?title=Healthy_life_years_statistics
[19] CMO Annual Report 2018. https://www.theguardian.com/society/2019/sep/15/inequality-healthy-life-expectancy-gap-widens
[20] There is also a gap of nine years life expectancy between the most socially advantaged fifth of the English population and the most socially deprived fifth of the population.
[21] British Heart Foundation. High blood pressure: how can we do better? Online: British Heart Foundation; 2016 [Available from: www.bhf.org. uk/healthcare-professionals/bp-how-can-we-do-better].

diseases do not receive the lifestyle advice and medical treatment they need: advice and treatment that could have prevented a fatal heart attack, stroke or cancer.

"Healthspan" is therefore really something of a misnomer since it only indicates being free from *visible* disability. Many people living their "healthy years" will have underlying early stages of a chronic disease: an undetected smoldering fire [14]. And whereas most people with visible disabilities such as musculoskeletal problems receive appropriate treatment, people with undiagnosed early stages of chronic diseases often do not, even though it is chronic diseases that are most likely to shorten lifespan.

Fortunately we have one major power defence against the early stages of chronic diseases. And that defence is a healthy lifestyle, especially diet and exercise. We all eat and move and how we do these things strongly influences our risk of chronic diseases. It is how to eat well to prevent chronic diseases that is the main theme of this book.

## Obesity

Even though the early stages of chronic diseases often go unnoticed, there is one very visible signal that indicates that all is not well. And that is obesity. Hippocrates once wrote, with great perspicacity, "corpulence is not only a disease itself, but the harbinger of others". He categorised obesity as a medical disorder that also leads to many other diseases (so-called comorbidities). Opinion today is divided about whether or not obesity should itself be called a chronic disease [15]. [22] However, the medical profession is united in the view that being overweight or obese (ie having a high body mass index, BMI) is a leading cause of disability, when taking into account both life-threatening chronic diseases and also common disabilities such as lower back pain. [23]

Obese people are at especially high risk of developing type 2 diabetes. Indeed, obesity is by far the most important risk factor for type 2 diabetes (far more important than genetic risk factors) [16]. Women with a BMI of 30 (which is classed as borderline obese) are 28 times more likely to develop diabetes than women of normal weight, and this risk rises rapidly as BMI increases [17]. Some types of cancer are also linked to obesity, and in the UK obesity now

---

[22] https://www.livestrong.com/article/13721733-is-obesity-a-disease
[23] HM Government. July 2019 Advancing Our Health: Prevention in the 2020s

rivals smoking as a cancer risk factor. [24] Obesity also increases the risk of many other chronic diseases such as CVD and dementia. The importance of obesity as a cause of health inequalities between socio-economic groups is less clear, at least in the UK. This is because although men from lower socio-economic groups have a higher prevalence of many chronic diseases than men from higher socio-economic groups, they are not more obese.

Many countries stand on the threshold of rampant levels of obesity. For the first time in human history, the majority of the human race is either overweight or obese. It is predicted that over one billion people, or approximately one in five of the world's entire adult population, will be obese by 2030 [18]. No country has successfully reduced their prevalence of obesity: the fight against obesity is not being won. Some current trends in the perception of obesity are worrying. Mark Pearson, deputy director of employment, labour and social affairs at the OECD, noted that obesity had become "the new normal" in Britain. This has profound implications for how health and disease are viewed. People in the UK "look around and they see this is normal, in a way that you don't see in other European countries," he said. [25] This normalisation is extremely concerning as it makes change far more difficult. [26] And some indicators suggest that fewer people are trying to lose weight [19].

Once obesity becomes normalised, society transitions into a post-obesity state where, rather than tackling obesity, the emphasis shifts to dealing with the consequences of obesity. This is a dangerous state to adopt. Apart from the health consequences of this to individuals, a post-obesity society is massively expensive for society and unlikely to be sustainable. The scale of the problem means that tackling obesity is unlikely to succeed without government initiatives. But governments are often slow to act. The former Chief Medical Officer in the UK Dame Sally Davies once said "healthy people are the number asset for a healthy nation" [20]. But this view often seems to be poorly

---

[24] https://www.theguardian.com/society/2019/jul/03/obesity-rivals-smoking-as-cause-of-cancer-uk-charity-warns

[25] https://www.telegraph.co.uk/news/2017/11/10/britain-sixth-fattest-nation-world-rising-faster-united-states/

[26] https://www.theguardian.com/commentisfree/2018/apr/10/fat-pride-obesity-public-health-warnings-dangerous-weight-levels
https://mothernaturesdiet.me/2016/12/06/are-we-normalising-obesity/
https://www.worldobesity.org/

reflected in government policies. Health initiatives are often too little too late - as demonstrated by the failure to prevent the current downturn in healthy life expectancy. The UK government's green paper on preventing ill health published in July 2019 demonstrated little interest in legislating to curb unhealthy eating even though its own figures show that a high BMI is the top reason for fewer healthy years [21].

## Taking personal responsibility

Medical interventions make a relatively small contribution to health - perhaps only 15% of preventable mortality in the US. It is social factors such as income, education, and employment that are more important [22]. This puts socio-economic inequalities centre-stage in the debate on health. Sir Michael Marmot in 2010 in his landmark report "The Marmot Review: Fair Society, Healthy Lives" highlighted the wide range of social factors that contribute to the huge health divide in the UK. [27] Widening inequities in UK society such as in education, employment, and economic prosperity are likely to be major contributors to the recent slowdown in cancer survival, the dramatic rise in poor mental health, and to the unexpected increase in CVD deaths in the UK among people aged 75 years and younger announced by the British Heart Foundation in 2019 - the first such rise in half a century [23].

Narrowing health inequalities has been a government policy for many years. But rather than decreasing, these are increasing [12]. UK governments have failed to implement meaningful and timely action. Budget cuts drive social inequities and are important barriers to improvements in health. A joint analysis by the respected UK think tanks the Health Foundation and the King's Fund estimated that by 2021 public health budgets in the UK will have been slashed by around 25% per head in real terms since 2015-16. [28] These echoes of the former USSR cutbacks are worrying. Mortality rates amongst the over 85's have been rising in England since 2010, and this has been directly attributed to reductions in spending on income support for poor

---

[27] The report was updated in 2020: https://www.health.org.uk/videos/watch-the-marmot-review-10-years-on.
[28] Health charities make urgent call for £1 billion a year to reverse cuts to public health funding. King's Fund. Jun 2019.
https://www.kingsfund.org.uk/press/press-releases/reverse-cuts-public-health-funding.

pensioners and social care [24]. Austerity is directly impacting on some of the most vulnerable members of our society.

The role of implementing UK government health policy falls on the NHS. Advances in medical interventions have hugely increased the ability to detect and treat heart disease, cancer and so on. Many people who only a decade ago would have died are now surviving these diseases. But although these advances improve lifespans they do little to improve healthspans since they are not designed to prevent the disease processes from being initiated. Extending healthspan is all about prevention.

Prevention is better than cure not only for the patient but also for society because in the long term it is far cheaper. It is now abundantly clear that keeping up with the ever-increasing costs of treating chronic diseases such as CVD, type 2 diabetes, cancers and dementia will soon bankrupt many health systems. A report by the American Heart Association summed it up: "What we spend on cardiovascular disease is not sustainable. But we can afford to prevent it. Ultimately, we can't afford not to." Despite this stark warning, current funding for prevention is dismal, and in the UK prevention receives a paltry 5% of UK health research funding. Funding for wider innovation in public health and social care has also remained scarce [25]. As a UK parliamentary report stated " The NHS spends many millions trying to keep people alive in hospitals for a few weeks at the end of their lives. Yet it spends less than 5% of its budget to prevent or delay diseases and impairments that degrade people's lives for many years" [26].

The cost of treating chronic diseases can be illustrated with coronary heart disease (CHD) [27]. The direct cost of CHD to the UK health-care system has been established by the British Heart Foundation Statistic Database to be around £3.2 billion in 2006, which represents a per capita cost of £50 with hospital care, representing 73% of these costs (British Heart Foundation Statistic Database 2008). However, looking just at health-care costs underestimates the total cost, as production losses because of death and illness in those of working age and from the informal care of people with the disease contribute greatly to the overall financial burden. Production losses because of mortality and morbidity associated with CHD cost the UK over £3.9 billion, with around 65% of the cost because of death and 35% because of illness of those of working age; informal care costs a further £1.9 billion/year. The overall cost to the UK economy of CHD was estimated at

22

nearly £9.0 billion when health-care costs, productivity costs and informal care are taken into account. [29]

To make a fundamental switch of focus from disease treatment, with its reliance on medicines and medical devices, to disease prevention will require a huge overhaul in the way health systems operate. So is there any likelihood that our current system based on treating disease - a National Disease Service - will re-prioritise and put maintaining health at its heart and so truly become a National Service for Health? I believe the answer is a cautiously optimistic yes. Although the NHS in the UK and other health systems around the world have deeply engrained cultures to prioritise treatment, there are signs of a slow reorientation of health care to prevention. The NHS Five Year Forward View report from 2014 stated that "the future health of millions of children, the sustainability of the NHS, and the economic prosperity of Britain all now depend on a radical upgrade in prevention and public health". In France, the new five year health plan implemented in 2019 puts prevention at the heart of the health system. [30] A cautionary note must however be injected. As the NHS Five Year Forward View report remarked "Twelve years ago, Derek Wanless' health review warned that unless the country took prevention seriously we would be faced with a sharply rising burden of avoidable illness. That warning has not been heeded - and the NHS is on the hook for the consequences." Let's hope that this time the warnings will indeed be heeded.

One stand-out prevention initiative in England is the NHS Health Checks programme. This GP-led initiative is designed to detect increased risk in 40-74 year olds of heart disease, stroke, type 2 diabetes and kidney disease, and to raise awareness of dementia. It does this by monitoring for early signs of increased disease risk such as elevated cholesterol and raised blood pressure. A recent evaluation found significant improvements in detecting increased risk for diseases especially CVD [13]. People who attend an NHS Health Check are more likely to receive advice and treatment for their risk factors and their risk of those diseases tested for by a health check decreased over six years' follow-up [28]. [31]

---

[29] British Heart Foundation Statistic Database 2008

[30] http://www.lefigaro.fr/conjoncture/2018/09/17/20002-20180917ARTFIG00342-macron-devoile-son-plan-pour-transformer-le-systeme-francais-de-sante.php

[31] https://www.medscape.com/viewarticle/916234?nlid=130896_5144&src=WNL_ukmdpls_1 90731_mscpedit_gen&uac=309816EK&impID=2045610&faf=1

Although this all sounds very positive, the Health Checks programme is under continual critical scrutiny, even attack. Many argue that the small gains in health are not justified by the programme's cost and pressure from some critics could lead to the Health Check programme being abandoned. I believe this would be a great loss to preventative medicine in the UK.

So why are current health gains with the Health Checks programme so modest? A major reason is that follow-up is dominated by medical interventions - especially prescribing statins for high blood cholesterol - rather than lifestyle approaches. GPs - the main managers of the health checks programme - receive very little training and typically (although there are exceptions) have little interest in lifestyle issues. Hence they have a preference, or even discrimination, towards medical interventions. A recent major report on the Health Checks programme was critical of the "marked absence of research on the impact of the programme on lifestyle behaviours" [13].

Since most GPs still operate within a health system structured to train doctors to treat disease with drugs, one possible solution is to develop more medications that help prevent diseases, just as statins do by reducing cholesterol levels. These "disease prevention drugs" are hugely attractive for drug companies since they are likely to be used over many years, resulting in large sales. As early pathological changes are identified in diseases such as Alzheimer's and CVD, drug companies are developing new drugs, not least because these early pathological changes may be more amenable to intervention. One example is the "polypill". Polypills contain various combinations of drugs used to lower blood pressure and fats in the blood and have been approved in more than 30 countries to prevent premature mortality from atherosclerosis. However, although they are seen as useful for some people [29], their wider benefits are still unclear and side-effects can be significant [30].

It is disappointing that there is a paucity of effective disease prevention drugs free from side-effects that can tackle the problems identified in disease prevention services such as the NHS Health Check. This contrasts with the medical advances, especially vaccines and antibiotics, which have proven so successful in helping defeat infectious agents. However, whereas infectious diseases are caused by specific viruses and bacteria and so can be specifically targeted with vaccines and antibiotics - so-called "magic bullets", chronic diseases, by contrast, wage slow, complex wars of attrition against our organs.

Few magic bullets can target this type of attack.

Some researchers are extremely critical of the huge amounts of money going into the persistent search for new and expensive medical interventions and drugs to solve the problem of chronic diseases. Medicalising chronic diseases by focusing resources into looking for cures through new medicines has been dubbed a "perpetual delusion" [31] and is leading to spiraling health costs [32]. Without greatly expanding support for lifestyle interventions, especially dietary advice, it is my view that the potential benefits of the Health Check programme will never be realised.

Even though a healthy lifestyle is a proven, safe and effective way to avoid the scourge of chronic disease, health systems change slowly. There is little doubt that a new *modus operandi* will take time to implement. GPs currently receive very little training in lifestyle-related approaches to disease prevention through diet and physical activity, and so are ill equipped to impart this information. So at the moment, self-help is the name of the game for disease prevention.

## Achieving more healthy years

Many studies have confirmed that adopting a healthy lifestyle is an effective way of extending healthspan. This can be illustrated with the results from studies of two large cohorts of Americans who have been used in many health studies. One is a cohort known as the "Nurses' Health Study" which recruited over 70,000 female nurses from 1980 until 2014. And the second is a cohort, the "Health Professionals Follow-Up Study", which recruited 38,000 male health professionals (such as dentists and optometrists) from 1986 until 2014. Participants were middle aged when initially recruited. The men lived 7.6 years more free from diabetes, CVD and cancer and the women 10 more years free from these diseases if they had adopted five specific healthy lifestyle factors compared to men and women not adopting any of these lifestyle factors [33]. These lifestyle factors were:

- not smoking
- keeping a healthy weight
- doing at least 30 minutes moderate to vigorous physical activity each day
- moderate alcohol intake
- eating a healthy diet

Another group who have been studied for the exceptionally long period of their lives spent disease-free are people who live in the so-called "Blue Zone regions" of the world. The Blue Zone regions include two Mediterranean islands (Sardinia in Italy and Ikaria in Greece), Okinawa in Japan, Loma Linda in California, USA, and the Nicoya peninsula in Costa Rica. These people commonly live disease-free until at least the age of 75 and are testimony to the potential of humans, even when relatively economically deprived, to live long and healthy lives. Being socially active, physically active and having a healthy diet probably all contribute to their many years of healthy life [34; 35]. Few of us live in the Blue Zone regions, but citizens around the world can learn from these people about how to delay entering the red danger zone of chronic illness and frailty.

Some people are tempted to apportion blame for their poor health on their genes and claim that a healthy lifestyle will make little difference, a stance reinforced by headlines such as "Thinness and obesity: it's in the genes". [32] Inheriting a good set of genes helps, of course, but for the vast majority of people lifestyle is far more influential. In the case of obesity, perhaps the most convincing evidence that nature (environmental factors) is far more important than nurture (our genes) is the fact that although our genes haven't changed over the last few decades, there has been a dramatic increase in obesity during this period. In England over the last quarter of a century or so (from 1993 to 2017) rates of obesity have almost doubled (from 15% to 29%) with similar increases in many other parts of the world. [33] For cancer, nearly half of all cancer deaths in the US have been attributed to potentially avoidable risk factors, especially smoking, rather than to genetic predisposition [36]. It is now clear that that environmental factors are the major cause of most chronic diseases.

## Nature versus nurture

Even when genes do increase the risk of disease, a healthy lifestyle may be able to negate this. This has been shown even for that most feared of diseases, dementia. In a study from the UK, almost 200,000 people over 60 were analysed for their "risk" genes for dementia and then followed for a number of years to see who developed dementia. The people who followed a healthy lifestyle including not smoking, regular physical activity, a healthy diet, and

[32] https://www.theguardian.com/society/2019/jan/24/thinness-and-obesity-its-in-the-genes
[33] Baker, C (2019) Obesity Statistics House of Commons Briefing Paper 6 August 2019

moderate alcohol all showed a similar reduction in their risk of dementia regardless of how many "risk" genes for dementia they had [37]. [34] This large study clearly demonstrated that a healthy lifestyle can trump risk genes for dementia.

Risk genes should not be completely discounted as they clearly do make some contribution to chronic diseases. This is more so with cancer than most other chronic diseases. But even in the case of cancer, it is estimated that four in ten cases could be prevented by lifestyle changes. [35]

Not surprisingly, adopting a healthy lifestyle as early as possible gives the best chance of being able to lead a long and active retirement. In one study of British adults, a healthy diet in middle age was a strong predictor of subsequent healthy aging - which in this study was defined as good cardiovascular, metabolic, musculoskeletal, respiratory, mental, and cognitive health [38]. "Old age is the verdict of life", said the British novelist Amelia E Barr. And our old age will be judged by the healthy behaviours we adopt in midlife to preserve physical and mental function.

## A healthy diet is key to more healthy years

In England, a poor diet is the leading cause of years lived with a disability (see Figure) [39]. In the UK as a whole, eating a poor diet reduces healthspan by two to four years. Smoking, by comparison only reduces healthspan by, on average, one to two years [40]. A poor diet is linked to many different risk factors for chronic diseases. For instance, poor diet can raise blood pressure, BMI, blood cholesterol and blood glucose levels, all factors that then increase the risk of CVD. There is no one single food in a poor diet responsible for these changes. In global rankings, salt is the main dietary cause of high blood pressure and the leading dietary cause of premature death. [36] This is followed in rankings by a diet low in whole grains - which may surprise many more familiar with the main diet message of the need to eat more fruit and veg (which came in third and fifth respectively in the rankings).

---

[34] https://www.theguardian.com/society/2019/jul/14/healthy-lifestyle-may-cut-risk-of-dementia-regardless-of-genes

[35] https://www.theguardian.com/society/2018/mar/23/four-in-10-cancer-cases-could-be-prevented-by-lifestyle-changes

[36] Https://www.Theguardian.Com/Society/2018/Nov/08/Poor-Diet-A-Factor-In-One-Fifth-Of-Global-Deaths-In-2017-Study

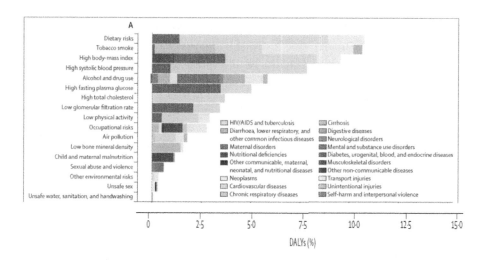

**Risk factors for disability in England for men and women combined**

Risk is expressed as the proportion of all years lost to disability - Disability-Adjusted Life-Years (DALYs). Risk factors are calculated independently of each other and so cannot be summed together. (Figure reproduced under the terms of Creative Commons) (Newton et al Lancet (2015) 386:2257)

A healthy diet may be only one part of the way to live longer and to live longer in good health, but it is the most important. And yet many people are confused by the dietary advice coming from the media and even from more official sources. The next chapter looks at ways to surmount this.

# 4. Barriers to healthier eating

## Overview

The gap between expressing willing to eat more healthily and actually doing so can be a chasm. Preventing us bridging the gap to healthier eating are the many influences on our food choices, which range from the obesogenic environment to the media and the internet. Despite these influences, the situation isn't immutable. Todays' wide range of eating habits show that we are now far more flexible than in the past about what we eat. Hence the very active food battles not only for our hearts and minds but also for our stomachs and wallets. One that unfortunately the junk food industry is currently winning. This chapter discusses some of the barriers thrown in our path towards healthier eating.

## The obesogenic environment

Participants on a crash diet programme broadcast by the BBC in 2018 had spectacular weight loss. [37] The programme's presenter duly went along to the NHS and said (I paraphrase): Hey look we've found the way to lose weight and you need to make it available on the NHS. The NHS's clinical director for Obesity and Diabetes was rather more circumspect. He pointed out that the participants' weight loss was in the context of massive support, not to mention the TV cameras pointing at them, and he estimated that it would require 20 hours per week support which the NHS would find difficult to afford. Diets can work if there is sufficient support - which is one of the main reasons for the success of Weight Watchers. This illustrates how important environmental influences can be on our eating habits.

Unfortunately, when it comes to influencing food choices, our environment is far more likely to encourage bad choices than good ones. From the home to the high street, this so-called obesogenic environment encourages excess eating. Food "deserts" - areas where there are relatively few outlets selling fresh food, and food "swamps" - areas with a high density of outlets selling

---

[37] Dr Javid Abdelmoneim The Big Crash Diet Experiment BBC 30 May 2018

fast food - can lead to poor quality diets [41]. Simply reversing these environmental influences can achieve positive results. When families were given housing vouchers to enable them to move from poor social housing areas to live in more affluent areas, family members lost more weight than similar families remaining in the poorer areas [42]. Proximity to more shops selling fresh fruit and veg and fewer selling junk foods was probably one reason for the weight loss. A second explanation may have been that living in the more affluent area reduced stress. A poll undertaken by the UK thinktank Demos in 2020 found that stress was the most important barrier to healthy eating, with just over half (51%) of consumers saying that they were too stressed to eat healthy foods [43]. In addition, at the physiological level, the stress hormone cortisol has been shown to be linked to weight gain. [38]

Adopting healthier eating habits is far from straightforward. The backdrop of day-to-day living - our surroundings, type of employment, money, housing, education and skills, transport environment, family, friends and community, and diet - all strongly influence how successful this will be. And it is not only obesogenic environmental factors that influence each decision we make about what to eat. Intermingling with these external influences is our own personal belief system. Everything from a taste preference developed in childhood to a concern for the global environment can impact on our eating decisions. Food is tied up with our sense of personal identity, our social interactions and our relationship with the planet. A sense of identity that comes from eating bacon as part of a "British breakfast" can easily over-rule advice to cut back because of its well-established cancer risks. For some, radical veganism may be more to do with a deep-seated view of social injustices in society rather than animal welfare.

Our social and cultural background also influence whether or not we eat more healthily. Employment and income influence how much we are willing to pay and how much free time we have to be able to devote to preparing healthy food, and our social and cultural background influence whether or not we have the cooking skills and taste preferences to eat more healthily. So each

---

[38] https://www.scribd.com/article/338357824/Why-Living-In-A-Poor-Neighborhood-Can-Make-You-Fat-Health-The-Sheer-Stress-Of-An-Environment-Contributes-To-Obesity-And-Diabetes

meal we eat reflects who we are. It is not only true that "we are what we eat" but also that "we eat what we are".

Because of the huge spectrum of influences on our eating that we bring to the table, it is hardly surprising that there are many paths to healthier eating and hence no simple, fool-proof way of changing our behaviour to eat more healthily [44]. It is for each individual to find the way that work best for them. The rest of this chapter considers some of the external influences.

The many external influences, both good and bad, on individual eating behaviour - sociocultural, political and global - have been called the "foodscape" [45]. At the heart of many liberal governments' policies is the view that food choice should be an individual's responsibility. But this is disingenuous since it is abundantly clear that the continual bombardment of food "advice" from the foodscape has created a high level of food confusion. This distorts the ability of individuals to make the healthy eating decisions that are in their best interests. In the opinion of Tim Lang, Professor of Food Policy at City University in London, and his colleagues, the present foodscape has created an "almost insurmountable barriers to making healthy dietary choices for many people" [46].

Hence Professor Lang and his colleagues argue that, for many people, without regulation it will not be possible to switch to a healthier eating pattern. Governments are not necessarily going to be helpful, however, often arguing that the level of nudging deemed necessary by many experts to promote healthy eating would create a nanny state. But fear of the nanny gives free rein to far too many negative influences. Over the last few decades, powerful commercial interests have created our food environment based on processed foods that poses, in the words of an influential report by the so-called EAT-Lancet Commission, "a greater risk to morbidity [disease] and mortality than does unsafe sex, and alcohol, drug, and tobacco use combined" [47]. These are all public health issues that governments are quite comfortable to act on as they are for our own benefit and, I believe, poor diet should not be excluded from this list. Action is particularly important for many in lower socio-economic groups who find it hard to imagine any other way of eating, and for whom poor diet will otherwise remain the number one killer [48].

There are many influencers in the world of food. Surveys often put family and friends as the strongest influencers on what we eat. As the food critic Frank

Bruni commented "Food is an aspect of culture that, because everyone necessarily participates in it to some degree, is more egalitarian than, say, ballet, or opera, or even theatre. It's easier and less intimidating to join the fray and weigh in with an opinion". [39] And these opinions are fed by many sources such as wellness blogs from celebrities, and newspaper and magazine articles. And further back in the chain of influencers are academics and the food industry. Each influencer comes with their own agenda. If from this potpourri of influences you feel that healthy eating messages are mixed and confused then you are not alone. As shown in the figure below, one UK survey identified confusion as the biggest barrier to being able to eat more healthily [41].

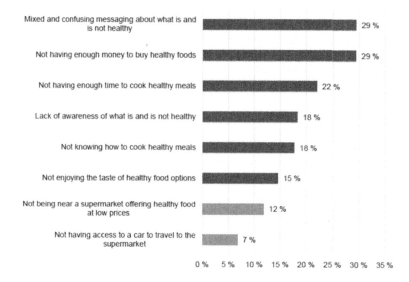

**Barriers to eating more healthily**

(Opinium survey commissioned by The Social Market Foundation. Reproduced with permission.)

# The food industry

The food industry must take some of the blame for the confusion around food advice, as there are many indicators that it has a policy of creating

[39] Quoted in https://culturedecanted.com/2014/10/19/eating-yourself-we-consume-identity-through-food/

uncertainty around evidence, making it harder for people to know what information is correct. Social media is widely used for this purpose. For example, a study from Australia found that the food industry was using Twitter to infer that health advocates who supported taxing sugary drinks were misinformed or not credible [49].

So how does food industry come up with a different narrative to healthy eating, when they are supposedly using the same research information as others with fewer conflicts of interest? One way is by sponsoring studies that are designed to reach conclusions that contradict more unbiased research. This then sows doubt about which is the correct conclusion. Although science may appear to be value-neutral, sadly this is not always the case, and it is possible to design studies that set up a false proposition so that it can easily be blown down - a "straw man" study. For example, a study may be designed so that it cannot conclude whether or not there is an association between consuming sugary drinks and obesity. So the conclusion of this study would be that "there is no evidence" for an association between sugary drinks and obesity. When nutritionists try and reach conclusions they usually pool the results of many different studies in a review. In this example, this would include both these "null" findings and other studies that did find an association between sugary drinks and obesity. Hence researchers writing a review may conclude that there is "no overall consensus" in a particular area, which is exactly what the food industry wants to hear. [40]

This tactic was demonstrated by comparing the conclusions drawn by reviewers either with or without declared conflicts of interest about whether drinking sugary drinks is or isn't linked to weight gain. Reviewers without any reported conflict of interest concluded that 83 % of the studies they examined did show that sugary drinks are a risk factor for weight gain. In contrast, the reviewers who reported a financial conflict of interest with the food industry claimed that the same percentage - 83 % - of the studies they examined had insufficient evidence to support a positive association between sugary drinks and weight gain [50].

---

[40] The strategies used are discussed in Schillinger D, Tran J, Mangurian C *et al.* (2016) Do Sugar-Sweetened Beverages Cause Obesity and Diabetes? Industry and the Manufacture of Scientific Controversy. *Ann Intern Med* **165**, 895-897.

For the scientific community, the evidence that sugary drinks increases the risk of obesity is now beyond reasonable doubt. Nevertheless, the sugary drinks industry continues its misinformation campaign to spread confusion in order to delay for as long as possible policies such as taxation that might harm its profits: a tried and tested tactic previously used by the tobacco industry.

## Advertising

Influencing what we eat is of course fundamental to the business models of the food industry. To achieve this, arguably none of the armaments at their disposal is more controversial nor as powerful as advertising. Advertisers have learnt the art of bewitching us so that we are prepared to suspend belief in what we know would be better for us. The junk food industries employ huge numbers of psychologists and marketing experts to "understand us better than we understand ourselves" to convince us to eat their foods even though we know they are unhealthy. The amount spent on ads for unhealthy foods far outweighs that spent on healthy foods. In the blue corner is the junk food industry with its multi-million pound advertising budget. In the red corner are the cash-strapped vegetable growers and public health advisors. Hardly an equal contest. So it's no wonder that the voice for healthy eating gets drowned out.

Regulation of food ads in the UK is another battleground for the food industry. Although it is the remit of the Advertising Standards Authority to monitor food ads in the UK, many health campaigners believe their powers go nowhere near far enough. Barbara Crowther of the Children's Food Campaign has pointed out that by the time the ASA reaches a decision it can be too late and the campaign has already been concluded. As she said, "Companies are not just breaching the rules, but clearly also ignoring the spirit of what those rules are there for, by deliberately targeting kids with apps, games and storybooks. We're pleased to see the ASA undertaking due diligence and upholding these complaints. However, it took six months for decisions to be reached, by which time the advertising campaigns had long ago concluded. The companies in question weren't penalised in any way, and children remained largely unprotected from the harmful effects of junk food marketing." [41] These concerns hardly inspire confidence that food ads are being sufficiently regulated.

It is unfortunate that some academics may be unwittingly aiding and abetting the ability of the food industry to influence what we eat. The extraordinarily complex way we arrive at a decision about when and what to eat has become a science unto itself, spawning a dedicated band of researchers who publish their findings in scientific journals with names like "Appetite" and "Nutritional Neuroscience". This neurosychological research can, unintentionally, be of great benefit for food advertisers - a process described by journalist George Monbiot as "brain hacking". [42]

---

### Advertising and communicable diseases

The major strategy to control communicable diseases such as malaria and yellow fever is to control the mosquito vectors that spread the disease from one person to another. Chronic diseases are (with a few notable exceptions such as cervical cancer) non-infectious since there is no vector spreading the disease. Hence, chronic diseases are frequently referred to as non-communicable diseases (NCDs).

But are chronic diseases really "non-communicable"? After all, there is a vector. And that vector is communication itself - in the form of advertising. Advertising is the main way that children and adults are exposed to new products from the junk food industry and are encouraged to make poor dietary choices. So in this respect chronic diseases can also be considered forms of communicable diseases.

There is an interesting implication here. Since eradicating vectors is seen as the most important strategy to control infectious diseases spread by mosquitoes, the same thinking could apply to chronic diseases today. Eradicating the advertising of junk foods would be an important step towards controlling the current epidemic of chronic diseases. Legislation is the poison needed to control today's vectors of chronic diseases: the advertising industry.

---

41 http://obesityhealthalliance.org.uk/2018/07/04/junk-food-brands-ignore-existing-weak-rules-continue-target-kids-statement-oha-childrens-food-campaign/
42 https://www.theguardian.com/commentisfree/2018/dec/31/advertising-academia-controlling-thoughts-universities

> It is not only communication via advertising that causes the spread of chronic diseases. Family and friends are amongst the strongest influencers on what we eat and so chronic diseases could also be called "socially infectious diseases". [43]

Another tactic used by the food industry is to sponsor surveys that "find" that we should be buying more of their products. For example, surveys by food supplement companies have led to the conclusion that many people are deficient in certain vitamins and minerals and therefore that we should be taking - you guessed it - more food supplements. Sometimes, other bodies indiscriminately report these studies. This can start a chain reaction of further quoting that builds up apparent credibility for the original study. The internet is a very powerful echo chamber for reinforcing and perpetuating this false information. And it does not seem to matter who is repeating the "information". As Vladimir Lenin is credited with saying "A lie told often enough becomes the truth". [44]

Political front organisations that disguise their true motives are a growing presence on the internet. The food industry is no different and a seemingly helpful website giving advice on food may not be all it seems. An investigation by the well-respected British Medical Journal found that staff at the Chinese branch of an organisation called the International Life Sciences Institute (ILSI) had successfully steered China's thinking on obesity prevention towards a focus on exercise and away from sugar reduction, which is in line with the industry's goals. ILSI's offices are located inside the headquarters of the Chinese Center for Disease Control and Prevention giving them "unparalleled access to government officials". [45] ILSI's mission statement declares that it "does not lobby, conduct lobbying activities, or make policy recommendations." However this does not only not tally with this incident but is further undermined by a detailed study of the organisation by researchers from Cambridge University who concluded "the International

---

[43] This has been defined and discussed at https://theconversation.com/beware-a-non-communicable-disease-may-be-socially-infectious-36477
[44] Prof David Katz has a very insightful article on this at
https://www.linkedin.com/pulse/how-health-nonsense-prevails-what-we-can-do-david/?
[45] https://www.theguardian.com/business/2019/jan/10/coca-cola-influence-china-obesity-policy-protect-sales-bmj-report

Life Sciences Institute should be regarded as an industry group - a private body - and regulated as such, not as a body acting for the greater good" [51].

## Taking responsibility?

In the 1980's and 1990's it seemed that finally the food industry had our interests at heart. Low-fat foods appeared everywhere and people worried about their weight and having a heart attack willingly turned to them. But we now know this was a big mistake. The fat in those low fat foods was mostly replaced with refined carbohydrates - ie sugar - that are just as bad for cardiovascular health and weight gain. A case of out of the fatty frying pan and into the carbohydrate fire.

Replacing fat with sugar is one the most widely used ways to reformulate food products. Reformulation is also undertaken to make a food or drink healthier by reducing a harmful ingredient. For instance, some junk foods are now being reformulated to reduce levels of unhealthy nutrients such as salt, sugar, saturated fat, trans fats or calories. Less commonly, reformulation is undertaken to increase the content of beneficial nutrients such as dietary fibre and whole-grains. [46]

A policy of reformulation was unilaterally initiated by some food manufacturers. But to speed up this process, in March 2011, the UK Government's Department of Health launched The Responsibility Deal. This was a public-private partnership that established voluntary agreements between the Government and the food industry to reformulate a range of food products. There was high hope for a win-win since reformulation by the food industry had already successfully reduced the salt content of a range of foods [52].

But it failed. Consider the case of salt. A significant reduction in salt intake occurred in the decade *before* the Responsibility Deal was introduced in 2011. But after the Responsibility Deal was introduced the reduction in salt intake actually slowed down - by almost a half. The authors of a study from Imperial College, a part of London University, estimated that this slow down was responsible for almost 10,000 additional cases of CVD and 1500 cases of gastric cancer [53].

---

[46] The definition excludes fortifying foods with vitamins or minerals.

Trans fats are another example. Many food industries reduced the trans fat content of certain foods, recognising their significant danger to cardiovascular health. But after its introduction, the Responsibility Deal did little to enhance this. The Responsibility Deal is a voluntary agreement and it failed to recruit the remaining food producers selling products high in trans fats, particularly those producing fast foods and takeaways. The authors of a study examining this concluded that the contribution of the pledges to reduce trans fats as part of the Responsibility Deal were negligible" [54].

Researchers from the Centre for Food Policy at City University in London have concluded that entering into this voluntary agreement was simply a policy used by the food industry to act as a delaying tactic to appear to be doing something and so to dupe successive governments. As they commented: "The Responsibility Deal approach is fundamentally flawed in its expectation that industry will take voluntary actions that prioritise public health interests above its own. Being government-led counts for little in the absence of sanctions to drive compliance. Instead the initiative affords private interests the opportunity to influence in their favour the public health policies and strategies that affect their products" [55]. In other words, food and beverage product reformulation is simply another corporate political strategy. It is procrastination to avoid the policies that do work - and so threaten sales - such as taxation. The Responsibility Deal was dropped in 2017.

Reformulation carries on to this day. You might think that this is a good thing. But it is also a brilliant marketing tool for the food industry: saying a product has reduced levels of something people want to eat less of, or has more of something desirable eg vitamin D, is a key marketing strategy [56]. At the end of the day, reformulating is a bit like adding a filter to a cigarette and declaring smoking to now be healthy. Reformulation is a smoke screen that the food industry uses in order to avoid making more fundamental and meaningful changes to their products. Reformulation legitimises eating junk foods rather than convincing people there is a need for a more fundamental change in diet. As Dr David Katz has pointed out, it's a bit like someone saying they will remove the lead from the bullet they are going to shoot you with, as they don't want you to get lead poisoning. But when they shoot you,

you are still going to die: lead poisoning is the least of your concerns. [47] In other words, a small reduction in one part of a junk food isn't going to make much difference when it's eating the junk food in any shape or form that is bad. Reformulation should mean replacing junk foods with whole foods! [56]

It is sometimes argued that government officials, dietitians, medical staff, academics and others seeking to switch people to eating more natural foods must work *with* the food industry to solve the problem of diet-related diseases. But there is a more radical school of thought that this is a trap set by the food industry to prevent, or at least delay, change. It would be naive to ignore the fact that profit is - and must be - the bottom line for the food industry. The business of the food industry is to sell their food, and as much of it as possible. In an analysis of industry self-regulation to reduce the obesogenic nature of their foods and drinks, a review concluded that most studies show self-regulation is ineffective. For example, children continue to be exposed to TV advertising of junk food and sugary drinks because of vague rules on advertising before the 9 pm watershed [57]. And a team of researchers writing in the Lancet concluded that in relation to the prevention of the harmful effects of the tobacco, alcohol, and ultra-processed food and drink industries, "despite the common reliance on industry self-regulation and public–private partnerships, there is no evidence of their effectiveness or safety" [58].

As the leading nutritionists Dr Kelly D. Brownell has eloquently put it: "When the history of the world's attempt to address obesity is written, the greatest failure may be collaboration with and appeasement of the food industry. I expect history will look back with dismay on the celebration of baby steps industry takes (such as public–private partnerships with health organizations, "healthy eating" campaigns, and corporate social responsibility initiatives) while it fights viciously against meaningful change (such as limits on marketing, taxes on products such as sugared beverages, and regulation of nutritional labeling)" [59].

There are solutions. For the junk food industry, obesity is the unfortunate "collateral damage" (as Michael Pollan has said) from their commercial war to increase sales. It is not in their interests to have this unfortunate side effect, but then again they have a legal duty to their shareholders to maximise profits,

---

[47]https://www.huffingtonpost.com/entry/mac-cheese-and-hot-lead_us_5971f0c9e4b0f1feb89b42a6

and the cheap sugar and fat in junk food is by far the most profitable way of achieving this. Like the tobacco industry, incentivising research into win-win solutions would be a far more constructive path (which at least to a limited extent vaping is for the cigarette industry and society). Unfortunately at the moment the food industry is adopting many of the past tactics of the tobacco industry, such as delaying tactics in order to hinder the introduction of taxation and other policies that research suggests would have a significant benefit to public health legislation, but also - the food industry fears - would dent sales [(60)].

For food companies there is often a conflict between the health information of its products a food company feels able to present to the public and its commercial obligations to its shareholders. In March 2018 the French government undertook an enquiry into the role of the food industry in the chronic disease epidemic and its preferred solutions. "We must have a sufficient level of profitability" said the food industry [(61)]. In France, as elsewhere, companies maximise their profits for their shareholders. It is an unfortunate reality that one of the most effective ways to add profit to a food product is to make it cheaper by substituting natural foods with less healthy industrial ingredients: a vitamin-fortified orange juice is more profitable than an orange, an orange juice drink made with flavourings even more so. One solution for this predicament is to create a legal status that requires an organisation both to make a profit and to serve a greater societal purpose. In the UK this has been developed with the B corporation movement, a voluntary certification system that legally requires companies to consider the impact of their decisions on their workers, customers, suppliers, community, and the environment. [48] A number of UK food companies have already joined this scheme. Companies should be proud to proclaim this. Another idea is to create league tables by ranking how healthy a food company is or isn't. [49]

## Government and the food industry

A straightforward way of transforming the food sector would be to make healthy natural foods more profitable for the food industry to sell. This is only likely to be achieved by taxing unhealthy foods. But the ongoing resistance in

---

[48] https://bcorporation.uk
[49] https://www.forbes.com/sites/hankcardello/2018/12/20/how-to-make-americans-healthier-rank-food-companies

the UK to extending the sugar tax to other products suggests that, at least in the short term, this is probably going to have only a limited effect on improving the food supply by switching the food industry to produce healthier options.

Although central government might be expected to take a lead role in promoting a nation's healthy eating, many experts consider the curbs on the junk food industry by the UK government are completely inadequate. Public Health England, an executive agency of the UK government's Department of Health and Social Care [50], has operational autonomy from the government and might be expected to take a robust stand in matters of public health. After all, according to its website, its priority is "making the public healthier and reducing differences between the health of different groups by promoting healthier lifestyles". [51] But PHE's strategy to promote the UK's childhood obesity plan was described by the respected medical journal the Lancet as "laughably passive" [62]. It's worth noting that the plan targets *childhood* obesity. Of course childhood obesity is very important as it greatly increases the likelihood of being obese in adulthood, but if you are already an adult this plan does not help you.

One of the main reasons why government is slow to interfere is that, as with the banks in 2008, the food industry is too big to fail. The Food and Drink Manufacturing sector is the largest manufacturing sector in the UK and in 2020 employed 430,000 people. [52] Restructuring this sector to produce healthier and more sustainable foods would take quite a few years. Governments eying the next general election rarely take this longer-term view if it threatens jobs in the short-term. And the economic might of the junk food industry extends to other associated businesses, especially advertising, which in turn supports the media such as TV stations that receive a lot of their revenue from advertising. So quibbling about some of the scientific evidence is really fighting a proxy war for the bigger issue. Junk food executives are just concerned about maintaining maximum profits, and politicians want to see their electorate employed, which may well be by the

---

[50] In August 2020, the UK government announced that PHE was to be disbanded

[51] https://www.gov.uk/government/organisations/public-health-england/about#responsibilities

[52] https://www.gov.uk/government/publications/food-statistics-pocketbook/food-statistics-in-your-pocket-food-chain#agri-food-sector-employees-gb-q4-2018

junk food industry. So tackling this requires making healthy foods more profitable to sell than junk foods.

## Academic nutritionists, government and the food industry

The US has some of the best IT specialists in the world and correspondingly the best IT industry; the best arms specialists and the best war machinery. It also has some of the best academic nutritionists. And yet it has one of the highest rates of obesity and diet-related diseases of all industrialised nations. Clearly, academic excellence on its own is not going to solve the problem of poor nutrition. The Covid-19 pandemic has also taught us that academic excellence in health is not in itself enough to create the healthiest societies. The UK and US were judged by a data base compiled by the US-based Johns Hopkins School of Public Health's Center for Health Security to have the top level of preparation for a pandemic, but the US and UK were amongst the countries with the highest deaths from Covid-19 [63]. [53] Political leadership trumps academic excellence.

Some academics claim that nutrition is up to the task of reducing diet-related chronic diseases [64]. But unfortunately this is not borne out by the facts: diet-related diseases are the number one cause of disability and premature death. And obesity rates continue to rise with no country successfully reducing them.

Most academic nutrition scientists see their principal role in the food debate as expanding the evidence base. This they do by undertaking research and reviewing the literature. But this limited sphere of activity is now inadequate. It would be a nonsense - and immoral - to discover a pill that cures cancer and then put the vast majority of future funding into continued research to look at how the pill works, rather than actually giving the pill to people with cancer. And yet it could be argued that this is pretty much the situation today around much (but not all) of academic food research. Most nutritionists agree that the "pill" has already been discovered: a diet based on natural, minimally processed foods. As researchers from Deakin University in Australia put it "dietary advice is relatively straightforward: eat less ultra-processed food and more unprocessed or minimally processed food". [54] Correspondingly, it has

[53] https://www.theguardian.com/commentisfree/2020/may/01/uk-global-leader-pandemics-coronavirus-covid-19-crisis-britain
[54] https://www.theguardian.com/science/2019/may/29/studies-link-too-much-heavily-processed-food-to-early-death

been strongly argued that there is an over-riding ethical duty to act on the currently available evidence and to avoid further "dither and death" and not to simply continue with more research [65].

There is a fundamental difference between a "minimally processed food pill" and a cancer pill that can explain why one to leads to action and the other does not. Money. When a cancer pill has proven its worth in clinical trials it is then in the commercial interests of the manufacturer - the pharmaceutical industry - and the medical interests of the medical provider, such as GPs, to prescribe this drug to their patient as soon as possible. But this is not the case with a food pill. There is no big commercial organisation set to profit from promoting a Med diet.

It is quite possible that many nutrition researchers would prefer to be doing research with more immediate benefit to the health of people. (I'm not aware of any surveys on this that I can use to support this proposition.) But one of the problems for academics is funding. Over the last few decades, government funding cuts for research have left private funding to fill the void. This has led researchers to follow the agendas set by private sector funders. What is in the best interests of the individual - a diet based on natural foods - is not in the best commercial interests of food manufactures who want to be providing their far more profitable highly processed foods. And for the private sector this means they are unlikely to fund areas that undermine their business model. [55] Occupational imperatives mean that most academics must follow the money.

Nutrition scientists usually leave implementing actions to policy makers. But this risks allowing the politics of food to be dominated by the interests of big business, which risks greatly weakening public health [66]. There is perhaps more hope at the local government level and with local food groups. The experience of the Brighton & Hove Food Partnership (a group started by local residents in 2003) demonstrates that the appetite for academics to engage with practical initiatives is there. When the BHFP contacted their local University of Sussex there was an "astonishing and immediate response"

---

[55] This is true in agri-business too:
https://www.theguardian.com/environment/2019/jan/31/us-academics-feel-the-invisible-hand-of-politicians-and-big-agriculture

which has had a major influence on their food strategy. [56] This a great example demonstrating that academics are delighted and keen to climb down from their ivory towers and use their expertise to engage with other sectors involved in the nitty-gritty of improving diets.

## Professional support

GPs top the rankings as sources of trusted medical advice. Their advice is reliable, appropriate and based on a thorough professional training. However, even though you are most likely to die from a diet-related disease, many GPs don't have the time, knowledge or inclination to talk about diet. The vast majority of GP training is about how to treat ill people, not how to prevent well people getting ill - which is mostly what a healthy diet does. UK GPs receive very little training in nutrition. Many see nutrition research as unreliable, not least because of the problems of designing high quality clinical trials (see ch. 5).

There are signs that attitudes of medical professionals to nutrition are changing. GPs with an interest in nutrition are no longer regarded by their colleagues as quite so strange. The BMJ - an influential source of information for GPs - has launched a sister journal focused on nutrition. [57] New medical students are taking more interest in nutrition. In the US, there is a programme that enables GPs to prescribe fruit and veg for people who would benefit. [58] This seems an excellent idea and would remove the obstacle of cost - which is often cited by poorer people as a major reason why they do not eat more fresh foods. Linking this with cooking skills would be even better. There is huge potential in this area. But there is still a long way to go, and it is little disconcerting to find that if you do a little internet search you may find yourself becoming more knowledgeable than your GP on an aspect of nutrition.

Although dietitians and nutritionists sometimes work alongside GPs, their influence on the public health debate remains quite low. Most dietitians work in hospitals or have private practices and deal with people on a one-to-one basis rather than in public health. How many people in the UK have heard of

---

[56] https://foodresearch.org.uk/foodvoices/measuring-the-impact-of-a-strategic-joined-up-approach-to-food-at-the-city-level
[57] BMJ Nutrition, Prevention & Health
[58] https://www.wholesomewave. org/how-we-work/produce-prescriptions

the British Dietetic Association or the Nutrition Society? These organisations have been around for many years and could be making a far bigger contribution to informing the public.

## Fake Nutrition

It seems that almost every day there are new stories in the media giving dietary advice. Although it is certainly not the case that all media stories about food set out to deceive, many give poor dietary advice that are based - at best - on flimsy evidence [67]. For instance, the claim that a diet high in saturated fat is *not* a risk factor for cardiovascular disease [68] has been strongly refuted by the world's leading nutrition experts, but this refutation has received far less publicity. [59] Similarly, media reports can give the impression that almost any food we eat either dramatically increases or decreases our risk of cancer; another claim soundly debunked [69]. Yet views such as these continue to be widely promoted. Their advocates may not deliberately set out to deceive, but the outcome is the same: the persistence of unsubstantiated claims that contradict the best available scientific evidence. It is fake nutrition.

Are there insights from fake news that can help solve the problems of fake nutrition? As Matthew D'Ancona explained in his enlightening book Post Truth, fake news creates a "collapse in trust" in sources of information. [60] After this loss of trust, rather than making decisions based on the information presented, people are more likely to accept ideas that simply resonate with their emotions. These decisions are often based on pre-formed opinions - a process known as confirmation bias.

There are significant parallels here with fake nutrition. Mistrust in media reporting of science and food is now widespread. An IPSOS survey for the UK found that seven-in-ten people think that the media sensationalises science [70]. In the US, the 2017 US Food and Health survey found that 78% of people encounter a lot of conflicting information about what to eat. [61] And yet the media is still hugely influential, and no more so than the internet. We prefer to have our views reinforced rather than challenged. This is the

---

[59] www.hsph.harvard.edu-nutritionsource-2014-03-19-dietary-fat-and-heart-disease-study-is-seriously-misleading-

[60] https://www.penguin.co.uk/books/1114599/post-truth/

[61] http://www.foodinsight.org/press-releases/survey-nutrition-information-abounds-many-doubt-food-choices

opposite of what was envisioned by many in the early days of the internet when it was assumed that the truth would shine through. But instead, social media has tended to reinforce a silo mentality where we visit web sites that support our views, and avoid those that challenge them.

The smorgasbord of dubious dietary advice has created a 'pick and mix' mentality: people select the advice that appeals and discard the rest [71]. Others ignore advice altogether, cynical of the swings between opposite conclusions. [62] Is butter good or bad for you? Many are confused, and well-meaning parents can feel perplexed about the best food choices for themselves and their family.

With our intellectual defences weakened in this way, it becomes all too easy to succumb to primitive hardwired urges for pleasurable sugary and fatty foods, and fall prey to the obesogenic environment of fast food outlets and junk foods [72]. The legacy of this confusion and distrust in nutrition information are national health services caving in under the burden of treating diet-related diseases such as type 2 diabetes, heart disease, dementia and cancer.

Just as fake news and fake nutrition both create a lack of trust, so perhaps the reasons why we respond to fake news could help direct public health campaigns. Two decisive events in 'post truth' society were Brexit and the election of Donald Trump. Both used fake information, yet both campaigns succeeded. The slogans -"Take Back Control" and "Make America Great Again" – were key to their success. Both drew on the powerful emotional need for group identity and a feeling of community.

Food has long played a fundamental role in establishing and reinforcing community, such as through "national dishes" or iconic meals like the Thanksgiving turkey meal in the US. Food has also been used to reinforce divisions between communities, such as when in the fifteenth-century reconquering Spanish Christians used pork dishes to identify Muslims. In her book on The Social Archaeology of Food, Christine Hastorf asserts, "perhaps more than any other human dimension, food creates community through its

---

[62] http://www.telegraph.co.uk/news/health/news/5377733/One-in-four-thinks-conflicting-messages-about-what-food-causes-cancer-should-be-ignored.html

web of symbolic meaning". [63] So could reinforcing group identity also be used as a powerful tool for implementing dietary change?

The need for a feeling of community is well-recognised and exploited by the food industry to sell products. Coca Cola ran an ad that exploited the feeling of rejection by the indigenous people of Mexico, by advertising Coke to "convey a message of unity" with the rest of society. [64] However, the ad was heavily criticised and the company was subsequently forced to withdraw it. On a more positive note, in French culture, the sense of community carefully cultivated at the family dining table, in the school dining hall and in local restaurants is fundamental to maintaining the country's strong tradition of eating healthy, pleasurable food together. In stark contrast, the UK government's plans to scrap school lunches for infants risks further diminishing our ability to instill healthy eating habits in school children. [65]

If, in a perverse way, the success of fake news reminds us of people's need to feel part of a community then maybe far more use could be made of this in nutrition campaigns, rather than just delivering information-based advice like the failed five-a-day campaign. [66] The fast food industry deploys insight into eating behaviours much more successfully than public health nutritionists. If industry can convince us to eat food we know is unhealthy, surely it shouldn't be so difficult for public health bodies to instill more community feeling into their campaigns to convince us to eat more healthy food?

## Celebrities

A big part of the value of communities is trust, and trust is a big part of the appeal of celebrity diets. If someone you like and trust believes in something, you are more likely to consider it favourably. It is also common to think that because a favourite celeb is successful they must be making good decisions, and so their decisions can be trusted. We become victims of the "halo effect", meaning that if a person is successful in one field of endeavor we are more likely to listen to them, even in a completely unrelated field. This can make

[63] Hastorf, C. The Social Archaeology of Food: Thinking about Eating from Prehistory to the Present

[64] https://www.theguardian.com/world/2015/dec/02/coca-cola-under-fire-over-ad-showing-coke-handout-to-indigenous-people

[65] http://www.bbc.co.uk/news/education-39961176

[66] http://www.telegraph.co.uk/news/2017/03/30/just-one-four-adults-eating-five-day-nhs-reveals/

celebrity endorsements of fad diets and junk food products particularly influential. Celebrities have "sell-ability" even if, when it comes to advice on eating, their credentials for selling are often of dubious depend-ability. And, in any case, we want to agree with the decisions of our favourite celebs. We don't want to think that the celeb we admire would say anything against our best interests. This would create cognitive dissonance, a highly undesirable state of affairs that creates serious mental discomfort and, as psychologists have shown, is a mental state we are keen to avoid [73].

Holding a strong view about diet is fine and most people recognise that they have only a limited perspective on a particular aspect, one based on personal experience. But promoting these views to a wider audience is a completely different matter. A little knowledge can be a dangerous thing. The Blind Men fable of men touching different parts of an elephant and coming to quite different conclusions about its identity is an apposite metaphor for our times (see ch. 8 for this in full). The clear conviction of one man touching just one part of the elephant that they are correct could explain why people with only a limited knowledge of a subject can feel so compelled to promote their own ideas. This conviction can be particularly strong in people in positions of prominence and power, which of course includes some celebs. This power can become intoxicating and lead to hubris, a dangerous combination of over-confidence, over-ambition, arrogance and pride [74].

Of course, some celebs use their high profile public positions to promote reliable public health messages. In the UK, notable examples are the celebrity chefs Jamie Oliver and Hugh Fearnley-Whittingstall, and their support for campaigns against childhood obesity. However, all too often, food industry campaigns or celebrities with dubious credentials, and equally dubious advice, swamp the media, drowning out the voices of medically and nutritionally trained professionals. Cancer patients are particularly vulnerable to fictitious claims of cures and there are increasing concerns that these risk eclipsing reputable information. [67]

---

[67] https://www.theguardian.com/science/2019/jul/14/cancer-fake-news-clinics-suppressing-disease-cure

# Tribes and norms

Having an association with a celebrity - even from just reading their blogs - creates a feeling of tribal belonging. We are tribal animals, and bonds in tribes are created by shared beliefs and values. Being accepted into a tribe was a huge survival advantage for early humans and agreeing with the tribal view was more important than if that view was correct. This priority has been brilliantly dubbed "factually false, but socially accurate". [68] Today, it is unfortunate that maintaining social accuracy can easily lead to eating a poor quality diet. This can be illustrated with English-speaking countries. English speaking countries have amongst the poorest diets: four of the top six highest ranked countries for obesity are the US (no. 1), New Zealand (no. 3), Australia (no. 5) and the UK (no. 6). [69] This demonstrates a clear association between having English as your mother tongue and your risk of obesity! Of course speaking English isn't the *cause* of obesity in these countries. The link here is not so much the language but rather the shared cultural values between English speaking countries.

One of these shared cultural values is the absence of a strong tradition of healthy eating. Without this pre-existing tradition to displace, the food industry readily and quite easily filled the void in these countries with its own brand of a food culture, one based on junk foods. With this has come the drive by the food industry to establish junk food as a normal way of eating. This has been remarkably successful, and we now have several generations for whom junk food has become the eating norm. Changing this norm to one based on unprocessed food is the challenge, especially in English-speaking countries where there is no clearly defined healthy norm to return to. Identifying fake nutrition is easier with a little knowledge of how reliable nutrition advice is developed, and this is the topic of the next chapter.

---

[68] https://jamesclear.com/why-facts-dont-change-minds
[69] OECD study figures for 2017 which track 35 industrialised nations. The other two are Mexico (no.2) and Hungary (no.4).
http://www.telegraph.co.uk/news/2017/11/10/britain-sixth-fattest-nation-world-rising-faster-united-states/?WT.mc_id=tmg_share_em

# 5. Overcoming the confusion in dietary advice

## Overview

To help counter the barrage of misinformation about what to eat, this chapter gives a brief overview of how nutrition research is undertaken so that you can make a more informed judgment about what to eat. The health benefits of what we eat are influenced by our own personal circumstances - such as our genes and current health - and the importance of taking these into account when making dietary choices is illustrated with a few examples.

## Introduction

The overabundance of dietary advice - some accurate, some less so - makes it hard for people to find trustworthy sources and reliable guidance when needed. The WHO calls this an "infodemic". Because of its perceived contrariness, the infodemic of dietary advice has translated into widespread scepticism and mistrust. A 2017 US Food and Health survey found that 78% of people encounter a lot of conflicting information about what to eat. [70] Well-meaning parents can feel perplexed and frustrated about the best food choices for themselves and their family.

This confusion is not new and can have serious ramifications, as one widely reported incident from the 1970's demonstrates. Seven-year-old Joseph Hofbauer received an untested nutritional therapy for his cancer. Not surprisingly, he died. With appropriate treatment Joseph would have had a 95% chance of surviving. But Joseph's parents had been persuaded that so-called "metabolic therapy" would cure their son. They were described as "concerned and loving parents", and cleared of any wrongdoing. [71] Sadly, they had simply misplaced their trust in phony advice.

---

[70] http://www.foodinsight.org/press-releases/survey-nutrition-information-abounds-many-doubt-food-choices

[71] http://www.leagle.com/decision/197969547NY2d648_1624/MATTER OF HOFBAUER

There is currently far more regulation of medical advice than of nutrition advice. In the nineteenth century, medical quackery was rife. So medical organisations such as the British Medical Association (BMA) in the UK and drug regulatory bodies established experimental approaches and regulations to ensure that the medicines and medical procedures people received had been subject to robust and honest scrutiny. Thanks to these approaches we can, by and large, now trust medical science with its reassuringly regulated codes of practice run by teams of highly respected professionals. The days of medical quackery are (almost) gone.

However, attempting to replicate these control measures for what we eat has been less successful. This is because of fundamental differences between medical interventions and diets. A medicine or medical device is an item developed by specialists that is completely novel to our body. By contrast, anyone can invent a diet. This has resulted in today's over-abundance of dietary opinions and it is often not easy to distinguish between charlatans and those giving unbiased informed advice.

Being cautious before believing one-off reports in the media about the latest food claim is one thing. But sifting through the super-abundance of nutrition "advice" that supports just about any personal belief is challenging. At present, there is no national regulatory body in nutrition in the UK whose primary role is to do this sifting for us. [72] So this chapter gives a brief overview of how nutrition research is undertaken with the aim to enable you to make a more informed judgment on what to eat.

## Nutrition research methods

A good part of nutrition research is based on epidemiological studies. These studies determine by how much eating a particular food or following a particular diet influences the health of an individual or population.

There are various types of epidemiological studies. In prospective epidemiology, a group of people (known as a cohort) records, usually by completing a questionnaire, what and how often they eat a range of foods.

---

[72] Current UK nutrition organisations either represent nutrition research (Nutrition Society) or are professional bodies (such as the BDA).
In the US, there have been calls to establish a National Institute of Nutrition
https://eu.usatoday.com/story/opinion/2019/08/19/america-should-establish-national-institute-nutrition-column/1819186001/

The cohort is then followed for a period of time to see if they develop a particular disease that can be related to what they were eating.

Due to the low rates at which chronic diseases develop, cohort studies for chronic diseases can take many years and this makes them expensive. Retrospective "case-control" studies circumvent this by evaluating what a group of people who have already developed a disease like cancer *used to* eat (the "cases") and compares them with the eating habits of another group who don't have the disease but are as similar as possible in other ways (the "controls").

Cohort and case-control studies are examples of "observational studies" - they observe free-living people in the real world. Which is a good thing. However, sceptics see observational studies as little more scientific than surveys, and they come with all the attendant baggage of surveys. For nutrition studies, one major issue is the assumption that people can accurately remember, and will be honest about, what they ate. Usually this information is obtained using self-reporting questionnaires about the types and frequencies of food consumption - Food Frequency Questionnaires (FFQs). These are subject to considerable bias and misreporting by participants, or simple because of lapses of memory. Some studies improve the reliability of the information they obtain from FFQs by backing up participants' responses by measuring markers of food intake in the blood (biomarkers).

Observational studies have other limitations. Most importantly, they can only demonstrate *associations*; they cannot prove *causation*. As the last chapter mentioned, there is a clear association between having English as your mother tongue and your risk of obesity. But it isn't speaking English that is the *cause* for this risk. An amusing example highlights the problem of distinguishing *causal* from *casual* relationships. The German researcher Helmut Sies, concerned about declining birth rates in Germany, found an almost perfect correlation between the declining number of pairs of brooding storks in West Germany and the declining birth rate of German babies [75]. Perfect! The declining birth rate must be due to there being fewer German storks to deliver the babies!

Also, lurking in the shadows of observational studies is the possibility of "reverse causality". This is when the outcome influenced the behaviour, and not the other way round - the behaviour influencing the outcome. For example, people who eat a lot of fruit and vegetables get less colon cancer. However, an observational study cannot prove that it was eating a lot of fruit and vegetables that was responsible for a person to reduce their risk of colon cancer. Reverse causality is possible - in other words that when people start getting colon cancer they then choose to eat less fruit and vegetables (perhaps because they find it more difficult to digest their food).

Since causation cannot be proven in observational studies, nutritional epidemiologists use the phrase "associated with" when describing their results. Using the phrase "associated with" may sound ponderous but failing to report that these studies only find associations and do not prove causality is extremely common. Unfortunately this type of misreporting isn't limited to the popular press, since it has been estimated that about a third of nutrition observational studies inappropriately report causality [76].

Studying free-living people is also complicated because of the many aspects of a person's life, apart from what they eat, that could potentially explain the results. Some of these variables - known as "confounders" in nutrition jargon - such as a person's education, income and other socio-economic factors, are normally taken into account during statistical analysis. However, there usually remains the possibility that unaccounted-for confounders may lead to an inaccurate conclusion. This is called residual confounding.

Too many variables are anathema to scientific research. The "scientific method" - the main way that most medical science has advanced - seeks to minimise the number of variables. This is achieved by conducting experiments under tightly controlled conditions, with the aim, ideally, of reducing the number of variables down to one. When this is achieved, only one variable can change when an action is applied and this can be measured. A change to more than one variable makes interpreting experimental data far more complicated.

Scientific method also uses the time-honoured paradigm of formulating a hypothesis, then designing an experiment to test the hypothesis, collecting evidence (data) from the experiment and then revising the hypothesis according to the results obtained. This iterative cycle of hypothesis - experiment - revise hypothesis is the most important way scientists arrive at their view of the world. Observational epidemiology is not based on the scientific method since it simply observes people living their normal lives and then tries to surmise links between their diet and their health. There is no scientific experiment. This is one reason why many in the medical profession have a low opinion of nutrition and also why nutrition still receives such little attention in medical training. This *status quo* has serious and negative repercussions for public health since the medical profession is powerful and influential (see ch. 4 for more on this).

## Randomised control trials

One approach that helps deal with the limitations of observational studies is the randomised control trial (RCT). RCTs are often considered to be the gold standard of experimental design for clinical studies (ie studies involving people). An RCT randomises participants into either the "test" group - those receiving the intervention under study, or the "control" group - those not receiving the intervention. RCTs test a hypothesis - such as whether or not a particular food or diet has a particular effect on health. Hence they obey the framework of the scientific method.

RCTs have also long been the standard way of evaluating pharmaceutical drugs. The effect of giving a drug to the test group is compared with a control group not receiving the drug. Importantly, the process of giving the drug to a person in the test group can be replicated in the control group by giving a placebo. This circumvents any "placebo effect" which is when the action of being given a drug, rather than receiving active ingredients in the drug, causes the effect.

RCTs in nutrition are not so easily conducted. For instance, it is usually impossible to design a placebo diet. Another problem is that foods are usually given to people who are already eating some of that food or nutrient. This contrasts with RCTs of drugs where the comparison is between receiving some drug (in the test group) versus receiving none (in the control group). An RCT in nutrition therefore usually simply compares the effect of eating more versus less of a food. This makes it far more difficult to demonstrate an effect. It's also a reason why studies with nutritional supplements often give variable results. The effectiveness of a nutritional supplement will usually depend on how much of the nutrient in question a person is already consuming as part of their everyday diet. If they do not routinely eat very much of the nutrient in question then the supplement will be far more beneficial than in a person already getting optimal amounts from their diet.

There are a number of other limitations of RCTs. One is that it is not always possible to evaluate an intervention with a RCT because either the required "control" group or "experimental" group is unethical. Imagine you agreed to take part in a RCT. Your study involves being taken 10,000 metres up in a plane. You see some of your colleagues are being given parachutes to wear. But you aren't. You are told the experiment is to evaluate survival from jumping out of a plane with a parachute, and this means that some people - including you - have been randomised into the control group ie those not wearing a parachute. Fortunately, it is unlikely that this RCT would have made it past the Ethics Committee! [73] But there are similar examples in nutrition too. For instance, it would be unethical to impose on a group of people a "test" diet that is suspected of increasing the risk of a disease - such as giving a group of people a diet high in processed meat simply to see if it increases their risk of cancer.

Another drawback for many RCTs is their duration. It takes a long time to complete a trial whose end-point is when sufficient numbers of previously fit people have developed a chronic disease such as cancer. This makes these trials expensive. Pharmaceutical companies are prepared to bear the expense of a long study since their drugs are highly profitable. This is not the case with dietary interventions since these are usually neither patentable nor profitable. So there is the temptation to keep the RCT short. But this may compromise the results. For instance, most RCTs of diets to reduce weight last only a few weeks or months, and so any important changes that occur over months or years and which influence the long-term success or failure of a diet will not be picked up. These longer-term changes could include a decrease in metabolic rate (which means that the same number of calories will increase a person's weight) or the longer-term inability to maintain the necessary behavioural changes. These longer-term changes are important since many weight loss diets fail for these reasons.

---

[73] The parachute example comes from Smith GC, Pell JP (2003) Parachute use to prevent death and major trauma related to gravitational challenge: systematic review of randomised controlled trials. *BMJ* **327**, 1459-1461

One way to shorten long study periods is to use people already at high risk of a disease, and so they are likely to develop a disease more quickly. One of the best known RCTs in nutrition, called the Predimed study, recruited people already at high risk of cardiovascular disease (CVD), rather than the general public, so that higher numbers of people reached the end point - getting CVD - than would have been the case if all members of the general public were recruited into the study.

Despite their limitations, RCTs are still usually considered the most reliable type of human studies in nutrition. It would however be a mistake to consign other types of study to the experimental dustbin. Even in the absence of a RCT, important public health decisions can still be made. There has never been a RCT to see if cigarette smoking causes lung cancer since it would clearly be unethical to select some people for the test group and oblige them to smoke (the control group would be those not smoking). Because of this, the epidemiological link between cigarette smoking and lung cancer in humans is based on observational studies. But few people dispute that smoking is a risk factor for lung cancer. This was however disputed for many years by tobacco companies, and this delayed the introduction of legislation resulting in many thousands of people dying unnecessarily from smoking-related diseases.

One reason why the observational studies that incriminated smoking as a cause of lung cancer were so convincing was because the "strength" of the association between cause (smoking) and effect (lung cancer) was high. With increasing smoking the risk of lung cancer rapidly increased. Another example of a strong association is between increasing weight and type 2 diabetes. The risk of type 2 diabetes increases rapidly with increasing weight indicating that being overweight is likely to be a cause of type 2 diabetes (see Figure next page) [77]. The term "diabesity" was coined to emphasise this strong link. There are also associations between obesity and many other chronic diseases but these associations are far weaker.

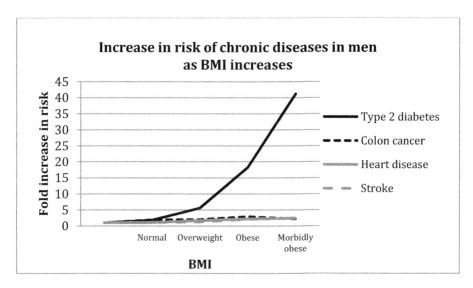

(Redrawn from data in [77] )

The strength of the association between a risk factor and a disease is one of a number of guidelines proposed by the English scientist Sir Austin Bradford Hill to judge whether or not it is reasonable that a statistical association found in an observational epidemiological study is causal [78]. It is a tribute to Hill that his guidelines, although proposed over 50 years ago, have stood the test of time. In all, Hill proposed nine guidelines and when most or all are met there is the likelihood that a diet is truly causing the protective or harmful effect. To date, this exercise has only been undertaken in a few cases. One example where all nine guidelines have been met is between better conformity to a Mediterranean diet and a reduction in cardiovascular events (such as a heart attack and stroke). This impressive demonstration is a strong reason for eating a Med diet to prevent CVD [79].

As well as epidemiological studies, Hill included laboratory studies in his guidelines. These provide experimental evidence – so-called biological plausibility - that can explain the effects observed in people. Today, studies that link peoples' diets with their health (ie epidemiological studies), biological approaches that consider physiological changes in the body, and studies in animals and cells that seek to understand mechanisms of action, are all thrown into the judgmental melting pot before a verdict about causality between a diet and a disease risk is reached [80].

This need for a multi-faceted approach to evidence gathering indicates that one small patch in the quilt of evidence should be considered insufficient to make a dietary recommendation. For example, extrapolating results from animal studies or other laboratory studies to then make recommendations for humans is fraught with problems. Similarly, associating a dietary intervention with a *marker* for a reduced disease risk, such as reduced blood cholesterol, is far less reliable as an indication that a dietary intervention is beneficial than by measuring the incidence of reducing the disease itself (such as CVD). The many media headlines that litter the popular press based on extrapolations from animal studies, or "biomarkers" for disease, to a health risk do the public few favours. Not only do they lead to a great deal of confusion but they also further increase scepticism of what most likely originated as a serious and balanced study. One extreme example is of a study reported in many British newspapers with headlines such as "Eating chocolate is as good for you as going for a run". The underlying research was actually a study in mice, *and not humans*, of a compound called epicatechin, *and not chocolate* (although there is some epicatechin in chocolate). A thorough debunking of this study was carried out by the NHS Choices website. [74] This website is a valuable tool for checking the reliability of media reports on health issues.

Using a multi-faceted approach to evidence gathering has enabled nutritionists to come to a broad consensus that eating a diet based on natural foods is optimal for health. This consensus comes from many epidemiological studies on dietary factors as well as a wealth of information on the mechanisms of action of dietary factors. It is a consensus that is taught in nutrition and diet courses in higher education and is disseminated by major health organisations. It has remained pretty much constant for many years. Unfortunately, many popular commentators fall well short of considering the many layers of nutrition research before giving their own dietary advice. So too do the media looking for a good headline. As unfortunately do many people looking for evidence to support their personal beliefs, rather than starting more objectively from the evidence.

---

[74] http://www.nhs.uk/news/2011/09September/Pages/dark-chocolate-and-fitness.aspx

# Putting risk in perspective

Knowing something poses a risk is not really that helpful without knowing by how much. Observational studies enable the statistical risk of someone getting a disease due to a particular way of eating to be estimated. This is relative to another group and so a relative risk (RR) is calculated. In cohort studies this is the ratio of risk among people with a particular feature of their diet, such as high meat consumption, to the risk without that feature (low or no meat consumption). An RR value above 1 indicates increased risk, for instance a value of 2.0 indicates a doubling in the risk, and an RR value below 1 indicates reduced risk. These numbers have been made more meaningful by translating them into years lost or gained from your actual age [81]. For example, smoking 20 cigarettes a day has been calculated to translate your actual age into a virtual age of eight years older and eating 50 g of processed meat a day as adding two years, whereas for every two portions of fruit and vegetables eaten per day you become one year younger. This idea can also be applied to specific organs in the body.

The importance of putting RR in perspective was demonstrated by US physician-scientists Dr Jonathan Schoenfeld and Dr John Ioannidis. They tested the validity of conclusions from a large number of studies that had examined the relationship between food ingredients and cancer risk [69]. More than three quarters of the ingredients tested in the studies were reported to either increase or decrease cancer risk. Schoenfeld and Ioannidis didn't choose these ingredients for their study because they were "superfoods" or because they were already suspected of increasing or decreasing cancer. In fact they randomly selected food ingredients from recipes in cookery books and then looked in the scientific literature for studies on these ingredients. It is implausible that so many common ingredients can influence cancer risk. When Drs Schoenfeld and Ioannidis examined the statistics, they found that many of the RR values were too small to make a plausible difference to cancer risk and that there were indications of "publication bias" - this is when there is a greater likelihood that positive findings (either an increased or decreased cancer risk) are reported than null findings. Lies, damned lies and statistics applies just as much to nutrition as it does to other fields, but this does not prevent these types of studies being widely reported in the media.

# Meta analyses

Drs Schoenfeld and Ioannidis in their analysis found that when the RR values from several individual studies were pooled together the estimates of cancer risk were more conservative and, they concluded, more reliable. Pooling the risk estimates from a large number of studies into a single figure is called a meta- analysis. Meta-analyses are widely used in nutrition research and are usually considered to give more reliable estimates of risk than single studies.

However, and as with all statistical analysis, this requires adequate competency in selecting studies; and many meta-analyses are poorly conducted. Meta-analyses appeal to researchers since they attract a lot of attention, and academic departments welcome this attention as it raises the profile of their department. Most scientific research requires funding for research equipment, which means writing a grant proposal and having it scrutinised by independent scientific referees to see if it is worthy of being funded. But this is not the case with meta-analyses since these are easily undertaken without external funding. Hence it is relatively easy for meta-analyses to be undertaken by groups who may lack the necessary expertise to design a sufficiently competent study - one that would pass scientific scrutiny from independent referees. The result can be a meta-analysis that draws a spurious conclusion.

One way this can occur is when studies differing in important ways are combined when they shouldn't be. A meta-analysis published in 2014 concluded that the risk of heart disease is not related to the type of fat in the diet - such as whether it is saturated or unsaturated [68]. But this meta-analysis did not consider what people replaced the saturated fat in their diet with. In particular, they did not distinguish between studies where people substituted the saturated fat in their diet with carbohydrates and studies where people substituted their saturated fat with unsaturated fat. There is considerable evidence to suggest that when saturated fat consumption is substituted with unsaturated fat (especially polyunsaturated fat) the risk of heart disease goes down but when the saturated fat is substituted with carbohydrate there is no change in risk. The authors' conclusion that saturated fat is no different to unsaturated fat was widely reported in the media under headlines such as "Butter is Back". But this advice has been widely criticised as incorrect by many authorative voices as "seriously misleading". [75]

# Why risk varies between people

Millions of people around the world struggle to control their weight. It is now clear, though, that a "one-size-fits-all" health campaign for weight reduction is not the solution [82]. Differences between peoples' genes, behavior, and their social and environmental backgrounds, all influence weight gain. Meaningful weight change for an individual means addressing the person as just that: as an individual.

But much of nutrition research is in the opposite direction, towards ever-larger numbers - as exemplified by meta-analyses. This can mask huge variations in risk between individuals within populations. A study that fails to differentiate high-risk individuals within a low-risk general population can produce a skewed overall risk estimate that mistakenly reassures high-risk individuals that their risk is the same as everyone else's. A one-size-fits-all policy in nutrition makes no more sense than calculating the average shoe size in a population and recommending that everyone wear that size. Even statisticians agree, "The mean is an abstraction. Reality is variation". [76]

Condensing down population-wide risk assessments into "one-size-fits-all" health campaigns means that we all receive the same advice: to get more exercise or eat more fruit and vegetables or avoid processed meat and so on. In some cases this is appropriate. Few would challenge a blanket statement that we should not smoke - even though not all people who smoke will die of a tobacco-related illness. (There is no test to find out if you will be in the lucky minority.) But unlike, say, where the risk of a plane crashing will equally affect everyone in that plane, risk is not spread equally between individuals when it comes to diet. For instance, some people are at high risk of adverse effects from alcohol because of an inherited inability to neutralise carcinogens formed from alcohol. So clearly these people should avoid alcohol. But for middle aged men- who represent a relatively high risk group for heart disease - the benefit of this type of advice is less clear since studies show that a modest alcohol intake can significantly reduce the risk of CVD [83]. Many in public

---

[75] https://www.hsph.harvard.edu/nutritionsource/2014/03/19/dietary-fat-and-heart-disease-study-is-seriously-misleading/
[76] From Blastland & Dilnot, 2008. The Tiger that Isn't: Seeing through a World of Numbers. Profile Books Ltd: London.

health recommend that the best amount of alcohol is none [77] but this may be doing a disservice to some individuals such as, arguably, middle aged men who enjoy a glass of wine.

The importance of considering your own circumstances is one of the themes running through this book and I will mention here a few more examples that crop up in more detail later in the book. Firstly, is the case of processed meat, which is an established risk factor for oesophageal cancer. But not all people may be at the same risk of oesophageal cancer from processed meat. People with a precancerous state called Barrett's oesophagus who eat processed meat appear to be at greater risk of it progressing to oesophageal cancer than people who eat processed meat but don't have Barrett's oesophagus [84]. A recent study estimated that eating a lot of processed meat increases the risk of oesophageal cancer by 81% [85]. But this study was based on the general population and it is quite possible that this figure is *much higher* in people with Barrett's oesophagus (and for the maths to balance out, this would mean lower in other people). So more targeted campaigns - such as encouraging bacon lovers with an increased risk of Barrett's oesophagus (for example, because of acid reflux) to get checked for oesophageal cancer - might be far more beneficial. People with elevated levels of insulin are also at increased risk of Barrett's oesophagus progressing to cancer compared to people with Barrett's oesophagus and normal insulin levels [86].

Another dietary factor that affects people differently is folic acid. Folic acid may help protect against colon cancer in people with no signs of this disease, but in people with precancerous growths in the colon known as adenomas, folic acid can make matters worse and increase the risk of full-blown colon cancer developing [87]. Folic acid truly is a Jekyll and Hyde character.

The circumstances in which women drink has also been found to influence cancer risk. Some studies such as the Million Women Study (which really did involve well over a million women) found no increased risk of these cancers for women drinking up to two units a day, so long as they were non-smokers [88]. But this study found that combining smoking with drinking dramatically increased the risk of mouth and throat cancers. It's thought that alcohol acts as a solvent that increases the absorption of carcinogens in cigarette smoke.

---

[77] Department of Health. Secondary 2016.
https://www.gov.uk/government/consultations/health-risks-from-alcohol-new-guidelines.

Another important group who tend to respond differently to some dietary factors than others are the overweight and obese. People who are overweight are at far higher risk of coronary heart disease from eating a high carbohydrate diet than people who are lean [89].

Even though population-wide 'big-is-better' public health approaches fail to take these differences between individuals into account, individuals can - at least to some extent. One way to garner personal health information in the UK is to have an NHS Health Check (if you are between 40 and 74). This measures basic disease risk factors such as blood pressure, cholesterol and sometimes blood glucose. For instance, there is strong evidence that if your blood cholesterol level is high then it is advisable to keep saturated fat intake low.

More and more people now also take genetic tests as part of the rapidly expanding field of personalised nutrition. This follows in the wake of personalised pharmacy where drug prescribing is being tailored to the genetic and physiological risk assessment of the individual. [78] The link between a person's genes and how they respond to diet has given birth to the new field of personalised nutrition. For instance, people with specific types of genetic changes (called SNPs - single nucleotide polymorphisms) are at greater risk of CVD than the general population if they consume high amounts of saturated fats [90]. Although some people are now starting to have their genes analysed to see if they should modify their diet, this is still very much in its infancy as few genes are sufficiently characterised to provide actionable information.

This book provides examples of where personal circumstances suggest that a particular way of eating might be advisable. A more general strategy - and one supported by a huge amount of evidence - is to hedge your bets with a proven healthy dietary pattern such as the Mediterranean diet. Observational studies often give widely varying estimates of the risks or benefits of eating specific foods such as carrots or coffee [69]. By contrast, there is far less variability between different studies when dietary patterns are considered [91]. Many

---

[78] A recent example is the finding that some people have protective factors that means they do not need to go on statins even though have high bp etc, and reverse- some people have risk genes and should go on even though lower bp...
https://www.theguardian.com/science/2019/jun/19/statins-cut-heart-risk-many-britons-study-dna-tests

different nutrients act together in healthy dietary patterns, and the outcome is far less likely to be influenced by specific variations between individuals. In nutrition-speak this suggests that there is a lot less confounding with dietary patterns than for individual foods. Confounders such the genetic backgrounds of the people taking part in the study or other aspects of their diets or lifestyles get ironed out with dietary patterns. We can now start considering what a healthy eating pattern consists of.

# 6. The building blocks of a healthy diet

## Overview

A healthy diet is composed of a balanced intake of protein, fat, carbohydrates, vitamins and minerals, dietary fibre and various plant chemicals called phytochemicals. These important components in a plant-based diet have led to the widespread view that the healthiest diets are based predominantly on plant foods.

## Making the calories count

One place to look for an answer to the question of what makes a healthy diet is with the diets of people in regions in the world where lives are long and healthy. We turn again to the exceptionally long-lived people of the "Blue Zone" regions. In many respects the diets in these regions are quite different. The Okinawans in Japan drink no alcohol, consume a lot of soya and have a high carb diet high in rice, whereas the Mediterraneans (from Sardinia in Italy and the Greek island of Ikaria), consume red wine and home-grown vegetables and eat a high fat diet rich in olive oil. These quite different diets demonstrate that a healthy diet can be high in carbs like the Okinawans or high in fats like the Mediterraneans. This conclusion is shared by some of the world's top nutritionists: "Current evidence indicates that no specific carbohydrate-to-fat ratio in the diet is best for the general population." they said in the top journal Science [92]. A similar conclusion was reached in a large and expensive study into weight control. This study conducted in the US and involving more than 600 people and costing $8 million concluded that the relative levels of fats and carbs was not of primary importance as a factor for weight control [93]. Both low fat/high carb and low carb/high fat diets achieved similar weight loss.

A reason why it doesn't matter too much whether we get our calories more from fat or carbs (within reason) is because when dietary fat and carbs are low our body's can make them. When glucose - the basic carbohydrate in the body - is too low we make it from fat and when fats are too low the body makes them from glucose (with the exception of two so-called essential fatty acids which we must get directly from our diet). There is an important caveat to this. And that is this ability to handle a broad range of dietary fats and carbs only applies to healthy individuals. There is growing evidence that diabetics and overweight people (often the two go together) do not retain this ability. This is because being diabetic or overweight leads to a reduced carbohydrate tolerance. Diabetics often benefit from low carb diets, and they are more likely to lose weight on a low carb diet. Some studies have found that low carb diets can reverse type 2 diabetes [94] and the role of low carb diets in treating type 2 diabetes is currently being intensively studied [95].

So if it isn't low carbs or low fat that makes a diet healthy for the general population, what is it? Simply describing a diet as low fat or low carb is a very incomplete way of describing its overall quality. For instance, it gives no information on what has replaced the fat or carbs. It could be something healthy; but equally well it could be sugar or processed foods or high amounts of meat. Hence low fat or low carb diets cover a broad spectrum from very healthy to very unhealthy. Of far greater importance than the specific proportions of carbs or fats in the diet is its overall quality. A study led by the eminent nutritionist Prof Walter Willett concluded that adopting a low carbohydrate diet increased the risk of dying if it resulted in a switch to fat and protein from animal products, and that the emphasis should be on plant foods [96]. The vast majority of nutrition experts agree that a high quality diet is one based on minimally processed foods from plants. As leading nutritionists David Katz and Stephanie Meller concluded "A diet of minimally processed foods close to nature, predominantly plants, is decisively associated with health promotion and disease prevention. [4]" [79]

The top plant foods are vegetables, fruits, whole grain products (such as bread, pasta, rice), pulses (ie dried beans) and nuts and seeds. Making vegetables centre stage and not worrying about calorie intake has proven to be a successful strategy for losing weight and, importantly, maintaining weight loss. By contrast, diets that focus on restricting calories usually result in compensatory physiological and behavioural mechanisms that prevent weight loss [97]. Most plant foods are highly nutritious, low in calories and effective at quelling appetite. Choosing highly nutritious plant foods but not obsessing

[79] https://www.theatlantic.com/health/archive/2014/03/science-compared-every-diet-and-the-winner-is-real-food/284595/

about calories is one of the key messages in this book, and can be summed up: *Don't count the calories; make the calories count*

Even though "eat a healthy diet" seems a simple message, achieving it is more of a challenge. The people of the Blue Zone regions eat a healthily because it is a natural part of their lifestyle and culture. [80] These aren't wealthy regions or with exceptional health services, nor do their populations necessarily have a heightened knowledge of what to eat to be healthy. For them, making the healthy choice is the easy choice, the default position. This can be more difficult in more industrialised societies with competing demands on time and the all-pervasive influence of the junk food industry. As Katz and Meller went on to say in their article: "Efforts to improve public health through diet are forestalled not for want of knowledge about the optimal feeding of *Homo sapiens* but for distractions associated with exaggerated claims, and our failure to convert what we reliably know into what we routinely do. Knowledge in this case is not, as of yet, power; would that it were so."

This chapter focuses on providing some of the knowledge by understanding a little about nutrients in our foods, is I believe one tool to help create some of the power needed for change. So I hope you will persist with a light serving of science in this chapter. Just as learning a foreign language requires an initial conscious effort to understand the vocabulary and grammar before speaking then becomes unconscious, so eventually the information in this chapter can lead to a natural approach to healthy eating. The rest of this chapter is a primer of the nutrient content of natural foods, which, I hope, will empower you to want to buy more natural foods.

## A balanced diet

A high quality diet provides all the nutrients for health without the need to consume excess calories. For the average person, this means a healthy diet will package all essential nutrients into about 2000 kcals [81] for women and 2500 kcals for men. Energetic people may need more calories. An optimal balance between nutrients and calories is easily achieved by consuming nutrient dense, natural foods since these foods mostly contain lots of nutrients per calorie.

---

[80] A lifestyle that also includes high levels of social contact and regular physical activity.
[81] One Calorie (note the capital C) is somewhat confusingly equivalent to one kcal, which is 1000 calories (small c).

It's ironic that cultures which most obsess about the composition of foods are often those with high levels of diet-related health problems. Food labels, the main source of information on food composition for pre-packaged foods, [82] are supposed to help, but their increasingly long lists enumerating calories, fat, salt, sugar, RDAs (Recommended Daily Amounts) and so on means they are in danger of becoming too difficult to decipher. [83] Eating a diet of natural, unprocessed foods is far simpler since there are no labels with nutrient content. So what is it about natural foods that make them so healthy?

Nutrients are categorised into macronutrients (proteins, carbohydrates and fats), micronutrients (vitamins and minerals), fibre and phytochemicals. To function healthily, the human body needs about forty nutrients. These nutrients are termed "essential" since our bodies cannot make them. Essential nutrients include nine of the twenty amino acids that we use to build proteins, a couple of fatty acids, and almost all of the thirteen vitamins and sixteen minerals we need to prevent disease. The rest of the nutrients that the body needs it can make for itself, although many are also found in the average diet. These include the eleven remaining amino acids, various fatty acids, glucose and vitamin D.

In industrialised countries, most diet-related health problems boil down to a combination of insufficient micronutrients, fibre or phytochemicals and/or too many calories from macronutrients. Macronutrients provide the fuel that drives the body's engine. Micronutrients, by contrast, are needed to keep the body in good repair, and so each time we eat a micronutrient-rich meal we are giving our body a mini-service. Unfortunately we often give more attention to servicing our cars rather than being more concerned about our bodies, as the author John Kendrick Bangs warned:

"What fools indeed we mortals are
To lavish care upon a Car,
With ne'er a bit of time to see
About our own machinery!"

---

[82] http://www.eufic.org/en/healthy-living/article/nutrition-labelling-qa
[83] https://theconversation.com/food-labels-too-complicated-for-most-shoppers-to-understand-new-research-121837
In many cases a far simpler labeling system would be sufficient such as a "quality logo" but these are not so common
http://www.eufic.org/en/healthy-living/article/quality-logos-in-the-european-union

# Macronutrients

Fat often gets a bad press but it is clearly essential that we get enough since every cell in our body is surrounded by a membrane rich in fat. Fat makes up 60% of the brain. Fat is also needed to help absorb the "fat-soluble" vitamins, namely A, D, E and K. Fat is the most concentrated source of energy providing nine calories per gram whereas carbs and protein provide four calories per gram. Some very healthy diets are high in fat such as the Med diet which provides about 35-40% of its calories (which is the same as saying energy) as fat.

Virtually all foods contain protein. Meat contains protein and fat, but very little carbohydrate. By contrast, unprocessed plant foods contain protein, fat and carbohydrates, with carbohydrates usually predominating. This is why meat has a higher proportion of protein per calorie than plant foods. Being omnivores, our protein options are broad: not just meat, but also seafood, legumes, nuts and seeds, eggs and dairy (milk, cheese, yogurt), to which can now be added fungi (such as Quorn), insects and artificial meat. Which of these we choose is based on taste, and ethical, environmental, health and financial reasons.

Excess calories from macromolecules - mainly fat and carbohydrates - are literally fueling the obesity epidemic. But important as this crisis is, it does nevertheless risk deflecting attention from the equally pressing problem of deficiencies in micronutrients (vitamins and minerals), fibre and various plant-derived chemicals called phytochemicals. Often, excess macronutrients go hand in hand with insufficient micronutrients, fibre and phytochemicals. Hence there are huge numbers of people who are both overfed and undernourished.

# Micronutrients

Lacking adequate micronutrients is much more likely to go unnoticed than consuming excess calories. A quick look in the mirror at your profile has an immediate impact. Undernourishment from a micronutrient deficiency is less easy to detect, at least in the early stages when there may be no symptoms. Lacking one or more essential micronutrients has been dubbed "hidden hunger" and is a major health crisis. Unlike measuring BMI, a person's vitamin and mineral status is not routinely tested for. Carrying out these tests would be a huge step towards transitioning the NHS to an organisation that prioritises disease prevention. Knowledge of micronutrient status should be up there with BMI or awareness of an allergy.

Vitamins and minerals are essential for many fundamental metabolic processes. Each performs specific functions and they are not inter-changeable. For example, vitamin B1 (also known as thiamine) is needed for the body to convert glucose into energy, vitamin D is needed for bone formation and so on. Our bodies cannot make vitamins (with the exception of vitamin D) and so we must obtain them from our diet. This is encapsulated in the word "vitamin" which derives from "vital amine". [84]

Government surveys in the UK generally paint a reassuring picture of micronutrient status in the UK population. But when they report average intakes, these population-wide statistics are hiding huge variability between groups in society since they do not take into account specific groups who, for one reason or another, may be vulnerable to deficiencies. The elderly are a group particularly vulnerable to deficiencies. A recent National Diet and Nutrition Survey (NDNS) in the UK reported elderly people living in the community were often deficient in vitamin D, the B vitamins thiamine and riboflavin, and the minerals calcium, magnesium and selenium [98]. In the general UK population, the most common deficiencies are for calcium, potassium and vitamin D.

As well as the elderly, another group vulnerable to a thiamine deficiency are the steadily increasing numbers of people who avoid most cereal products (such as bread and pasta) because of gluten intolerance. These food products are the main source of thiamine in the average UK diet, so it's not surprising that many gluten-intolerant people are thiamine deficient. Fortifying gluten-free alternatives with thiamine and other vitamins would be an obvious solution, but, unfortunately, this is not usually done. Followers of the paleo diet also avoid cereal products, leaving this group vulnerable to thiamine deficiencies. Pork is an especially good dietary source of thiamine, but many people do not eat pork. Also, if you prefer your pork as sausages rather than fresh meat, then you are waving goodbye to most of the thiamine, since, in the UK, pork sausages are preserved with sulphites that destroy the thiamine.

---

[84] It's now known that not all vitamins belong the chemical family known as amines.

Ready meals that include sausages are very popular. Many older people rely on ready meals for a large part of their daily vitamin intake but it is concerning that pork sausages are not going to be providing much-needed thiamine. Some countries, such as the US, take a more sensible approach and have banned the use of sulphites in sausages for this very reason. Isn't it time that the UK also removed sulphites from sausages and other foods where it is not necessary?

Various micronutrient deficiencies are common in people with coeliac disease. This may be because coeliacs avoid vitamin and mineral fortified wheat products, or because of the malabsorption of some micronutrients such as iron, calcium, folate and fat-soluble vitamins especially before a diagnosis is made - which on average is fourteen years.

Obese people are also more likely to be micronutrient deficient. Many obese people don't consume enough iron, calcium, magnesium, zinc, copper, folate and vitamins A and B12, probably because of their poor diet [99]. What's more, body fat acts like a sponge for the fat-soluble vitamins A, D and E making them less available to the rest of the body. Although this book strongly advocates diet over supplements, the problems obese people have eating a healthy diet means that this is one case where a multivitamin supplement may be advisable [99].

## Micronutrients and chronic diseases

Lack of a particular vitamin causes a so-called deficiency disease such as rickets, scurvy or pellagra. Even if the early signs of these deficiency diseases may be missed, eventually their deficiency will lead to a medical diagnosis and the appropriate treatment. Much less well known is that some micronutrient deficiencies also increase the risk of *chronic* diseases [100]. A person not consuming enough of a micronutrient to prevent a chronic disease is sometimes referred to as having an "insufficiency" for that micronutrient. There are many examples. B vitamin insufficiency is linked with mild cognitive decline, insufficient vitamin B9 (which occurs naturally in plants as compounds called folates) increases the risk of CVD, vitamin D insufficiency affects the correct functioning of the immune system and thiamine (vitamin B1) insufficiency is linked to type 2 diabetes [98]. Minerals are also linked to preventing chronic disease. For instance, selenium, copper, zinc and magnesium all have roles in the aging process by reducing inflammation and ensuring the correct functioning of the immune system [(101)].

Early stages of these chronic diseases can easily go unnoticed since the initial effects may be relatively mild, diffuse and easily missed. Apathy, a decrease in short-term memory and muscle weakness can all be caused by insufficient thiamine - but these are also symptoms that could have many other causes and if this is due to insufficient thiamine this can easily go unrecognised and so untreated. After all, a feeling of apathy or being a little forgetful from time to time is nothing unusual. But ensuring enough thiamine is crucial. [85] The brain needs thiamine to be able to convert glucose into energy, and without adequate thiamine, brain cells die. The brain also needs thiamine to make acetylcholine, the main neurotransmitter that is deficient in patients with Alzheimer's disease. Thiamine levels are frequently low in patients with Alzheimer's disease and the early stages of cognitive decline, and there are trials underway to see if taking thiamine derivatives can reduce the symptoms of this disease.

Micronutrient insufficiencies probably also play a major role in cancer risk. For instance, both experimental and clinical studies indicate that inadequate intake of folates increases the risk of some cancers like breast cancer [(102)]. Multiple micronutrients are linked to cancer risk. A few years ago, the eminent scientist Dr Bruce Ames postulated an interesting theory linking micronutrient deficiencies with increased cancer risk [(103)]. Cancer starts with damage to DNA. It is well established that radiation and chemicals can damage DNA and so increase cancer risk. Ames demonstrated that insufficient micronutrients also damage DNA in the same way and he went further to suggest that these insufficiencies may be a far more significant cause of DNA damage than radiation or chemicals. A long list of micronutrient deficiencies mimic radiation exposure including deficiencies of various B vitamins, vitamins C and E, iron, and zinc. Folate (a type of B vitamin) deficiency is common in people who do not eat enough fruits and vegetables, and is linked to increased risk of colon cancer and acute lymphocytic leukaemia. Dr Ames hypothesised that when micronutrient intake is inadequate, the micronutrients available are prioritised for immediate use rather than to be used for processes that would have longer-term benefits

---

[85] Hoffman, R. (2017) Are you getting enough vitamin B1 to help fend off Alzheimer's? https://theconversation.com/are-you-getting-enough-vitamin-b1

like keeping DNA intact and so preventing cancer [103]. This prioritisation - triaging - has the consequence of increasing the risk of cancer over time. The triage hypothesis has been extended to other chronic diseases. Suggesting that micronutrient deficiencies are a fundamental cause of the epidemic of chronic diseases is a radically different perspective to the usual one that points the finger at obesity as the main cause.

## Micronutrient requirements

In the UK, the advisory amount of a micronutrients is usually expressed as its Reference Nutrient Intake (RNI). Most RNIs are based on the amount needed to prevent a *deficiency disease*. For instance, there is a fairly well established amount of vitamin D needed to prevent rickets. Establishing how much of a micronutrient is associated with helping prevent a *chronic disease* is more difficult. For instance in the case of vitamin D, there is uncertainty of the level needed to maintain a good immune system - another well-established role for this vitamin. This is because many other factors also contribute to good immune function. The same argument applies to the amounts of other vitamins needed to prevent chronic diseases. Because of these complexities, it is perhaps not surprising that few RNIs for micronutrients take into account their roles in chronic diseases. This is of concern since some researchers believe that the amounts of micronutrients needed to prevent many chronic diseases are higher than those needed to prevent deficiency diseases [104].

Another challenge with setting RNIs for micronutrients is that individuals can have widely different requirements [105]. This can be due to genetic differences between people, disease or medications. For instance, levels of thiamine in diabetics can be up to 50-75% lower than normal. A person with heart failure or a person taking the drug furosemide are two situations that decrease thiamine status in the body and hence increase requirements.

Vitamin deficiency diseases are sometimes seen as something that was left behind in the Victorian era and so today they receive relatively little attention. [86] But their widespread occurrence in some vulnerable groups like the elderly and their fundamental role in chronic diseases shows that this greatly undervalues their importance. Reference intakes for calories, sugars, salt and fat appear on the labels of most packaged foods, but there is no legal

---

[86] Although some like rickets are increasing again.

requirement to include any of the twenty nine vitamins and minerals. This probably contributes to the poor awareness of the dangers of low micronutrient intakes compared to, say, the dangers of excess calories or salt. Although mandatory labeling is one route, I do not believe that more labeling on packaged foods is the most practical guide on how best to eat [106]. Recommending diets with high nutrient profiles is a more straightforward approach [107].

## Dietary fibre

The chances are you do not consume enough dietary fibre: only 7% of UK adults are eating recommended amounts [5]. [87] UK adults eat 18 grams per day on average which is little more than half the recommended amount of 30 grams per day [108]. Figures are similar in many other western countries. Many avoid high fibre foods suspecting they will taste like cardboard. Most fibre is lost during food processing and junk foods typically contain hardly any. Because the typical "western diet" includes a lot junk food and other processed foods it is not surprising that fibre intake is inadequate.

Most people know that dietary fibre is a good thing, but only vaguely understand what it is and why it is healthy. The benefits of dietary fibre were already recognised by the time of the ancient Greeks, the physician Galen describing it as "food that excites the bowel to evacuate". This not very enticing view of fibre as a broom that cleans the gastrointestinal tract persisted until the 1970s. But fibre is far more than just a cleansing agent. It lowers the risk of colorectal cancer and possibly other cancers such as breast, pancreatic and oesophageal [88], and it also protects against stroke and type 2 diabetes [109]. Although eating at least 30 grams per day is best to minimise your risk of colorectal cancer, a study funded by the American Institute for Cancer Research found that if your intake of fibre is very low, even just getting up to the UK/US national average intake of about 17-18 grams per day will still dramatically reduce your risk of cancer. [89]

It is not mandatory for packaged foods to label fibre and so few do. Calculating your daily fibre intake is not a realistic proposition. So the best

---

[87] https://www.bbc.com/news/health-46827426
[88] https://www.sciencedirect.com/science/article/pii/S1078143917305367
[89] AICR/WCRF report (2018) Wholegrains, vegetables and fruit and the risk of cancer

way to avoid becoming fibre deficient is to select a range of fibre-rich foods. This section discusses what dietary fibre is and which foods are good sources.

## What is dietary fibre?

Plant cells are surrounded by a cell wall. (This is not the case with human cells.) This wall gives plant cells a rigid structure and acts as a barrier to protect the contents inside. Chewing can mechanically break down plant cell walls to a small extent. But this is where the digestion of the cell wall ends, since unlike for other nutrients (like protein and fats) there is no further digestion of plant cell walls in the stomach or small intestine. It is the digestion-resistant bits of plant cell walls (along with some other indigestible parts of plants) that we call dietary fibre [110].

There are many different types of dietary fibre and classifying dietary fibre has proven to be a challenge. It is sometimes simply divided into "soluble" and "insoluble". A more recent approach distinguishes different types of dietary fibre according to how they act in the body. In the small intestine (upper gut) dietary fibre acts as a physical agent, whereas in the large intestine (lower gut) some is broken down (fermented) to various bioactive products by gut bacteria. Based on these properties, three main types of dietary fibre are now recognised: viscous, fermentable and insoluble.

## Viscous fibre

High amounts of viscous fibre are found in oats (as a substance called beta-glucan), barley, aubergines, okra, most fruits, sweet potato, squash and legumes. This fibre forms gels in the intestinal tract. These gels reduce the amount of cholesterol that is absorbed and less LDL ("bad") cholesterol in the blood reduces the risk of CVD. The viscous fibre will be most effective at reducing cholesterol absorption if it is present in the gut at the same time as the cholesterol. So eating oats in the morning is not likely to have a large impact on cholesterol eaten during an evening meal. Viscous fibre also slows down glucose absorption and so can reduce the blood sugar surge that comes after eating a meal. Bread is mainly starch and gets broken down to glucose and typically causes a big surge in blood glucose. But eating fibre-rich dried fruits was shown to halve the rise in blood glucose caused by eating bread [111]. Reducing glucose levels is important both for lowering the risk of type 2 diabetes in healthy people and for helping people already with diabetes manage their condition. These effects of viscous fibre on cholesterol and glucose absorption illustrate how one food component can influence the absorption of another and that this will be most effective when both are present in the gut at the same time.

Another benefit of gel-forming fibres is to distend the stomach since this sends signals to the brain to register a feeling of fullness (satiety) [112]. This is a very important mechanism for appetite control and demonstrates how eating foods high in viscous fibre can help in weight control.

## Fermentable fibre - other mouths to feed

Since it is able to evade the onslaught of digestive enzymes in the small intestine, dietary fibre can make its way unscathed to the colon (large intestine). Here, some of the fibre is digested. It is not digested by enzymes produced by human cells, though, but by enzymes released from the trillions of bacteria that live there. These are known as the gut microbiota. The fibre that can be broken down in the colon by bacterial enzymes is called fermentable fibre since it is broken down in the absence of oxygen by the process of fermentation. Fermentable fibre is found in high amounts in oats, barley, onions, artichokes and legumes.

The colon is the compost heap of the body, full of bacteria that ferment waste scraps of food to useful products essential for our health. One particularly useful breakdown product of fermentable fibre is a short-chain fatty acid called butyrate. Butyrate is important because it keeps the cells that line the colon healthy and reduces their chances of becoming cancerous. Butyrate has many other actions as well, including regulating fat and carbohydrate metabolism, suppressing inflammation and even switching genes on and off.

The gut microbiota makes up more than half of the trillions of cells in the human body. We may think we have the upper hand in this relationship, but it is more finely balanced than we may care to think. The relationship has evolved as one of mutual benefit ("mutualism"). And to maintain the peace, each party must fulfill its side of the deal. For their part, gut bacteria expect adequate fibre. Gut bacteria are sometimes referred to as probiotics and hence the fermentable fibres that feed them are called "prebiotics". Eating a western diet is unlikely to provide adequate prebiotics and this can lead to a violent response from otherwise friendly colonic bacteria. If these bacteria do not receive enough prebiotic food they will look for alternative sources. One is the mucus that lines the colon [113]. This mucus layer normally acts as a protective barrier between the bacteria in the cavity (lumen) of the colon and the underlying colon cells. But hungry bacteria will digest this mucus barrier. Some types of colonic bacteria then exploit this breach in the barrier to invade into the underlying colon cells. This generates an inflammatory defensive response by the body to try and control the invading bacteria. So a normally beneficial coloniser has become a dangerous enemy. This starts a protracted war between gut bacteria and the body and the protracted inflammation arising from this is thought to contribute to many chronic diseases in the body. [90] This is a key event in understanding chronic diseases and is discussed more in chapter 10.

The composition of the gut microbiota is strongly influenced by diet. A diverse diet generates a diverse gut microbiota [114]. This diversity improves resilience and general health, since one species can compensate when another needs support, just as biodiversity improves resilience in a natural ecosystem such as a rainforest [115]. A potential threat to gut resilience is switching to a low carb diet since this can have a dramatic effect on the gut microbiota and potentially on health as well. Going on a low carb diet is likely to lead to a significant drop in dietary fibre intake since low carb diets advise against eating grains which are an important sources of fibre. A drop in fermentable fibre in the diet can reduce the production of beneficial butyrate in the colon. [91] The long-term health consequences of this are not known, but some studies suggest that eating too few carbs increases the risk of premature death [96].

## When is starch not starch?

The answer is: when it is resistant starch. Resistant starch is a form of fermentable dietary fibre. Unlike ordinary starch, resistant starch resists digestion by enzymes in the small intestine. Instead it travels unscathed to the colon where it is then fermented by bacteria. Resistant starch has the same *chemical* composition as normal starch (both are composed of chains of glucose molecules) but it has greater resistance to being broken down by digestive enzymes. In whole grains there are components of the whole grain that can act as physical barriers to protect the starch from attack by digestive enzymes. In other cases, the resistant starch may resist digestion by changing its physical structure into enzyme-resistant crystals and coils. Helical coils

---

[90] https://www.nytimes.com/2018/01/01/science/food-fiber-microbiome-inflammation.html
[91] https://www.medicalnewstoday.com/articles/323171#The-health-benefits-of-eating-carbs

form when starchy foods such as pasta are heated and then cooled down. This is an interesting example of how cooking can affect the healthiness of a food.

Like other forms of fermentable fibre, resistant starch is fermented to butyrate. Studies suggest that a diet high in resistant starch may lower the increased risk of colon cancer that comes from eating too much red meat. The mechanism proposed to explain this is another illustration of how foods may interact in the gut. Gut bacteria can ferment red meat to carcinogens, increasing the risk of colon cancer. It has been suggested that when resistant starch is included in the diet this is preferentially fermented, and so less red meat is fermented into carcinogens [116]. Resistant starch may also be useful for people with irritable bowel syndrome, and as it induces satiety it may benefit weight control.

High amounts of resistant starch occur in less ripe bananas, pasta, pulses and potatoes. Swallowing starchy foods like potatoes or bread without chewing them also reduces the glucose surge that normally comes after eating them [117]. Not very tempting maybe, but it does illustrate how retaining an intact food structure affects digestion.

## Insoluble fibre

Insoluble fibre is the third type of dietary fibre. It occurs in high amounts in wheat, rye, most vegetables, legumes, nuts and seeds. Plant cell walls consist mostly of insoluble fibre especially in the form of cellulose. Insoluble fibre is not fermentable even by our gut bacteria and the actions it exerts are due to its physical nature. It does this by creating large, soft faeces and by speeding up the passage of waste through the digestive tract. This enhanced speed reduces the time cells in the colon are exposed to carcinogens, reducing the risk of colon cancer.

Because non-fermentable fibre passes through the intestine relatively intact, the body does not absorb any of its calories. This fibre is sometimes known as "bulking" fibre. If you are concerned about your weight, it is reassuring to know that a large part of plant foods rich in non-fermentable fibres are going to come back out again in the faeces, carrying with them a massive population of bacteria (about a quarter to half of the solids in faeces are bacteria), undigested food and various waste products such as broken down red blood cells [118].

## Getting your fibre

Dietary fibre is found in all plant foods including grains, vegetables, fruits, legumes, nuts and seeds. Although, as highlighted above, particular foods are often high in one or other dietary fibre, most plant foods are a mixture of several types. And since each type of fibre offers unique health benefits the aim should be to eat a wide variety of fibre-rich foods and not to rely on a single source. In general, the least processed form of a food provides the most fibre. For example, whole grains provide more fibre than refined grains, and whole fruit supplies more fibre than juice. Processing natural plant foods into more refined products such as junk foods can lead to the complete loss of fibre. This is a major reason why the typical western diet high in processed foods is poor in fibre. The loss of dietary fibre during the food manufacture of junk foods has serious implications on health as will be discussed in the next chapter.

Some people rely on supplements or a food such as All Bran as their main source of fibre. Although fibre supplements boost fibre intake, natural foods high fibre also supply a bevy of other protective nutrients such as phytochemicals and these are less likely to be present in fibre supplements. So the best aim is to get fibre within an overall healthy eating pattern. It is to phytochemicals that we now turn.

## Phytochemicals - Nature's food additives

We are indebted to plants for their phytochemicals. These are the "plant chemicals" that give the plants we eat their brilliant colours and delicious flavours and which makes eating food plants such a delight. [92] Food plants produce phytochemicals for different reasons of course. Since they are literally rooted to the spot and unable to move, it is phytochemicals that serve to attract friend and repel foe. The colours of flowers attract pollinators, and the flavour molecules of fruits entice animals to consume them and so disperse their seeds. Toxic or bitter-tasting phytochemicals, some we find tasty, serve to repel microbes and insects so preserving the plant from attack. So phytochemicals are the natural chemicals that give plants their colours, flavourings and preservatives. Phytochemicals are Nature's food additives.

---

[92] Phytochemical simply means "plant chemical" although all other components of a plant such as its macromolecules are also chemicals.

Unlike their industrial artificial substitutes, Nature's food additives are full of healthful properties. Anyone eating a healthy plant-based diet is eating hundreds if not thousands of different phytochemicals every day. It was only a few years ago that nutritionists were dismissing phytochemicals as having little nutritional value. Plants, it was said, produce phytochemicals for their own benefit, but they are of no use to us. Indeed phytochemicals were somewhat disparagingly called non-nutrients. But there is now a huge amount of evidence that some of our organs, such as the eye, require specific phytochemicals to function correctly, and that more generally our health benefits enormously from consuming a diet high in phytochemicals. The tide has turned, and it is now clear: phytochemicals - "fightochemicals" - fight disease.

Another group of nutrients found in plants that fight disease are vitamins. There are, however, important differences between phytochemicals and vitamins. Vitamins perform very specific functions in the body and insufficient consumption of a vitamin results in a specific deficiency disease, such as rickets (a deficiency in vitamin D), or to an increased risk for a chronic disease. Phytochemicals on the other hand are usually more interchangeable and perform more generalised roles in the body. This means that many different phytochemicals can perform the same role and so if we don't get enough of one we can substitute another. Perhaps the best example of this general and interchangeable role is when phytochemicals act as antioxidants. A person's diet influences the types of phytochemicals they consume but it is the overall amount of antioxidant phytochemicals that matters more than the type.

Many antioxidant phytochemicals belong to a large family of phytochemicals called polyphenols. There is now evidence that polyphenols act as "life extenders". This not inconsiderable benefit was demonstrated in a study examining the health benefits of the plant-based Mediterranean diet (Med diet). This study found that the group of people consuming a Med diet richest in polyphenols had a 37% reduced risk of dying prematurely compared to those consuming a similar diet but with the least polyphenols [119].

A few polyphenols do have more specific roles against diseases. For example, lignans are a group of polyphenols found at high levels in some grains (and so in bread) and in seeds such as flax and sesame and which may help protect against breast cancer. Some studies suggest that women already with breast cancer who consume foods rich in lignans are far less likely to die of their disease [120].

Despite the huge growth in phytochemical research over the last few years, these substances still remain relatively unknown beyond the world of nutrition science. However, there are now so many interesting claims for their health benefits that phytochemicals warrant far more attention. Thinking of phytochemicals as Nature's food additives - colours, flavourings and preservatives - is a simple way of becoming familiar with these important chemicals.

## Phytochemicals as colours

The bright reds, oranges and yellows of many vegetables and some fruits are due to a family of phytochemical pigments called carotenoids. The best-known member of this family is orange coloured beta-carotene, which is found in carrots. Some other examples of carotenoids and their main dietary sources are shown in the table.

**Some commonly consumed carotenoids**

| Carotenoid | Converted to vitamin A? | Some dietary sources |
|------------|------------------------|----------------------|
| alpha-carotene | yes | carrots |
| beta-carotene | yes | carrots, spinach, tomato |
| lycopene | no | tomato |
| lutein | no | broccoli, green beans, green pepper, cos lettuce, spinach, corn |
| zeaxanthin | no | corn |
| beta-cryptoxanthin | yes | oranges, red pepper |
| capsanthin | no | red pepper, paprika |

A few types of carotenoids are converted in the body into vitamin A. This is the main way that vegans obtain vitamin A since vitamin A itself is only found in animal products. Much of the current interest in carotenoids is related to their powerful antioxidant properties. Two carotenoids perform an essential antioxidant role in the eye to help maintain good eye health. These are the yellow carotenoids lutein and its close relative zeaxanthin (named after *Zea mays* the Latin for sweet corn (Am. maize), a particularly rich source of zeaxanthin).[93] Retinal cells in the eye have devised a way of selectively sucking up these two carotenoids from the surrounding blood. Once in the retina, lutein and zeaxanthin accumulate in the part of the retina responsible for acute vision called the macula where they are thought to protect against photo-oxidative light damage and reduce the risk of age related macular degeneration (AMD).

There are many studies underway to see if supplements of lutein and zeaxanthin can help reverse early stages of AMD once it has already formed and there have been a few promising results [121]. However, meta-analyses, which combine the results from a large number of studies, have found that there is little evidence that taking these carotenoids in supplements prevents the progression of AMD [122]. It is possible that other substances in the diet are also needed for optimal eye health and this could explain why studies with these carotenoids alone is not sufficient to protect the eye. Lutein is also found in high concentrations in the brain and there is increasing evidence that lutein helps prevent cognitive decline [123].

The specific roles for lutein and zeaxanthin in the body align them more with vitamins than with phytochemicals and so there are now moves to classify these carotenoids as essential nutrients. This would lead to assigning lutein and zeaxanthin Recommended Nutrient Intake (RNI) values as is done for vitamins and minerals. It is because there are currently no RNI values for lutein and zeaxanthin that it cannot be stated if some people are consuming insufficient amounts of them. Studies do however suggest that the so-called western diet - which is a diet rich in processed foods and low in natural foods and so low in carotenoids - increases the risk of macular degeneration [124; 125]. One researcher has gone so far as to say that the western diet is entirely responsible for AMD and that eating a healthy diet would make AMD "entirely preventable" [125]. The trend to replace artificial colours with natural ones means that some carotenoids are now added to processed foods. However there is no evidence that these are effective substitutes for their

---

[93] A third carotenoid called meso-zeaxanthin may also play a role.

natural equivalents [126]. Overall, it does seem that the importance of dietary lutein and zeaxanthin does not receive enough publicity.

The most widespread of all phytochemicals is the green pigment chlorophyll. Within each molecule of chlorophyll there is an atom of magnesium and when chlorophyll is broken down in the body the magnesium is released. This is why green vegetables are a good source of this essential mineral, one that many people do not get enough of.

---

**The remarkable similarities between chlorophyll and haemoglobin**

Chlorophyll and haemoglobin are crucial to making plants and animals tick. Chlorophyll plays a central role in photosynthesis, the process that generates energy molecules for plants. The by-product of this process is oxygen. Haemoglobin in human red blood cells carries oxygen from plants around the body. The chemical structures of chlorophyll and haemoglobin are remarkably similar, the main difference being that at the heart of chlorophyll is an atom of magnesium and at the heart of haemoglobin is an atom of iron. The similarities between the structures of chlorophyll and haemoglobin led a group of Dutch researchers to suggest that chlorophyll in green vegetables may protect against the cancer-producing properties of haemoglobin in people. This is discussed more in ch. 12.

---

Photosynthesis is a complex process that involves lots of electrons flying around. These electrons can cause damaging oxidation reactions that harm cells. [94] So as the rate of photosynthesis in a plant increases so too does the risk of damage from oxidation. In order to protect themselves against this damage, plants package the machinery of photosynthesis with defensive antioxidant carotenoids (in structures called chloroplasts). A dark green vegetable is a sign that it contains a lot of chlorophyll and so has a high capacity for photosynthesis. Because there will also therefore be a correspondingly high risk of oxidative damage, dark green vegetables also contain high amounts of antioxidant carotenoids. Hence dark green

---

[94] These are unpaired electrons and occur in free radicals. They can remove an electron from another molecule, which is an oxidation reaction.

vegetables are excellent sources not only of magnesium from the chlorophyll but also of carotenoids. Dark green kale for example contains high amounts of the carotenoid lutein.

A third group of pigments in food plants are anthocyanins. These are responsible for the red and purple colour of many berries and the colour of red wine, and they are also present in the skin of aubergines and in red onions. Anthocyanins reduce risk factors for cardiovascular disease like high cholesterol levels [127].

## Phytochemicals as flavourings and preservatives

As fruits ripen, their seeds mature and become ready to be dispersed. A fruit signals this readiness to consumers (both animal and human varieties) by changing its colour from green to oranges and reds and by producing attractive aromas. This is typified by the ripening of a tomato (botanically a fruit), which develops its red colour and appealing aroma. Consumers then act as vectors for dispersing the seed, and the fruit rewards this service rendered with a deliciously sweet energy-rich sugary flavour.

One widespread group of phytochemicals responsible for flavours and aromas are the monoterpenes. Perhaps the most familiar of these is a molecule called limonene, which is found in citrus peel. It has a pleasant lemony flavour and aroma. There is some evidence that limonene may help protect against breast cancer but more work is needed to substantiate this [128]. Limonene is a very common flavouring and scent in foods.

Monoterpenes are also major contributors to the characteristic tastes and smells of herbs and spices, but here their main role is as anti-feedants to protect the otherwise defenceless plants from predation. Many other taste molecules also mainly act as anti-feedants to deter predation. Two groups of vegetables, namely members of the cabbage (brassica) family and members of the allium family (such as onions, garlic and leeks), produce sulphur-containing phytochemicals. These act as anti-feedants to insects. By contrast, we often find them tasty and some are very good for our health. Brassicas and alliums only generate their characteristic strong sulphurous odours when they are chopped and the more cabbages and garlic are chopped, the more sulphurous they become. This is because chopping breaks open the cells of the plants and this starts chemical reactions that convert relatively non-sulphurous precursor molecules into far smellier products. For a growing plant, it is insect attack that breaks open the cells. The sulphurous anti-feedant molecules are then generated which helps ward of attack. This means that the plant only produces the sulphurous products when they are needed.

For the cook, the most dramatic experience of this chemical reaction is when an onion is chopped since this leads to the production of a lachrymatory (tear-generating) factor. More important for health are the reactions that occur when brassicas are chopped or chewed. Brassicas contain a group of precursor sulphur molecules called glucosinolates and when these are activated they are converted into isothiocyanates (thio = sulphur). The best-known example of an isothiocyanate is a phytochemical called sulphoraphane, which is produced in high amounts in broccoli. There is good evidence that sulphoraphane has anti-cancer properties.

## The benefits of bitterness

Another common taste in the plant world is bitterness. Although it is thought that humans evolved to dislike bitterness in order to avoid eating potentially toxic plants, moderate levels of bitterness add interest and complexity to foods. Cultural conditioning during childhood is an important influence on what is considered an enjoyable level of bitterness in foods, and this is expressed in terms of an individual's "bitterness acceptance threshold". People also vary in their bitterness *detection* thresholds. Many foods are prepared in ways to keep bitterness to acceptable levels. For example, green tea is brewed in water at about 80°C in some cultures in the Far East, rather than with boiling water, to reduce the extraction of bitter compounds. Many Mediterranean greens, both cultivated and collected from the wild, such as wild chicory, wild rocket and dandelion, are sought for their bitterness. These greens are eaten raw in salads, sometimes by complementing the bitterness with a sweet dressing. If the level of bitterness is too high, the greens can be lightly boiled to leach out some of the bitter compounds. Bitter wild greens remain a source of food in more traditional Mediterranean societies and villagers in a rural area of Crete who consumed a lot of wild greens were found to have far better cardiovascular health than otherwise similar villagers who ate fewer wild greens [129].

Fruits that are too bitter to be eaten raw, such as quince and bitter (Seville) oranges, are cooked with sugar and made into preserves, making for an interesting overall taste. As tastes become more sophisticated there is an increasing desire for bitter tastes, and according to a recent Waitrose report there is an increasing trend for bitter foods such as high-cocoa chocolate and kale. [95]

It's been said that good medicine tastes bitter. Hippocrates, in the 5th century BC, was one of the first to use a medicinal bitter substance, which he described as "a bitter powder extracted from the willow that relieves pain and reduces fevers." In 1763, Reverend Edward Stone described the bark of the white willow as "a very effective remedy" to treat fever. We now know that the active substance in willow was the bitter phytochemical salicylic acid. Today 45,000 tons of aspirin, a salicylic acid derivative (which breaks back down to salicylic acid in the body), is produced each year [130].

Research is now revealing some intriguing ways how bitterness in plant phytochemicals confers health. Although we only detect bitterness through taste receptors on our tongues, other parts of the body also have receptors for bitter compounds. When bitter compounds bind to these receptors they can trigger beneficial physiological responses. An interesting example of this is in the airways. Some bitter compounds relax the airways and protect against airway constriction in experimental models of respiratory diseases like asthma and COPD [131]. These studies have not yet translated into new bitter medicines for asthma but this is a very active area of research. Because it is based on plant foods, the Med diet is rich in bitter compounds and eating this diet is associated with a reduced incidence of asthma [132]. Although it is tempting to think that at least some of this benefit is due to the bitter compounds binding to receptors in the airways this has not been possible to establish because of the many other potentially beneficial substances in a Med diet.

**How phytochemicals can improve stress resistance**

As well as binding to receptors, bitter compounds may benefit the body in a completely different way. This mechanism has fundamental implications for health. It starts from the somewhat paradoxical idea that toxicity in phytochemicals can be a good thing. This does however depend on the dose of the phytochemical since the beneficial effects only occur when the phytochemical is consumed in low amounts. Higher amounts of the

---

[95] Waitrose & Partners Food and Drink Report 2018-19

phytochemical are toxic. The differential effect of a high versus a low dose was encapsulated by Paracelsus 'the father of toxicology' in the sixteenth century in his famous aphorism "The dose makes the poison". Perhaps a more accurate aphorism to emphasise not only the dangers of a high dose but also the benefits of a low dose is "that which does not kill us makes us stronger".

So how can a low dose of a bitter phytochemical make us stronger? A considerable body of research has shown that low amounts of some phytochemicals induce mild levels of stress in the body and this benefits the body by making it more resilient to disease. This phenomenon is known as hormesis. Aspirin is a drug with these wide ranging benefits in the body. Aspirin is derived from the phytochemical salicylic acid and when aspirin is ingested it gets broken back down to salicylic acid, which is the active form of aspirin. In 2012, researchers from the University of Dundee in Scotland led by Professor Graham Hardie demonstrated that salicylic acid activates an enzyme called AMPK [133]. AMPK is a master switch responsible for a huge range of beneficial responses in the body including making the body more resilient to disease - a so-called hormetic response.

There is now increasing evidence that one of the main mechanisms underpinning the hormetic benefits of many bitter phytochemicals is their ability to activate AMPK [134]. This is related to the bitter phytochemicals acting as mild poisons. The process starts with bitter phytochemicals poisoning small structures in cells called mitochondria. Mitochondria are the powerhouses in cells that generate ATP - the cell's main energy currency. When mitochondria are poisoned, levels of ATP fall. AMPK is an enzyme that helps restore ATP levels. So when ATP levels fall AMPK is activated. Since ATP is generated in mitochondria, AMPK can only help restore ATP levels if the mitochondria are only partially poisoned but not killed. Too much of the poison and the cell dies. So a low non-fatal phytochemical dose enables the cell to benefit by activating AMPK triggering many beneficial effects in the body, whereas a high phytochemical dose can kill the mitochondria, which has a detrimental effect. This differential effect of a benefit with a low dose and a detrimental effect with a high dose is hormesis.

An interesting Mediterranean food that contains bitter phytochemicals that activates AMPK is the olive. Olives are inedible in their natural state because of their bitterness. Palatability is only achieved by processing olives - this processing removes most but not all of their bitter compounds (the simplest being prolonged washing in water). Extra virgin olive oil (EVOO) is produced by squeezing olives, which again removes most but not all of the bitter compounds. The main bitter phytochemical in olives and EVOO is called oleuropein. Extracts of EVOO rich in oleuropein have wide-ranging beneficial anti-cancer and anti-aging effects and these have been linked to activating AMPK [130].

Oleuropein is only found in olives and no other foods. So this important hormetic compound, oleuropein, will only come from eating olives or EVOO. EVOO is one of the defining plant foods of the Med diet. As discussed in chapter 12, EVOO may be essential to achieve the full health benefits of the Med diet, and oleuropein and its hormetic effects may be one reason for this.

Bitter compounds are just one example of a far wider range of mild assaults on the body that by not killing us make us stronger. Other examples include exercise, low-level exposure to toxins and calorie restriction. All of these mild stressors can increase resilience in the body and all can act by activating AMPK (other mechanisms are also involved). These mild stressors act a little like vaccines to immunise the body and provide an insurance mechanism against a future more serious disease.

It is not only humans that respond to external stressors. Plants also experience stress. Plants become stressed when they do not have enough water or nutrients, when they are exposed to overly intense sunlight, or when they are attacked by pathogens. Plants often respond to these stressful conditions by producing more phytochemicals [135]. During intense sun exposure, the outer skins of plants produce more phenolic compounds and carotenoids. This is not so much to act as a sun-cream to block out the sunlight but rather because these phytochemicals act as antioxidants to protect the plant from photo-oxidation.

The heat and drought and other environmental conditions that stress plants would also have been unfavourable for early humans because it is likely to mean a reduced food supply. So it would be highly beneficial if humans could recognise the phytochemical stressor signals in food plants and adapt physiologically to these new more challenging conditions. It has been proposed that humans have evolved to do just that. This is achieved by "reading" the environment through eating stressed plants and then adapting by up-regulating physiological processes that increase resilience. This concept is termed "xeno-hormesis" - the idea of a hormetic adaption to a foreign (ie plant) signal (xeno = foreign). This process may still occur to a significant extent in some human societies that must resort during drought years to eating wild greens, which have managed to survive by adapting to the stressful conditions. These plants have been labeled "famine foods".

Attractive as this idea of signaling between plants and humans is, is there any evidence that hormesis and xenohormesis actually exist? One candidate xenohormetic phytochemical receiving a lot of attention is resveratrol. Grapes produce resveratrol when they are stressed in response to exposure to intense sunlight or to infection by the mould *Botrytis cinerea*. Most resveratrol is consumed in wine. Experimental studies have found that resveratrol has wide-ranging benefits against cancer, dementia, type 2 diabetes and even aging [136]. Like many hormetins, resveratrol activates AMPK. (Although also like many hormetins this is not its only action in the body.) Clinical trials with resveratrol have shown promise but remain inconclusive and many scientists dispute its relevance to human health [137]. The ups and downs of resveratrol are well illustrated by the interest in this phytochemical shown by the pharmaceutical industry. The pharmaceutical giant Glaxo Smith Kline bought the rights to develop resveratrol as an anti-aging drug for $720 million but a few years later in 2013 this project was closed down as there was insufficient evidence for the efficacy of resveratrol. However if the benefits of resveratrol are through long-term xenohormetic effects, these may only appear after many years. These long-term mild benefits may not be of so much interest to a drug company although maybe they can be achieved by regularly drinking red wine.

## Organic plants and stress

Plants can find life particularly stressful when they are grown organically. Organic fruit and veg receive no artificial pesticides and so they are obliged to muster their own defence systems. They must also search harder in the soil for nutrients such as nitrogen because these are not provided in artificial fertilisers. These daily stressors can trigger the production of stress compounds, and this may account for why organic fruit and veg have higher amounts of phytochemicals than fruit and veg grown using conventional agricultural practices [135]. For instance, the phytochemical salicylic acid is produced when maize is stressed because of an increase in salinity. This then triggers a protective responses by the plant, namely greater salt-tolerance [135]. The xenohormesis paradigm predicts that because fruit and veg accumulate stress compounds when grown organically, consumers who eat these organic foods will increase their resilience to diseases such as cancer. Unfortunately the debate about whether or not organic fruit and veg are healthier is unresolved, since studies in humans are complicated by many confounding factors such as other healthy lifestyle features of people who tend to eat organic foods [138].

## Foods not phytochemicals

Despite the huge catalogue of health benefits ascribed to phytochemicals, some scientists remain sceptical. A main concern is that many phytochemicals are rapidly broken down in the body. Most vitamins by contrast remain more or less intact in the body for quite long periods. Countering this argument, it is now clear that many of the broken down forms of the phytochemicals (phytochemical metabolites) are still effective at reducing chronic diseases.

Related to this, when studying phytochemical effects in the body it is rarely taken into consideration that different people break down phytochemicals to different extents. When evaluating the health benefits of phytochemicals, it is also important to take into consideration other foods in a person's diet. For example, many herbs contain phytochemicals that influence the rates of uptake and breakdown of other phytochemicals in the body [139]. A good example of a substance able to do this is piperine, which is found in black pepper. There is quite good evidence that piperine increases levels of the anti-inflammatory phytochemical curcumin (found in the spice turmeric) and of resveratrol in the body, probably by decreasing the rate at which they are broken down [137; 140].

Natural food plants contain high amounts of phytochemicals but many are lost or at least dramatically reduced in industrial versions of natural foods. Orange squash contains hardly any of the phytochemicals found in an orange. Few phytochemicals are available as supplements to compensate for these lost phytochemicals and even if more phytochemicals were available this is a poor substitute for the huge variety found in a plant-based diet. So the best way to ensure adequate intake of these life-extenders is from a diet rich in unprocessed or minimally processed plant foods [141]. Every time a choice is made to eat a more processed version of a plant food, this risks losing health benefits, as the next chapter will demonstrate.

# 7. The risks from industrialised foods

## Overview

Not only does the average western diet contain too little fruit, vegetables, fish, legumes and whole grains, it also includes too much industrialised food. One of the great success stories of the food industry has been to normalise eating the highly processed foods that they manufacture so profitably. But the low costs for the food industry and at the checkout are paid for by a huge cost to society. The true costs are displaced to organisations that must deal with the aftermath: to our health systems for the costs of treating the chronic diseases that come from eating too much junk food and to society in general for the cost to the environment. In this chapter we look at some of the reasons why junk food is unhealthy.

## The rise of junk foods

It is not difficult to see where we went wrong by adopting our current western diet. Through human history there have been three major dietary transitions, periods when one diet was replaced by another. Early humans hunted and gathered what they could from Nature. The prerequisite for survival was to find food that was nutritious and to avoid foods that were toxic. The wrong choice made by an early human could mean death and so end their genetic lineage. This process of natural selection enabled humans to evolve over hundreds of thousands of years to make the most of available foods and to provide the nutrients needed for a healthy body.

Then, about 12000 years ago, humans realised that food supplies could be made more reliable by purpose-growing crops and keeping animals in captivity. And so arose the age of agriculture. The fundamental idea of food as sustenance was maintained because the plants and animals chosen were still those that were the most nutritious as well as being easy to produce.

Now we are in the third major transition where, increasingly, our food comes not from plants and animals but from products manufactured in factories. Behind every industrial process is the drive for profit. So we now have a disconnect: food produced for sustenance has been replaced with food produced for profit.

A key industrial strategy to maximise profits is to replace expensive ingredients with substitutes that are cheaper and extend shelf life. And so arose junk food. Why use natural fruit extract when you can use a "Nature-identical" artificial flavouring at a fraction of the cost? Why use natural fats when you can replace them with trans fats that greatly increase shelf life? Unfortunately we now know that the answer is because very many artificial ingredients and foods arising from industrial processes are bad for health. But why is this? Why does natural usually mean healthier?

## Junk foods are "ultra-processed foods" (UPFs)

Take some potato starch, add sunflower oil, cheese flavour and various other flavourings, a hotchpot of other ingredients and some clever processing and you have Walkers quavers cheese snacks. [96] Most junk foods are made like this, from highly refined ingredients concocted by industrial processes into, in the words of food writer Michael Pollan, "food-like substances". Many contain materials foreign to the average domestic kitchen such as protein isolates, modified starches and hydrogenated fats. Cosmetic additives such as colourings, flavourings, artificial sweeteners and emulsifiers are used to imitate the sensory qualities of natural foods or to disguise undesirable qualities in the final product. Because junk foods are created and assembled in processing plants with an array of industrial ingredients, the Brazilian nutritionist Carlos Augusto Monteiro and his colleagues call them "ultra-processed foods" (UPFs) [142]. This term has stuck with many nutritionists and it is the term I use here. [97]

Examples of UPFs include confectionery (Am. candy), commercial puddings, fruit yogurts, cakes and biscuits (Am. cookies), ice cream, processed meats, sausages and patés where the meat has been reconstituted, breakfast cereals, instant packaged soups and noodles, sweet or savoury packaged snacks, industrial pizzas and sugary drinks such as sugared milk and fruit drinks [143].

---

[96] For the ingredients of 10 common junk foods see
https://www.theguardian.com/lifeandstyle/2018/apr/12/ultra-processed-truth-10-bestselling-foods-cherry-bakewell-fray-bentos-pies
[97] For a critique of the term UPF see Fraanje, W. & Garnett, T. (2019). What is ultra-processed food? And why do people disagree about its utility as a concept? (Foodsource: building blocks). Food Climate Research Network, University of Oxford.

The end product rarely resembles the starting material, because the structure of the food has been fundamentally changed during processing. A cornflake bears little resemblance to an intact kernel of corn. Sugary drinks are a concoction of chemicals and water. Many fast foods are UPFs, but not all, since it is possible to buy healthy fast food based on fresh ingredients - fast food street vendors in SE Asia and elsewhere are testament to this.

The term *ultra* processed food was coined to distinguish these foods from other foods that are also processed. Canned vegetables and beans, canned fish, fruit in syrup, cheeses, freshly made bread, and salted or sugared nuts and seeds are all processed products. But these are not usually classified as *ultra* processed foods because they still retain some or most of their original composition. (Culinary products, such as salt and cooking oils, and unprocessed foods are also excluded from the UPF category.) The difference between UPFs and processed foods in Monteiro's classification is that processed foods at least started from natural foods, even if some of the nutrients may have subsequently been removed during processing. UPFs by contrast are made predominantly or entirely from industrial materials and are devoid of any resemblance to natural foods.

## The appeal of UPFs

UPFs are conceived in industry boardrooms and born in industrial processing plants. These babies of industrial food production make industry nerds drool at the marvels of manufacturing technology as viewers of the BBC series Inside the Factory will have witnessed. Just as the food industry loves UPFs for their low cost and high profit margins, retailers love them too for their long shelf lives. The shopper is enticed by intense marketing, attractive packaging and the fact that UPFs are ready for you: ready to eat, drink or heat. It's no wonder that in many places UPFs have virtually replaced fresh foods, foods that are "handicapped" by a short shelf life, less appeal to the shopper and a far lower profit margin for the food industry. Strategies that promote diets based on unprocessed or minimally processed foods are strongly resisted by the food industry.

If you like UPFs, you are not alone. Eating ever more UPFs is the single biggest trend in eating around the world. The average Brit now gets over half their calories from UPFs - the highest in Europe [144; 145; 146]. [98] It is clear that UPFs are part of daily life for many people in the UK, just as they are in many other parts of the world. [99] In the UK, younger people (18-29 years) get the most calories from UPFs (58%), but even the fifty year olds and older still obtain about 50% of their calories from UPFs [146].

UPFs are easy no effort food. It's food that gives instant gratification and because there's no cooking it's non-judgmental with no risk of being criticised for lousy cooking. But this way of eating sidesteps most of the social benefits of eating. If a natural home-cooked meal is a healthy embrace prepared with love then junk foods are more like a quick money transaction for a short-term fix. But "laced mutton" is no substitute for a lovingly prepared lamb stew.

## Evidence that UPFs are unhealthy

The campaigning paediatric endocrinologist Dr Robert Lustig once said that, because it is mostly diet-induced, type 2 diabetes should be called "processed food disease" (in today's parlance he would mean UPF disease), and that the huge shift in diet from consuming mainly natural foods to consuming mainly UPFs is an experiment that has gone horribly wrong, and should be stopped. And stopped right now [147].

Most junk foods manufacturers would no longer have the audacity to claim their products are healthy by making a virtue of their sugar content. The slogan "A Mars a day helps you work, rest and play" has passed its use by date. But although it is a truism to say that junk foods are bad for health, establishing watertight scientific evidence for this has been challenging for nutritionists. Which is great news for the food industry. A problem for nutritionists has been defining junk foods. It is obviously a prerequisite to know which foods to define as junk foods in order to analyse their health effects. Which is why the definition of UPFs devised by Dr Monteiro and his colleagues has proven such a boon to nutrition research. Coming to a consensus on which foods to categorise as UPFs now allows studies by

---

[98] The precise estimate varies a little between research groups because of using slight differences in their definitions of UPFs (eg NDNS includes canned vegetables)

[99] According to nationwide food surveys based on intake, household expenses, or supermarket sales, in European countries, the US, Canada, New Zealand, and Latin American countries, UPFs represent between 25% and 60% of total daily energy intake. See Srour, B. et al Ultra-processed food intake and risk of cardiovascular disease: prospective cohort study (NutriNet-Santé) BMJ 2019;365:l1451

different researchers to be directly compared and pooled to make the conclusions more robust. [100] And the consistent conclusion is that UPFs are indeed bad for your waistline, your heart and your brain.

One line of evidence suggesting that obesity is linked to eating UPFs comes from studies showing that the availability of UPFs in a country and the proportion of people in the country who eat UPFs are strong predictors for the rate of obesity in that country [144; 148]. Just a 10% increase in consumption of UPFs is associated with an 18% increased risk of obesity in people in the UK [149], and in a study of Canadians, those eating a diet with the highest proportion of UPFs were 32% more likely to be obese compared to individuals eating a diet containing the least UPFs [150]. Defenders of UPFs will point out that these studies only demonstrate an association and do not prove cause-and-effect: namely that it is the UPFs causing the obesity. This is quite right. For more definitive proof we need to turn to the gold standard for establishing a causal link, the randomised controlled study (RCT) (see ch. 5). RCTs look for factors that link cause and effect; experiments are conducted under carefully controlled conditions and so minimise the likelihood of spurious associations (known as confounders). Researchers from the National Institute of Health (NIH) in the US carried out an RCT to examine the links between eating a diet of UPFs and obesity, the first such RCT ever undertaken [151]. Twenty adults staying in a completely controlled environment known as a metabolic unit were randomly assigned to eat either a diet of UPFs or to eat a "control" diet of unprocessed foods, both eaten as three meals plus snacks across the day. Participants were allowed to eat as much as they wished. After two weeks on one of the diets, they were switched to the other for a further two weeks. This type of crossover study improves the reliability of the results since each person takes part in both arms of the study and acts as their own control. The study found that, on average, participants ate 500 calories more per day when consuming the diet of UPFs, compared to when eating unprocessed foods. And on the ultra-processed diet, they gained weight - almost a kilogram. This is the best evidence so far that eating UPFs directly leads to obesity. [101]

---

[100] UPFs are one category in the so-called NOVA classification system. However there is not universal agreement on which "junk" foods to define as UPFs.
[101] https://theconversation.com/ultra-processed-food-causes-weight-gain-firm-evidence-at-last-116980

We can gain weight quickly and so it is feasible to isolate people for a few weeks to see if they gain weight on a diet of UPFs. This is clearly not realistic for chronic diseases such as cancer since these typically take many years to develop. For these studies, free-living people are studied. These so-called "observational" studies rely on people accurately communicating their diet to researchers. [102] And they also rely on the researchers being able to rule out other factors that could explain links between eating UPFs and the health change such as which socio-economic group a person belongs to, their age, sex, BMI and calorie intake. A number of these observational studies that have taken these and many other possible confounding factors into account (it is not possible to consider every possible factor) have reported their findings in top ranking journals. All have shown that over-eating UPFs increases the risk of chronic diseases and of dying prematurely compared to people who eat a healthier diet. This consistency between studies greatly increases the likelihood of cause and effect. In a French study called the NutriNet-Santé study (so-called because participants were recruited from the internet), a group of middle-aged adults who ate the most UPFs were found to have a 10% higher risk of overall cancer and the women in the study had a 10% higher risk of breast cancer [152]. The risk of dying prematurely from heart attacks and stroke was also increased by over 10% for every 10% increased intake of UPFs [153]. In a group of Spanish adults, eating more than four portions of UPFs increased the risk of dying earlier - especially from cancer - by 62% [143]. Similar results were found in a study of a nationally representative sample of US citizens (called the National Health and Nutrition Examination Survey (NHANES)) [154]. People eating the most UPFs had a 31% higher risk of dying prematurely compared to people eating a diet low in UPFs. Taken together, these and similar studies strongly suggest that a diet high in UPFs increases the risk of dying prematurely from a chronic disease such as cancer or heart disease.

It's not only physical health that suffers. Although eating UPFs might make you happier in the short term, over the longer term there is an increased risk of depression. The middle-aged adults in France taking part in the NutriNet-Santé study were 21% more likely to suffer from depressive symptoms for every 10% increase in eating UPFs [155].

---

[102] A more object record of people diet is possible in some circumstances by looking at biomarkers in the blood. But at the moment there are no biomarkers for UPF consumption.

The consistent finding from these studies is that UPFs cause harm, and this has been sufficient for some nations, including France [156] and Brazil [157], to evoke the "cautionary principle" of potential harm and to advise their citizens in food guidelines to minimise consumption of UPFs. [103] If the junk food industry wants to claim that eating their products is not linked to health risks then they should provide the evidence to justify this, rather than there needing to be more studies showing that they are unhealthy. Of course, it's unfortunate for this industry that obesity is the collateral damage from eating their products since it's clearly not in their interests to contribute to the obesity epidemic, and they certainly don't like being held responsible for it. And the junk food industry is fighting back. Many articles critical of Monteiro's UPF classification system have been published, but it was found that of 38 authors writing critical articles on this UPF classification system, 33 were found to have links with the UPF industry [158]. [104]

The die-hards and the food industry often argue that it is the overall diet that matters and not one type of food. The picture they paint is of junk foods being consumed as an occasional treat. However, this is somewhat disingenuous since many UPFs are engineered with flavourings and textures that induce cravings and these, along with intense advertising, encourage them to be eaten in high amounts. There is currently an active debate as to whether or not ingredients like sugar, fat and salt should be classified as addictive like, say, nicotine. Others suggest it is the *act of eating* itself that is addictive, as a behavioural response to, for example, a stressful day - so called "eating addiction" [159]. However, far fewer people are likely to binge on broccoli than sugary and fatty foods after a hard day at the office and so it is highly unlikely to simply be the act of eating that is addictive.

Because UPFs are such a common part of the western diet, there have been attempts to estimate how much a person can eat without this causing adverse health effects. Dr Anthony Fardet from the National Institute of Agronomic Research in France (INRA) estimates that keeping UPF consumption below 15% of total calories (about 300 calories) a day - rather than the 50% or more

---

[103] This cautionary principle is reminiscent of that used by the AICR/WCRF in recommending that processed meats are best completely avoided.
[104] https://www.theguardian.com/food/2020/feb/13/how-ultra-processed-food-took-over-your-shopping-basket-brazil-carlos-monteiro

in the average adult UK diet - will not significantly increase the risk of obesity [160]. This is equivalent to the calories in two cans of regular Coca Cola or a medium order of chips (French fries). However, obesity is only one of the health risks that comes from eating UPFs. There is little understanding about where the bar should be set for junk foods in relation to other chronic diseases. A common belief is that healthy eating some of the time can offset less healthy choices the rest of the time. But, I will argue, for most people the bar should be shifted much further than they think towards healthy foods.

## Some reasons why UPFs are harmful

The main culprits in UPFs convicted of harming health are salt (which raises blood pressure increasing the risk of CVD), and sugar and fat (whose calories cause weight gain). Many countries are required by law to label sugar, salt, fat and calories on packaged junk foods. [145]. However, many observational studies still find an association between UPFs and poor health even after having taken sugar, salt, fat and calories into account. Hence there must be other factors in UPFs that also account for their harmful effects. So sugar, salt, fat and calories are only part of the far more complicated picture that explains why UPFs are unhealthy.

What additional reasons could there be? One of the aims of renaming junk foods as UPFs was to shift thinking of them simply as harmful packages of sugar, salt and fat and towards thinking more about what happens during the production of UPFs. During the processing of UPFs there are losses of nutrients, the additional of potential harmful substances and significant changes in physical structure. It is these changes that must bear a significant part of the responsibility for the detrimental health effects of UPFs.

### 1. Loss of beneficial nutrients

During the manufacture of ultra processed ingredients from natural foods, most nutrients are stripped away. When these ultra processed ingredients are reconstructed into a UPF, sugar or fat are usually added. Hence these calories from sugar or fat are associated with few nutrients in the overall food product - they are "empty" calories. So eating a UPF does not make the calories count since there are no associated nutritional benefits. This is the opposite of natural unprocessed foods where the calories are associated with other components with nutritional value. Here the calories do count.

Another way empty calories in UPFs are expressed is to say that UPFs have a low nutrient density. This means that it is very difficult when eating a diet high in UPFs to consume adequate healthful nutrients without at the same time consuming excess calories. To achieve recommended levels of nutrients from a diet high in foods full of empty calories would require consuming levels of calories well above recommended levels. Even consuming excess calories, many people still do not consume adequate nutrients. This consumption of high-calorie, nutrient-poor foods is generating a new type of malnutrition: one where people are both overfed (and so risk becoming obese) and undernourished [99; 100; 161]. Most people have quite low levels of physical activity and so cannot afford to consume empty calories.

People busy eating UPFs often limit their intake of healthy foods for fear of eating too many calories, or simply because they don't have any appetite left for them. Because the average Brit gets more than half their calories from UPFs, staying within the recommended calorie intake risks serious nutrient deficiencies. So it is not surprising that many people eating a diet high in UPFs fail to achieve adequate micronutrient intake if they stay within the recommended calorie intake [162; 163]. Using data from the U.K. National Diet and Nutrition Survey for 2008–2014, researchers found that over 90% of people in the UK categorised as consuming the most UPFs were not consuming recommended levels of dietary fibre and potassium [145]. Similar trends were seen in US adults. The average content of protein, fibre, vitamins A, C, D, and E, zinc, potassium, phosphorus, magnesium, and calcium decreased significantly as consumption of UPFs increased [164]. Gaining weight prompts many people to diet, but reducing calorie intake on a nutrient-poor diet risks micronutrient deficiencies and so it is not surprising that many people on diets become micronutrient deficient [165].

Health bodies have long recognised that vitamins and minerals are lost during food processing, and so some must be added back by law. Bread is a significant source of dietary micronutrients, and there is a modest attempt in the UK and other countries to compensate for those lost from wheat grains during milling or processing into cereal products. In the UK, refined wheat products must be fortified with calcium, iron, and the B vitamins niacin and thiamine. However, these are not necessarily like for like replacements. Iron has been added to flour and cereal products for many years, but the form of iron added is more like iron filings and is very poorly absorbed by the body

(166). Hence there is no guarantee that this mineral will actually be of much benefit when it is added back.

There are also concerns about thiamine fortification. Inadequate thiamine causes the deficiency disease beriberi. This disease is uncommon in western countries, but insufficient amounts of thiamine can lead to apathy, a decrease in short-term memory and muscle weakness, and may even be linked to an increased risk of Alzheimer's disease [167]. Unlike most other vitamins, there is evidence that thiamine is poorly absorbed when taken as a supplement. [105] Thiamine is destroyed during the production of some UPFs. Governments may point out that vitamin deficiency diseases in their country are very low and so their current strategies of micronutrient fortification are working. But, as I discussed in the previous chapter, this skates over the heightened risk of specific vulnerable groups in society such as the elderly in relation to thiamine deficiency [98; 168].

The food industry has not been slow to exploit a marketing trick here, and sometimes market their snack bars or other UPFs as being "fortified" with a nutrient or two. This has been shown in studies to favour purchasing these products over healthier alternatives [169]. But a couple of added-back vitamins are a poor return on the very many nutrients likely to have been lost during the manufacture of these products.

## 2. Salt

Salt is the main dietary cause of high blood pressure - the number one cause of premature death. Public health campaigns to reduce salt have had some success. However, many UPFs still have a high salt content and in the UK people who eat a lot of UPFs have a higher than average salt intake [145]. Of course, UPFs are not the only dietary source of salt. This may explain why there is less of an association between high salt intake and eating UPFs in most other countries that have been studied (such as the US and Canada). In these countries, other foods in the overall diet are probably also important sources of salt. Salt added directly to food could also be an important source of salt in these countries.

---

[105] Scientific Opinion of the Panel on Food Additives and Nutrient Sources added to Food (ANS) on a request from the Commission on benfotiamine, thiamine monophosphate chloride and thiamine pyrophosphate chloride, as sources of vitamin B1. The EFSA Journal (2008) 864, 1-31.

## 3. Synthetic chemicals

Most UPFs contain complex cocktails of synthetic chemicals. Some are added during the production of UPFs to improve taste or texture whereas others are byproducts that form during manufacture. Some are regulated, but this is not the case for all and some don't even need to be labeled on the packaging.

<u>By-products formed during the manufacture of UPFs</u>

One of the most notorious group of by-products that form during the industrial manufacture of some UPFs is trans fats. Industrial trans fats form when vegetable oils are converted into semi-solids by an industrial process called partial hydrogenation. Industrial trans fats find their way into many UPFs such as deep-fried fast foods, bakery products, packaged snack foods and margarine. The food industry loves trans fats because they are so stable. They are highly resistant to oxidation compared to other fats and so far less likely to go rancid which means an increased shelf life.

Trans fats also form during deep-frying - a common cooking method for many UPFs such as chips. Many fast food outlets have adopted healthier processes such as using more stable oils but these are more expensive [170]. Some small takeaway shops operate under very tight profit margins and inadequate regulation means that levels of trans fats in takeaway foods are only weakly scrutinised. In one survey from the UK, kebabs were particularly high in trans fats, sometimes exceeding recommended daily levels in a single serving [171].

The detrimental effects of trans fats on health should be far too high a price to pay for their convenience. The pros and cons of many nutrients may be vigorously debated. Not trans fats. They are universally condemned because of their links with coronary heart disease (CHD) [172]. You might think that because of their harm to health, industrially produced trans fats would be banned. This is the case in some countries such as Denmark. But it is not the case in the UK where regulation is still on a voluntary basis. Many food manufacturers in the UK such as margarine manufacturers have changed their production processes to reduce levels of trans fats. But trans fats continue to be consumed. According to calculations from UK researchers, a complete ban on trans fats in the UK would save over 7000 lives per year from CHD [173]. This would particularly benefit people from lower socio-economic groups who are more likely to consume foods higher in trans fats. An evaluation of the current voluntary agreement to reduce trans fats in the UK concluded that its effectiveness "appears to be negligible" [54]. It is clearly time for regulation.

Various other potentially harmful byproducts form during the manufacture of UPFs. For instance, processing breakfast cereals and carbohydrate-rich snacks involves extrusion and high temperatures, processes that leave high amounts of substances called AGEs in the finished product [174]. AGEs promote harmful inflammation in the body and are linked to a wide range of chronic diseases (see ch. 10). One AGE called acrylamide is a suspected carcinogen as judged by the European Food Safety Agency. It is present at high levels in various UPFs such as crisps and biscuits. Eating high amounts of UPFs has been linked to an increased risk of cancer [152] although it is not known to what extent acrylamide is responsible for this.

UPF additives

Many substances are deliberately added during the production of UPFs to enhance taste and texture, and these may contribute to the harmful effects of UPFs. We will consider three: artificial sweeteners, phosphates and emulsifiers.

Consuming sugar-sweetened beverages (SSBs) is strongly associated with an increased risk of obesity and type 2 diabetes [175]. Drinking sugary drinks (including fruit juices) is also associated with an increased risk of overall cancer and more specifically with breast cancer [176]. Hence the sugar in SSBs is now the target for government taxes and public awareness campaign.

Because the case against SSBs is now very strong, manufacturers are increasingly replacing the sugar in SSBs with artificial sweeteners. But these do not always fare any better. High consumption of sugar damages the body's ability to absorb sugar (in the form of glucose). The body is said to have a decreased tolerance for glucose. In a series of experiments, the artificial sweeteners sucralose, aspartame, and saccharin were also found to reduce glucose tolerance in healthy humans [177]. This glucose intolerance is linked to type 2 diabetes and many other diseases. This is unfortunate since switching from sugar to artificial sweeteners was designed to avoid this. Gut bacteria are known to influence glucose tolerance and it is thought that the artificial sweeteners may be disrupting the balance and diversity of gut microbiota, and promoting the growth of types of bacteria that produce inflammatory substances [114]. Although this study needs confirming, this finding prompted one group of scientists to claim that "contrary to popular belief, artificial sweeteners may actually be unhealthier to consume than natural sugars" [178]. It is not only SSBs that are the problem as artificial sweeteners are added to many other "diet" products, most of which are classified as UPFs.

Phosphates are another cause for concern. "Why phosphates will be the next taboo ingredient" runs one headline. "Is phosphate the new sodium?" runs another. [106] However unlike sodium chloride - aka salt - few people are aware of phosphates in food and even fewer know that high amounts can pose a serious health risk. Artificial phosphates are added in high amounts to many UPFs and other processed foods. They are added to cola drinks to stop them turning black and to meats, poultry and fish to retain water and make them juicier after freezing and reheating. Canned fish and baked goods also often contain phosphates [179].

Phosphates also occur naturally in many common protein-rich foods such as dairy products, fish, meat, sausages, nuts and eggs. However, whereas only about half of naturally occurring, so-called organic phosphates, are absorbed by the body, the artificial forms, inorganic phosphates, added to UPFs and other foods are almost completely absorbed. This matters since high levels of phosphates in the blood increase the risk of CVD by causing calcium deposits and hardening of the arteries around the heart.

People with chronic kidney disease are less able to excrete excess phosphates and have long been advised to limit phosphates in their diet. However, with the rise in UPFs, estimated daily intake of phosphates has more than doubled since the 1990s, and these high levels of phosphate are posing a health risk even for people with normal renal function. At the moment, phosphates added to many foods are not labeled, although this may change over the next few years. In the meantime, packaged foods that do label phosphates will show as ingredients containing the prefix "phos".

Emulsifiers crop up in many UPFs such as reduced-fat products and ice cream. Like artificial sweeteners, these too can reduce gut biodiversity and promote inflammation. This area of research is still in its infancy, but it could emerge that many products common in processed foods may endanger our

---

[106] https://www.washingtonpost.com/lifestyle/wellness/why-phosphate-additives-will-be-the-next-taboo-ingredient 2017/03/29

health by negative impacts on the gut microbiota. The good news is that changing to a more gut-friendly diet can result in significant improvements in the gut microbiota in only a few days [114].

## 4. Loss of food structure

Renaming junk foods as ultra processed foods shifted the focus from *what they contain* (such as high amounts of sugar, salt and fat and low amounts of many nutrients) to *how they are produced*. Producing UPFs not only influences nutrients but also physical structure. The blob of processed ingredients born on the factory conveyor belt needs clever technological trickery to transform it into a product that is digestible, visibly attractive and with a desirable texture. Food texture matters to food manufacturers. Not for them a biscuit without a satisfying crunch nor a chocolate without a melting texture.

Food texture for a food technologist may be all about sensory appeal, but it also influences health. For thousands of years humans have been altering the structure of food to improve digestibility. Wild grasses were ground down by Neolithic man before being cooked [180]. The process of bread making - turning barely digestible raw dough into a loaf of bread - happens millions of times every day and benefits many millions more. Grinding and cooking break down the structures of unprocessed foods and provides greater access to digestive enzymes. These enzymes can then liberate more molecular food fragments to be absorbed by the body. These changes to the physical structures of foods improve the availability - so-called bioavailability - of important nutrients.

The food structures of natural foods are lost in UPFs. And whereas some lost nutrients can be replaced in UPFs, this is not the case with food structures. The loss of food structures in UPFs is a defining feature of food processing and unrectifiable. The health benefits conferred by the food structure of natural foods is lost when these natural structure are altered by processing. The superior health benefit of whole grains versus refined grain products is a good example.

Many UPFs have artificially created food structures. But these do not confer the same health benefits as natural food structures. So why does the baked crispiness of a biscuit not confer the same health benefits of the crunchiness of a whole grain or apple? The difference is that the physical structure of a biscuit is uniform, whereas the physical parts of food plant divide it into many structural compartments. For instance, a wheat grain consists of several distinct compartments: an outer fibrous wall, the "bran", which protects the compartment containing the embryo (germ), and a separate compartment called the endosperm that contains the embryo's starchy energy supply (see Figure). The intactness of the compartments influences how we digest the plant food. In intact wheat grains, the fibrous cage enclosing the starch protects the starch from being broken down into glucose by digestive enzymes. Whole grain bread retains many intact wheat grains, while grinding the grains into whole meal flour breaks down the protective fibrous cage. So even though the fibre is still a constituent in whole meal flour, it is now distributed throughout the flour and so no longer acts as a barrier protecting the starch from digestive enzymes. It is no more protective than if the fibre had been removed. Hence whole grain bread raises blood glucose levels to the same extent as bread made from more refined flour.

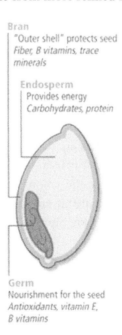

**A whole grain**[107]

---

[107] (https://commons.wikimedia.org/wiki/File:Grain.gif)

The extent to which a food increases "blood sugar" (ie glucose) levels is expressed by the food's Glycaemic Index (GI). GI is measured on a scale of 0 -100: the higher the GI value the greater the rise in blood glucose. [108] Whole grain breads have a relatively low GI value (53), but wholemeal bread, even though it retains all the fibre, has a higher GI (74), which is the same as the GI value of white bread, which is low in fibre. This is because even though none of the fibre is lost in wholemeal bread it has been dispersed and its original physical structure is lost. So the structure of the food matrix can be more important than the overall fibre content, at least as far as controlling blood sugar is concerned. Fibre eaten as a bran food or supplement does not reproduce the structural benefits that dietary fibre in unprocessed foods bring by protecting nutrients from digestion. [109] The low GI values of whole grains are an important reason why they are recommended in dietary guidelines.

Nutritionists refer to the rigid structures of a food plant as its food matrix and it is where most of the dietary fibre is found. During food processing much of the food matrix is lost and hence most UPFs contain very little dietary fibre. Antioxidants and other phytochemicals are tightly bound to the plant's fibrous matrix [181]. The matrix protects these molecules during digestion by chaperoning them through the upper gut, protecting them from digestive enzymes. Many of the phytochemicals are then released from the fibre in the colon by enzymes produced by the gut bacteria. Hence many matrix-bound phytochemicals are absorbed across the colon rather than across the small intestine. The health consequences of this are little studied. It does however suggest that complex naturally occurring fibre, with its bound phytochemicals, is not the same as industrially produced bran products since the industrial processing strips off many of phytochemicals and other nutrients. (This is why bran cereals are fortified with vitamins to add back some of those lost during the manufacture of the bran.)

The food matrix explains why fruit juices are less healthy than eating intact fruits. Chewing an apple only partially releases its sugars since a lot of the sugar is protected by fibrous components of the plant cell walls and so passes

---

[108] https://www.health.harvard.edu/diseases-and-conditions/glycemic-index-and-glycemic-load-for-100-foods
[109] However, fibre has other health benefits.

110

through the small intestine unabsorbed. Juicing and refining on the other hand remove cell walls liberating high levels of sugars from fruits. These so-called free sugars are readily absorbed in the small intestine. So, fruit juices have higher GI values than intact fruits. For example, the GI of apple juice is 41 compared with 36 for an apple, and the GI of orange juice is 50 compared to 43 for an orange. Health-wise this has important consequences. High levels of blood glucose trigger spikes in insulin and raised glucose and insulin spikes are linked to an increased risk of type 2 diabetes [175]. Consequently, NHS advice in the UK is to limit fruit juice consumption to one portion (150 ml) per day, preferably with a meal (as this may itself slow down sugar absorption), whereas there is no limit for fruit consumption. Although spikes in glucose and insulin occur with natural fruit juices, these are still preferable to artificial sugar sweetened beverages (SSBs). SSBs carry a far greater risk of type 2 diabetes, and have few, if any, of the redeeming nutritional benefits of natural fruit juices such as micronutrients [175].

There is some clinical evidence that less refined fruit juices are healthier. One study found that people drinking cloudy apple juice had lower levels of blood glucose than after drinking a more refined juice made from concentrate [182]. The cloudy apple juice was found to contain about twice the concentrations of a phytochemical called phloridzin. Phloridzin is a potent blocker of glucose uptake from the gut and this may help explain why there was less glucose absorption from the cloudy apple juice. Perhaps a glass of cloudy apple juice, as well as an apple a day, may help keep the diabetes doctor away. Current government recommendations make no distinction between less refined juices and juices made from concentrates, which may be missing a trick.

Fibre-rich natural foods are sometimes shunned because they take longer to chew than UPFs. To chew through a whole orange with its intact food matrix takes far longer than gulping down the equivalent calories as orange juice. If you have the teeth, fibre-rich foods are worth persisting with. The time needed to chew has hidden benefits since it gives time for satiety mechanisms to kick in before too many calories have been consumed. We are told fast foods make us fat because of their calories. But we also usually eat them fast and so consume more calories before satiety mechanisms kick in [183]. [110] This

[110] Hoffman, R. (2019) Ultra-processed food causes weight gain – firm evidence at last

was demonstrated in the randomised control trial carried out at the NIH on UPFs mentioned earlier in this chapter. The study found that when participants ate a meal of UPFs they consumed on average seventeen calories more per minutes than when they ate a nutritionally equivalent meal of unprocessed foods. The participants eating UPFs then went on to consume 500 more calories than when they were eating unprocessed foods [151]. [111]

An interesting message emerging from this and similar studies [184] is that, in order to regulate calorie intake, we should retain the natural matrix of unprocessed foods. This obliges us to eat more slowly, allowing time for the body's satiety mechanisms to kick in time and so prevent excess calorie consumption. This mechanism does not operate with UPFs since the food matrix is lost during manufacture. To reduce calorie intake, we need slow food not fast food.

It is also possible that the dangers of fat in UPFs may extend beyond the absolute amount of fat and include how the fat is arranged within the overall food matrix. This is discussed in the Dairy section of chapter 12.

It can be a real challenge for many people to find the time to sit down and slowly eat a meal of unprocessed foods. Some countries, however, vigorously defend the tradition of sitting down to meals and eating a succession of dishes in a leisurely - and pleasurable - way. It is noteworthy that in some of these countries, such as France, obesity levels are well below those of other comparable countries. Slow eating whole foods may be an important antidote to the weight gain caused by grabbing a quick meal of UPFs.

If eating a diet centered on natural unprocessed foods makes the calories count, then eating a diet centered on junk foods fails to make the calories count. To rephrase Michael Pollan's famous aphorism "Eat food, mostly plants, not too much" we could say, "Eat mostly plants. Minimise UPFs." This chapter has also emphasised that looking at the broader way nutrients in foods interact is more important rather than focusing on individual nutrients. This theme is developed in the next chapter.

---

https://theconversation.com/ultra-processed-food-causes-weight-gain-firm-evidence-at-last-116980

[111] Fibre is an important satiety factor in unprocessed foods. Most UPFs contain little if any fibre (most or all of it is lost during their manufacture) and so are easier to eat fast. But this difference cannot explain the results of this study since the researchers equalised the fibre content of their two diets by adding a fibre supplement to the ultra-processed diet.

# 8. We eat meals not nutrients: why this matters

"The problem with nutrient-by-nutrient nutrition science is that it takes the nutrient out of the context of the food, the food out of the context of the diet, and the diet out of the context of the lifestyle." (Marion Nestle)

## Overview

There's a sketch in a Monty Python film of a waiter serving a restaurant meal. This is a meal with a difference though since the meal simply consists of a few pills. Served alongside the pills is a photo of the dish the pills are there to replace. The ultimate dénouement in junk food maybe, but one where our current path of industrialised food could all too easily lead. So what is wrong with this, you may ask. In this chapter I will attempt to answer that question.

## Why measuring nutrients is not very helpful

In the 1930's, the Hungarian biochemist Albert Szent-Györgyi found that a newly isolated compound called hexuronic acid prevented guinea pigs from developing scurvy-like symptoms. This discovery earned Szent-Györgyi the Nobel prize, and paved the way for vitamin C, as the compound was renamed, to be used to treat scurvy. Preventing or curing deficiency diseases such as scurvy by providing the deficient vitamin or mineral has been a great achievement of nutritional medicine.

The amount of a vitamin or mineral needed to prevent a deficiency diseases helps set its recommended nutrient intake (RNI) value, and today RNIs are a standard part of dietary guidelines. Of course, few people go through the day calculating their intake of a particular vitamin or mineral. RNIs for protein, carbohydrate or fat are of even more doubtful use to the general public because there is a lot of flexibility in the daily amount of these nutrients that are compatible with a healthy diet (see ch. 6). Both a relatively high carb diet and a relatively high fat diet can be healthy. The NHS statement that "the average man aged 19-64 years should eat no more than 30g of saturated fat a day (20 g for women)" [112] or that "adults should have no more than 30g of free sugars a day, roughly equivalent to 7 sugar cubes" is really not much use to most people. [113] (Who uses sugar cubes anyway these days?) So absolute amounts carry little meaning, and although RNIs are helpful for nutritionists, they are of little use to non-nutritionists.

Giving specific advice about how much of a nutrient to consume can confuse, and increase the risk of a person excluding healthy foods from their diets. A person may reduce their intake of dairy produce, especially full fat, in order to reduce their saturated fat intake. But reducing dairy risks overly reducing this important source of calcium and iodine. Concerns about saturated fats have led to a profusion of low fat products where the saturated fat is often replaced with sugars and trans fats, although both of these in excess are health risks. By avoiding foods high in saturated fats, many people have found themselves eating less healthy, not healthier, foods. These concerns about nutrient-based dietary advice have led many nutritionists to conclude that advice about what to eat should be based on foods not nutrients. [114]

## The limits of supplements

Supplements are the ultimate in nutritional reductionism. Millions of people take nutritional supplements hoping they will boost their health or even cure them of certain diseases like arthritis or depression. But compensating for a nutrient-deprived western-style diet with supplements is a poor trade-off. The relationship between diet and health is far more complex than simply popping a supplement for an ailment.

Claim and counter-claim about nutritional supplements ping-pong between whether or not they are beneficial. Whilst this may simply influence whether or not you choose to buy them, the consequences can be far more significant. An infamous example concerns the antioxidant beta-carotene. In the late

---

[112] *https://www.nhs.uk/live-well/eat-well/eat-less-saturated-fat/*
[113] *https://www.nhs.uk/live-well/eat-well/how-does-sugar-in-our-diet-affect-our-health/*
[114] For instance, the 2018 WHO guidelines recommend that no more than 10% of calories should come from saturated fat but, it was suggested, this statement should be replaced with food-based advice 185. Astrup A, Bertram HC, Bonjour JP *et al.* (2019) WHO draft guidelines on dietary saturated and trans fatty acids: time for a new approach? *BMJ* **366**, l4137.

1980's there was a good deal of excitement in the nutrition world that dietary beta-carotene might prevent lung cancer. Studies had found that people who ate a diet rich in beta-carotene, such as from eating carrots, had a lower risk of getting lung cancer. A trial was undertaken giving purified beta-carotene (together with the antioxidant vitamin E) to smokers and asbestos workers - two groups at heightened risk of lung cancer. To the surprise of virtually the entire nutrition community, rather than decreasing the risk of lung cancer the beta-carotene supplements increased the risk [186].

Joining beta-carotene on the list of dubious antioxidant supplements are vitamins with antioxidant actions, namely vitamins A, C and E. Various reviews and meta-analyses of different studies have concluded that consuming antioxidant vitamin supplements has no benefit and in some cases may increase, not decrease, the risk of premature death [187; 188]. Again this contrasts with dietary sources, since diets rich in antioxidant vitamins are associated with reduced mortality.

Nutrition research is littered with similar examples where the benefits of a whole diet are not reproduced when the putative beneficial ingredient is isolated and given as a supplement. And like beta-carotene, in some cases the isolated nutrient may not just be neutral but a risk to health. Folic acid has a Jekyll and Hyde character since it can both increase and decrease cancer risk depending on the circumstances. It is not recommended that cancer patients and cancer survivors and those over 50 routinely take folic acid supplements [87]. Folic acid given in supplements is often not completely broken down in the body and the remaining intact folic acid circulating in the blood stream can increase cancer risk. Folic acid is the synthetic form of an important group of naturally occurring micronutrients called folates that are present at high levels in green leafy vegetables. There is no evidence for harm from natural dietary folates [87].

Some countries supplement flour with folic acid to prevent foetal abnormalities and this is also advocated for the UK [189]. Because of its possible adverse effects it has been suggested that a better approach might be to supplement flour with one of the naturally occurring forms of folate instead. [115]

Surprisingly, the benefits of omega-3 fish oils supplements are also far from clear cut, despite their much-touted role in protecting against heart attacks or stroke [190]. Recent studies, including a meta analysis from the highly regarded "Cochrane Library", found they were of no benefit in reducing the risk of heart disease [191]. Similarly, in a large RCT of over 25,000 healthy middle-aged Americans, omega-3 supplements were found to be of no benefit in reducing CVD or cancer [192]. This contrasts with the well-established benefits of omega-3 rich oily fish for preventing CVD.

A major problem with omega-3 fatty acids is that when they are taken out of their natural milieu they become highly vulnerable to oxidation. Using poor quality processes to isolate the fats or not storing them correctly greatly increases the risk of these fats oxidising. This is of real concern since studies have found that in some countries the majority of omega-3 fatty acid preparations being sold are thought to be oxidised [193]. Oxidised omega-3 fats increase inflammation and oxidative stress in the body and there is currently much debate not only if omega-3 supplements are of any value but also if they may cause actual harm [193]. The omega-3 fats in fish and other natural sources are naturally protected from oxidation by antioxidants and the widely recommended advice to eat oily fish at least once a week is far less controversial.

Many phytochemicals are also far less effective when they are no longer part of their natural milieu. Pomegranate juice has benefits against cancer and CVD but these effects are much reduced when the main putative active component (a substance called punicalagin) is isolated from the juice [194]. The spice turmeric has interesting anti-inflammatory properties, and although this is often attributed to its main component called curcumin, a detailed review concluded that there is no good evidence that curcumin on its own has any therapeutic benefits and that other substances in turmeric may be important [195; 196].

---

[115] Searby, L. (2014) Folates not folic acid for flour fortification, urge researchers. nutraingredients.com

Figuring out why single substances given as supplements often show no benefit is often challenging and this is why taking supplements is discouraged by many nutritionists. It is possible that supplements do in fact have a benefit under some circumstances and it is the scientific evaluation that is failing to pick this up. Looking back on early evaluations of supplements, it's fair to say that some were not well conducted. Some studies simply did not last long enough to be able to see any health benefit. Medicines usually act rapidly to treat acute medical problems and so clinical evaluations can be quite short term. But chronic diseases develop of many years and so a study with a supplement is unlikely to pick up a benefit if the study only lasts a year or so. In addition, if a participant in a study already has early pre-clinical stages of the disease then it may be too late to expect any benefit since the horse - the stage of the disease a supplement is able to prevent from progressing - may already have bolted. In fact it is common to recruit participants at high risk of the disease in question, some of whom are likely to already have preclinical stages of the disease in question. This is done to increase the numbers of people getting the disease in the control group.

Another issue with evaluating supplements is that when a participant takes a supplement they are simply adding to the pre-existing amount of that nutrient already in their body. This so-called pool size can vary widely between participants but is often not taken into consideration. Some studies that have taken into account the pre-existing pool size find that it is indeed an important consideration, and that supplements are of greater benefit to patients who before the trial has started are deficient in the nutrient being tested (ie they have a small pool size). This situation is quite different with pharmaceutical agents. In these studies, none of the patients has any of the test drug at the start of the trial and so all participants in the trials start on a level playing field - which makes interpreting studies with drugs far easier and also makes it far more likely that an effect will be seen.

Not distinguishing between the natural form of a nutrient that occurs in foods and a synthetic form - the form usually used in supplements - is another problem. As mentioned earlier, folic acid does not seem to be broken down effectively in the body and may be toxic - which is not the case for naturally occurring folates [197]. Vitamin D is another interesting case. Because vitamin D deficiency is common in developed countries, taking a supplement is sometimes warranted. But too much vitamin D is toxic and so achieving optimal levels through supplementation is not easy. As well as dietary sources, vitamin D is produced naturally under the skin in response to sunlight. Production by the skin is carefully regulated by the body to ensure optimum levels are achieved and there is a "safety mechanism" that prevents excess production.

If these discussions seem a bit removed from your own concerns, for the user there are other issues. Taking a supplement can lull a person into thinking that, though not perfect, it gives licence to continue eating a poor diet. Sadly this is not the case. It is overly optimistic to expect that a single supplement is the solution to the multifactorial problem of a chronic disease. This would be like expecting a scalpel to be all that's needed to perform open-heart surgery. Developing heart disease can result from multiple pathological changes, including high blood pressure, elevated cholesterol and inflammation, amongst others. A single nutrient such as an omega-3 fat is unable to remedy all of these. If you are fortunate enough to have the factors under control that omega-3 fats don't target then an omega-3 fat may possibly be of benefit. But this is a lottery. Multiple nutrients are needed to tackle all the pathological changes associated with a chronic disease. For the majority of people, money spent on supplements would be far better spent on improving the quality of their overall diet.

## Foods not nutrients

Nutrients interact in complex networks and this highlights why we need to ensure all nutrients are at optimal levels in our body.  This inter-dependence was demonstrated in a study on the benefits of eating fish, a rich source of omega-3 fats and of selenium. Improvements in the cognitive function of a group of elderly men and women was found to depend on both the selenium and omega-3 fats from eating fish [198]. It is possible that the cognitive improvement was reliant on the selenium protecting the omega-3 fats from oxidation. Although eating fish automatically provides both, many people may take omega-3 supplements because they are concerned about their diet, which may include insufficient selenium. Hence, rather than benefitting from the omega-3 fat supplement there is an increased risk that it will be converted into harmful oxidation products.

Another example is in the field of cancer where there are many well documented cases of phytochemicals interacting to prevent a tumour from developing [(199)]. One way phytochemicals help prevent cancer is by acting as antioxidants. Antioxidants often work together in complex networks where the overall antioxidant activity of a mixture of antioxidants can be greater than the sum of their individual effects (a synergistic effect, discussed further below) [(200)].

These examples show why it is so important to ensure that all members of a nutrient community are present in adequate amounts. Foods, not supplements, are the most reliable way to achieve this. Nutrients are gentle entities and most work collectively with other nutrients to help prevent disease. They are not the same as powerful medicines, which usually act alone to eradicate disease.

The food source of a nutrient is critical for understanding whether or not it will benefit health. The relationship between nutrient and food is somewhat analogous to syntax in language. Consider the word "can". Without knowing its context, the word "can" could mean "a can" or "I can". Understanding nutrients in context is equally important in order to ensure that statements about diet are correctly expressed. For instance, saturated fat from dairy produce is not associated with the risk of heart disease to the same extent as saturated fat from meat (see ch. 12). In the words of Marion Nestle, taking "the nutrient out of the context of the food" can influence its apparent health effect. Incomplete information can be deceptive, and failing to describe nutrients accurately in relation to their food source is responsible for many confusing messages in nutrition.

Because of the shortcomings of nutrient-based dietary advice, many nutritionists now prefer to link food groups, such as fish, with health rather than individual nutrients, such as saturated fat. A study of US adults identified various food groups responsible for nearly half of all deaths (those from heart disease, stroke and type 2 diabetes) [(201)]. The main culprits were suboptimal intake of nuts and seeds, vegetables and fruits as well as high intake of sugary drinks and processed meats, and insufficient omega-3 fatty acids from seafoods and high salt. This information is far clearer than if it was expressed as specific nutrients. A meta-analysis looking at food groups found that people with an optimal intake of whole grains, vegetables, fruits, nuts, legumes, and fish, and a reduced intake of red and processed meats and SSBs reduced their risk of premature death by 80% compared with people who consumed only low amounts of these foods [202].

## Meals balance out nutrients

The argument that food groups are of far greater relevance than nutrients can be taken to the next level by considering the overall meal. Salt is linked to an increase in blood pressure, but there's less risk from eating a few salty olives if this is compensated for by reducing salt elsewhere in the meal. Balancing the foods in a whole meal or through the day is the way to stay healthy. This is why most dietary advice talks about *daily* (or even weekly) intakes.

Taking the perspective of a complete meal into account also makes it easier to consider how nutrients interact. These interactions are not only because of the various nutrients but also the order in which they are consumed. Drinking alcohol before food leads to lightheadedness far more quickly than alcohol drunk after eating. This is because a full stomach empties more slowly which in turn slows down alcohol absorption from the gut into the blood. Eating a sugary dessert at the end of a meal after a savoury course may have less impact on blood sugar levels than eating the same sugary food as a snack on an empty stomach. This is because ingredients in savoury dishes such as onions contain fibre and various phytochemicals that may reduce glucose absorption from the carbs [203] (see ch. 12). The ability of vegetables to block glucose absorption was shown in a study of a typical Asian meal. Eating vegetables before the meat and rice considerably reduced the surge in blood glucose and this may be of benefit to diabetics [204]. Eating veg first might not seem very desirable but traditional ways of doing this include starting a meal with a vegetable soup or with crudités. The importance of the order of a meal was recognised by UNESCO for the "gastronomic French meal" which is eaten to celebrate important events such as birthdays. In 2010, UNESCO added this meal to its list of Intangible Cultural Heritages of Humanity. The meal is a series of courses eaten consecutively and along with honouring social aspects of the meal, UNESCO also recognised that the meal "should respect a fixed structure commencing with an apéritif (drinks before the meal) and ending with liqueurs, containing in between at least four successive courses, namely a starter, fish and/or meat with vegetables, cheese and dessert. "[116] The UNESCO designation was not primarily concerned with health but

---

[116] https://ich.unesco.org/en/RL/gastronomic-meal-of-the-french-00437

nevertheless preserving the way a French meal is constructed may have important, albeit little studied, health benefits.

## Holistic nutrition

Like much of science, nutrition research is dominated by a reductionist approach. Reductionism studies complex entities by breaking them down into simpler constituents. It was reductionist thinking that led nutritionists to hope that beta-carotene could explain the benefits of eating a diet rich in carrots. A more holistic approach considers the whole diet. A reductionist approach can be productive in some cases - as isolating vitamins and using them to cure people with vitamin deficiency diseases has shown. Similarly, salt and trans fats have been targeted in public health campaigns with some success in reducing their harm.

Unfortunately this approach has serious limitations when trying to prevent chronic diseases. History has shown that a reductionist approach focusing on "good" versus "bad" nutrients is unlikely to solve the problems of complex chronic diseases. In the early 1970's it was concluded that a high fat diet was a major cause of chronic diseases. So in 1977 the U.S. Senate Select Committee on Nutrition and Human Needs called on Americans to eat less total and saturated fat and to eat more, supposedly healthier, carbohydrates [92]. Today, the proportion of fat in the US diet has decreased to about 34% of total calories from about 42% in the 1970s. But during this time the US has also seen a huge rise in obesity and type 2 diabetes. This is probably because dietary carbohydrates increased substantially to compensate for the reduced calories from fat. This illustrates how targeting single nutrients in public health campaigns can dramatically fail. Despite this, many publicly promoted diets continue to focus on demonising one type of nutrient such as saturated fat or fructose.

The limitation of the reductionist approach is often depicted by "The blind men and an elephant", a parable which originates from India and was popularized by American poet John Godfrey Saxe in the mid-20th century: " Six blind men were asked to determine what an elephant looked like by feeling different parts of the elephant' s body. The blind man who feels a leg says the elephant is like a pillar; the one who feels the tail says the elephant is like a rope; the one who feels the trunk says the elephant is like a tree branch; the one who feels the ear says the elephant is like a hand fan; the one who feels the belly says the elephant is like a wall; and the one who feels the tusk says the elephant is like a solid pipe. A king explains to them: 'All of you are right. The reason every one of you is telling it differently is because each one of you touched the different part of the elephant. So, actually the elephant has all the features you mentioned.' "

Feeling the different parts of the elephant is analogous to the reductionist approach of examining only individual nutrients. Considering the meal is being able to see the whole elephant. This is the holistic perspective. Holism asserts - in Aristotle's famous dictum - that "a whole is more than the sum of its parts". This could be paraphrased in nutrition to "A food or a meal is more than the sum of its nutrients", and, holism asserts, the whole meal cannot be understood by simply studying each nutrient independently.

Underpinning this is the idea that nutrients interact synergistically. Reductionism contends that the outcome of 1+1 always equals 2, whereas holism evokes synergy and that the outcome from 1+1 can be greater than 2. The reductionist might view dietary nutrients as interlocking cogs that together form a complex mechanism, like a mechanical watch. The holist declares that nutrients are not immutable cogs in a mechanism but instead are subject to continual change. Rather than cogs, nutrients are more like paints that combine into new colours out of which a new painting emerges. A reductionist might argue that the painting can still technically be reduced to each pigment in the picture. But a holist would argue that using this approach it is impossible to delve down into the painting's beauty: it would be like preferring the analysis of a painting's pigments to an appreciation of its overall beauty.

## Holism and evolution

The term "holism" was coined by the South African statesman Jan Christiaan Smuts. In his 1926 book *Holism and Evolution* he linked the ideas of holism and evolution by defining holism as "the tendency in nature to form wholes that are greater than the sum of the parts *through creative evolution*." This link of holism with evolution is very interesting. Evolution underpins much of our understanding of biological systems. As the evolutionary biologist Theodosius Dobzhansky said in his 1973 book "Nothing in Biology Makes Sense Except in the Light of Evolution". The unprocessed plants and animals we eat as food are wholes, the products of creative evolution. The combinations of nutrient constituents in organisms have been optimised through creative evolution in order to confront and protect the organism from the challenges of life. For instance, all organisms must produce antioxidants to protect their cellular constituents. Polyunsaturated fats, present in all higher organisms, are particularly prone to oxidation and so parts of organisms rich in polyunsaturated fats are also high in antioxidants. The brown skin covering an almond or walnut is high in antioxidant phenolics that protect the fats inside from oxidation. Walnuts are particularly rich in an omega-3 fatty acid called alpha-linolenic acid, which is very susceptible to oxidation and walnut skins are also particularly rich in antioxidants.

Many of these same challenges also confront us, and when we eat natural foods - a fruit, a nut or a fish - this protection is also passed on. When we consume an organism's polyunsaturated fats we are also consuming its protective entourage of antioxidants. We are not only benefiting from each individual nutrient constituent but also from the millions of years of R&D that has combined them in ways that optimise the health of the organism. Eating gives us the holistic benefits of nutrient combinations optimised through evolution. Being guided by foods rather than nutrients ensures that nutrients are presented together as Nature intended.

Looking through this evolutionary lens also shows us why most industrial foods are less healthy. As food production moved from farm to factory, industrial processing removed much of the creative evolution of natural foods. A UPF is the extreme example of a food which is no longer a "creative whole", a product of evolution, but rather a reconstructed entity, a product of industrial R&D. UPFs have evolved not through natural selection and survival of the fittest but through commercial selection and manufacture of the most profitable. They arise from reductionist thinking, products built from synthetic building blocks such as additives and flavourings, not for evolutionary advantage but for profit.

From a nutritional perspective, the complex structure of an organism is its food matrix, a structure designed by creative evolution and built by Nature. The food matrix we eat influences many aspects of nutrition, including satiety and the interactions and the bioavailability of nutrients such as phytochemicals and carbohydrates [205]. These influences would be hard to recognise from a reductionist analysis. For instance, the influence of carbohydrates on blood sugar isn't simply due to how much glucose there is in the food but how the glucose is contained within structures in the food matrix.

Looking beyond nutrition, reductionism and holism represent two different views of the world. Reductionism represents a desire to categorise, simplify and "take back control". Holism is more tolerant of complexity. The reductionist conventional farmer kills pests with pesticides in fields bounded by fences; the holistic organic farmer integrates control with Nature in fields bounded by jumbled hedgerows. There is now a strong case to be made for returning to more holistic natural foods and letting go of reductionist UPFs. To achieve this may well need a change in mindset that goes well beyond just food. In the next chapter we consider this whole "dietary pattern" approach to eating by discussing the Med diet. This holistic perspective is widened even further in the final chapter of this book when we discuss farming and the Med diet.

# 9. The healthy Mediterranean Diet

## Overview

So far we have considered why natural foods are the best way to obtain all the nutrients needed for a healthy diet. Many diets can achieve this, but none rivals the Mediterranean diet when it comes to the overall package of health, taste, and convenience. The Med diet includes many different types of foods and it is the overall diet in all its diversity that is optimal for health. There is no evidence that low fat or low carb versions have these health benefits. In this chapter we look at what a Med diet really is, and see that as well as the food on the plate there are many other lifestyle factors that probably contribute to the overall benefits of this most healthful of diets.

## The Med diet around the world

In the 1950's, the American nutritionist Ancel Keys described a diet he had observed Mediterranean peasants eating, especially those living in Crete and Southern Italy. He coined the term "Mediterranean diet" (Med diet) for this diet. Today, the diet Keys described is referred to as the "traditional" Med diet to distinguish it from the "Med diet" now eaten by many people in Mediterranean countries and in other parts of the world. Even though today the Med diet is popular well beyond the shores of the Mediterranean, in some Med countries its popularity has dramatically declined. This is particularly the case in Greece, one of the diet's original heartlands [206]. Indeed, some people in non-Mediterranean countries now eat a diet closer to a Med diet than many living in Mediterranean regions. Swedish and Dutch children are more likely to eat a Med diet than their Greek counterparts. [117] Even worse is that Greek children are now amongst the most obese in Europe. It isn't a Med diet making them fat, though, but their switch to a Western diet with its many processed and refined foods. Obesity is also worryingly common in children

---

[117] https://www.theguardian.com/society/2018/may/24/the-mediterranean-diet-is-gone-regions-children-are-fattest-in-europe.

in some other Mediterranean countries like Spain, Italy and Cyprus and this also is linked to a big rise in their junk food consumption. [118]

## What is the Med diet?

The Med diet was originally based on a "holy trinity" of Mediterranean crops: olive trees, wheat and grapes. Olive trees were grown for their olives from which oil was extracted, grains were cultivated for producing bread and other foods and were made mainly from unrefined or partially refined wheat, and vines were grown mostly to produce wine. These foods still underpin Mediterranean cuisine.

Of course, today's Med diet consists of a far wider variety of foods. It is largely defined by various food *groups*, such as fruits and vegetables, rather than by *specific* foods, such as oranges or carrots, and also by how frequently these food groups are eaten over the course of a week. The food groups are: a large variety of fruits, vegetables and whole grains eaten daily, pulses eaten at least twice a week, nuts and seeds (often eaten as snacks), daily consumption of dairy produce (traditionally made from sheep or goat milk rather than cow's milk), fish at least twice a week and a small amount of meat, eaten once or twice a week. Modest amounts of wine are often drunk with the main meal of the day, and olive oil (preferably extra virgin), rather than butter or vegetable oils, is used for frying and dressings. Herbs and spices are also widely used. The Med diet does not exclude sweet treats but these are usually fruit or fruit-based rather than concoctions of sugar. These different food groups are discussed in more detail in ch. 12.

| **Foods and food groups in the Med diet** |
| --- |
| • Olive oil (preferably extra virgin) as added fat |
| • Daily consumption of vegetables |
| • Daily consumption of fruits |
| • Daily consumption of unrefined cereals |
| • Twice weekly consumption of legumes |
| • Nuts and olives as snacks |
| • Twice weekly consumption of fish |

---

[118] https://www.theguardian.com/world/2018/may/25/people-just-have-less-time-now-is-the-mediterranean-diet-dying-out

- Daily consumption of cheese or yogurt
- Monthly or weekly consumption of meat or meat products
- Daily moderate consumption of wine, if it is acceptable on religious and social grounds

The Med diet is often represented in a pyramid such as the one shown here [207] (see Appendix for a larger version)

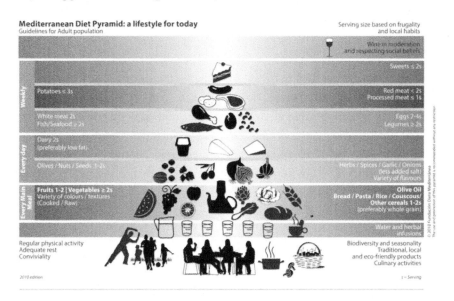

Because the Med diet is defined mainly by food groups rather than by specific foods, it is perfectly acceptable to replace foods not typically Mediterranean with more local fruit and veg. Apples and cabbages can be as much a part of a Med diet as apricots and courgettes. Consuming local produce brings the added benefits of lowering transportation costs and supporting local farmers. Choosing more local varieties also helps make a Med diet more culturally acceptable to people living in non-Mediterranean countries. With global warming, traditional agricultural boundaries are moving, anyway, and more and more Mediterranean crops are now being grown where previously this was not commercially viable. Vineyards flourish in the north of England and there are even apricots orchards in southern counties of the UK. [119]

Some foods, though, do still need to be imported to sustain a Med diet in countries such as the UK. Principal among these are olive oil and wine, some types of pulses such as chickpeas, and various preserved products such as olives, anchovies and capers. Unlike a lot of exotic produce, these non-perishable products can be transported relatively cheaply and in a relatively environmentally friendly way since they do not need the refrigeration or rapid air transport of more exotic fresh foods imported from further afield.

## A diverse diet

One little-recognised feature of the Med diet is the diversity of its foods. This diversity is important since it helps safeguard against micronutrient deficiencies and ensure that all necessary micronutrients are consumed. Eating a Med diet quickly ensures this because it includes optimal amounts of macronutrients like fats and carbohydrates, micronutrients (vitamins and minerals) and fibre [208]. When eating a Med diet, there is absolutely no need to compensate for the risks of nutrients deficiencies with dietary supplements (as is the case for a vegan diet, for example).

So-called "diet diversity scores" estimate the diversity of a person's diet and several studies (including of non-Med diets) have linked a higher diet diversity score to a lower risk of disease. This benefit is independent of the actual *amount* of healthy foods eaten. By reducing the risk of a micronutrient deficiency, a diverse diet reduces the risk not only of classic vitamin deficiency, which are now less common in the west anyway, but also of the far more common chronic disease (the role of micronutrients in chronic diseases was discussed in ch. 6). Although the healthier diets of people in higher socio-economic classes is usually assumed to be due to their higher consumption of fruit and veg and other healthy foods, it may be due as much to the far greater diversity of their diets compared to those typically eaten by people from lower socio-economic groups.

Studies have found that the overall Med diet, with all its food groups, is far more protective against disease than any single food group within the Med diet. Making a habit of eating a diverse diet also makes more sense than a

[119] https://www.theguardian.com/money/2012/aug/06/britain-grows-apricots-large-scale

sudden - but often temporary - craze for the latest "superfood" to hit the headlines since this risks excess consumption. Beetroot hit the headlines recently as a source of blood pressure-lowering nitrates, but eating large amounts of beetroot may not be such a good idea for people with low blood pressure. A balanced Med diet irons out the storms of excess and the lulls of deficiency helping keep our bodies on a more even keel.

## Processed foods in the Med diet

The short winters and long growing season in the Mediterranean made it possible for the traditional Med diet to be mainly based on fresh foods. This does not mean that all processed foods are excluded. Some foods are fermented (such as yogurt and olives), salted (capers, olives, some fish such as salt cod and anchovies) and dried (herbs and spices) to improve storage, which also often had the coincidental benefit of improving taste and healthiness. Unlike UPFs though, these naturally processed foods still resemble the foods from which they are derived. Naturally processed foods usually retain their fibre and most of their phytochemicals. The rationale for processing Mediterranean foods is quite different to that of the junk food industry whose products are created from cheap ultra-processed ingredients for profit.

Unfortunately, a few modern processing techniques have crept into the production of some Med foods which do compromise the food's nutritional value. These foods are best avoided. More refined types of olive oil are a good example: these oils have lost most of their healthful phytochemicals and it is preferable to choose extra virgin olive oil, which is far less processed (see ch. 12). Also detrimental is an industrial process called the California method, which is used to produce a type of black olive. In this process, green olives are aerated to turn them brown-black. The aeration oxidises phenolic compounds causing a browning oxidation reaction (in the same way that slicing an apple and exposing the flesh to air turns it brown). The black colour produced in the olives is then fixed with ferrous gluconate. Unfortunately, a very beneficial phenolic called hydroxytyrosol is destroyed during the oxidation process. So although these black olives are usually the cheapest, they are unlikely to have the same health benefits of more naturally processed olives [209]. "Ferrous gluconate" is listed on the label and lets you know if this process has been used.

## A typical day's Mediterranean meals

The cultural and geographical diversity of nations around the Med has resulted in quite diverse Med cuisines. Nevertheless, traditional Med diets across the region share similarities as well as differences. For breakfast, there will be no UPFs, so this means no boxed cereals or sugary drinks. Tea (often herbal) or coffee and lots of water are drunk. Bread (from unrefined flour, often sourdough), cheese and fruit are commonly eaten. There are also more country-specific traditions. In Egypt, for example, a stew of broad beans (*ful medames*) is common. At a traditional Cretan breakfast, barley rusks (*paximadia*) often replace bread. Barley has a low glycaemic index, and the tradition of dipping the rusk in olive oil further reduces its glycaemic index. In Spain, grilled bread smeared with tomato and olive oil (*pan con tomate*) is popular.

For lunch and the evening meal, fresh seasonal ingredients are eaten raw or cooked with their flavours being enhanced with preserved Med ingredients from the larder. Again, no UPFs. Starting from fresh raw ingredients is extremely important for creating healthy Mediterranean meals. Vegetable or legume-based dishes dominate, mostly prepared as salads, soups and stews and doused in copious amounts of extra-virgin olive oil. Acidic condiments such as vinegar and lemon juice are common and these can help reduce the glycaemic index of the meal. Many people eating a traditional Med meal have their own vegetable garden, which provides an abundance of fresh, varied and usually organically-grown produce.

As with other cuisines, Med cuisines have been influenced by other countries. These influences have had both positive and negative health benefits. Invasions by Byzantines, Arabs, Venetians and Ottoman Turks influenced Cretan cuisine by introducing the use of healthy spices such as cumin, coriander and saffron. Less healthy modifications were introduced more recently into Greek cuisine by the Greek chef Nicholas Tselementes (1878-1958). After working abroad, he returned to Greece and modified traditional dishes with French influences such as adding a béchamel sauce to moussaka. It was Tselementes who promoted the use of butter in Greek dishes. Although these modifications have now become a part of Greek cuisine, olive oil is the authentic fat of Greek cooking.

# Health benefits

The health credentials of the Med diet have been hard earned after extensive scrutiny in hundreds of scientific studies. Every year a team of twenty-five of the world's top nutritionists evaluate diets from around the world. And for the three years 2018-2020 they have voted the Med diet the healthiest in the world. [120] There is convincing evidence that eating a Med diet reduces the risk of many different chronic diseases including coronary heart disease and stroke, type 2 diabetes, cancer and dementia. Eating a Med diet not only benefits healthy people - so-called primary disease prevention. It also benefits people who are at greater disease risk because they have elevated risk factors (such as being obese), or because they have already had a previous incidence of the disease such as a previous heart attack. This is called secondary prevention. There is generally less evidence that a Med diet on its own can reverse a chronic disease once it is already clinically diagnosable, although a Med diet may help manage disease symptoms.

The most convincing benefits of a Med diet are for preventing CVD (heart disease and stroke). CVD is the number one cause of premature death in the UK and many other western countries (see ch. 3). All types of epidemiological studies have confirmed this, including observational studies, prospective studies, randomised control trials, meta-analyses and even meta-analyses of meta-analyses! The stand-out study is the Predimed trial. This was a randomised control trial that recruited over seven thousand participants from various clinics in Spain between 2003 and 2006 (Predimed is an acronym of Prevención con Dieta Mediterránea) [210]. People were eligible to participate in the study if they were at increased risk of CVD because of their age (they were all middle-aged or elderly), and because they had other risk factors for CVD such as high blood pressure, elevated cholesterol, smoking, a family history of heart disease and/or being obese. Participants were randomly assigned to one of three intervention groups: one group was advised to eat a Med diet supplemented with extra-virgin olive oil (EVOO); the second group to eat a Med diet supplemented with nuts; and the third group was advised to eat a low fat "control" diet (which was the diet recommended by the American Heart Association). To encourage adherence to their relevant diets,

---

[120] *https://health.usnews.com/best-diet/best-diets-overall*

participants in the EVOO group were given free EVOO (one litre per week, with participants encouraged to consume at least 50 ml per day and the rest for other family members); participants in the nuts group were given free mixed nuts (30 grams per day consisting of 15 g of walnuts, 7.5 g of almonds, and 7.5 g of hazelnuts plus extra allocations for the family); and to balance things up participants in the control diet group received non-food gifts. There were no restrictions on how much participants ate, and there were no efforts to increase their physical activity. The trial was stopped early - after just under five years rather than the planned six years - for ethical reasons because it was apparent that participants in the groups receiving the Med diet supplemented with either EVOO or nuts had a 30% lower risk of having either a stroke or heart attack or of dying from one compared to people in the control group. This study has received both huge praise and huge scrutiny. It was identified that a small number of participants had not been randomly allocated but were family members. This led the authors of the study to retract their original paper in 2018, re-analyse their data and republish the study with a new, corrected statistical analysis [211]. This did not result in any changes in the authors' findings, and the Predimed study remains a landmark study on the cardiovascular benefits of the Med diet.

People who survive a first heart attack or stroke have an increased risk of a second event since atherosclerosis, the underlying disease, has not usually been cured. This makes the findings of a second study, one conducted between 1988 and 1992 in the French city of Lyon, particularly important. In this randomised control trial, participants who had survived a first heart attack were randomised to either a "Mediterranean-style" diet or a control diet. [212] There were about three hundred participants in each group. Participants in the Med diet group were encouraged to eat more fruit, vegetables, bread and fish and to replace red meat with chicken. Participants in the "intervention" group were also provided with their main fat in the form of a special margarine made with oleic acid (the main fatty acid found in olive oil) and the omega-3 fatty acid alpha-linolenic acid. The control group ate the low fat diet recommended at the time by the American Heart Association. So although the intervention group was advised to eat a diet similar to the Med diet there was no emphasis on consuming olive oil itself. Nevertheless the results were impressive. After two years there was a 73% reduction in coronary events and a 70% reduction in total mortality. So as not to deny these benefits to the control group, the study was stopped early.

It is not only epidemiological studies that validate the health benefits of a diet. As I mentioned in ch. 5, the British epidemiologist Sir Austin Bradford Hill identified that, ideally, nine criteria should be fulfilled in order to provide the best evidence for a causal link between a diet and a health outcome. It is to the great credit of investigators of the Med diet that its cardiovascular benefit have been shown to meet all nine of these criteria - a feat never before shown in such detail for a diet [79]. Aside from epidemiological evidence, one of the most important criteria is biological plausibility - in other words that there are plausible biological reasons that have been experimentally proven that help explain why the diet should work. Numerous foods and nutrients in the Med have been shown to have biological properties (such a lowering blood pressure or cholesterol levels) that could plausibly contribute to the clinical benefits of preventing a stroke or heart attack. It is highly unlikely that these clinical benefits come from a single nutrient or food. It is far more likely that it is the additive effects of many small benefits from many foods and nutrients that together create a clinically significant benefit. Attempting to mine down to the seam of a specific beneficial food is only likely to reveal fool's gold.

Impressive though the cardiovascular benefits of the Med diet are, recent evidence suggests that its benefits can be improved even further. Obesity is probably the most important public health issue of our time and a successor to the Predimed study, the Predimed-Plus study, has been set up with the aim of combining the health benefits of the Med diet with weight loss. As well as encouraging adherence to a Med diet, this study includes a programme that aims to increase physical activity and help people avoid the high calorie foods (such as UPFs) that increase the risk of CVD [213]. Participants are supported to achieve these aims with motivational behaviour change techniques. Early results are promising. Participants receiving the Predimed-Plus programme are losing more weight and achieving greater reductions in risk factors for CVD (such as abdominal obesity and triglycerides in the blood) than the participants in the control arm - which is advice to eat a Med diet [214]. So a Med diet with a weight loss programme may be even better than the Med diet alone.

Studies have found that some people who eat a Med diet lose weight even without any conscious efforts to do so. [121] This may seem surprising since the Med diet is quite high in fat. The reason may be because the high amounts of plant foods and fibre in the Med diet are quite satiating which helps keep calorie intake in check. Maintaining a healthy weight is very important since it reduces the risk of many other diseases, especially type 2 diabetes. The benefits of a Med diet for controlling type 2 diabetes were confirmed in the Predimed-Plus study since diabetic participants who lost weight were found to significantly improve their blood sugar levels (glycaemic control) and insulin sensitivity. Many studies have now found that eating a Med diet reduces the risk of type 2 diabetes in healthy people, as well as helping diabetic people better manage their symptoms [215]. In fact, the Med diet was voted the best diet of all thirty-five evaluated for type 2 diabetes by the panel of twenty five experts in 2020. The Med diet is not the best diet for losing weight however and so the anti-diabetic effects of the Med diet are probably more to do with the diet's overall composition rather than simply causing weight loss. A comprehensive review has found that the best ways to reduce the risk of type 2 diabetes are to eat whole grains, cereal fibre (rather than fibre from fruits and vegetables), to drink moderate amounts of alcohol and to not eat red meat, processed meat or bacon, or drink sugar sweetened beverages [216]. These are all components of a Med diet.

For cancer and the Med diet, the evidence is more moderate. The Med diet reduces the risk of getting and dying from cancer when all types of cancer are pooled together in studies [217]. For individual types, there is particularly good evidence for protection against breast cancer, but when other cancers are considered separately the evidence is weaker. This does not mean that the Med diet has no role to play in these cancers but it may be that dietary factors are less able to counteract cancer-causing factors such as smoking than it is to reduce the internal pathological changes that drive diseases such as CVD and type 2 diabetes. This is discussed more fully in ch. 11.

Another chronic disease of huge societal importance is dementia. CVD is the major cause of vascular dementia, and so it is not surprising that a Med diet reduces the risk of vascular dementia. Even more significant is the mounting evidence that a Med diet can reduce dementia caused by Alzheimer's disease

---

[121] Some studies are summarised at *https://health.usnews.com/best-diet/best-diets-overall*

and also the mild cognitive impairment that represents the preclinical stage of this disease [217; 218; 219]. This is hugely important not only because Alzheimer's disease is a major cause of fewer healthy years and premature death but also because there are currently no recommended treatments for mild cognitive impairment. There is increasing interest in the Med diet in preventing dementia. In the UK, GPs have been recruiting participants from Birmingham, Norwich and Newcastle to see if a combination of eating a Med diet and greater physical activity can reduce dementia. Preliminary results are expected in 2021 [220].

## Med-icine?

Although Hippocrates is attributed with saying "Let food be thy medicine and medicine be thy food", there is evidence from his writings that he recognised that food and medicines are not the same thing [221]. Similarly the Med diet should not be thought of as a medicine to treat disease but rather as a diet to *prevent* diseases. Sometimes it can also slow disease progression, but it rarely cures people of chronic diseases (although modern medicines are often not particularly good at this either).

It is in this mainly preventative capacity that a Med diet is recommended by various health advisory bodies. In the UK, these include NICE (National Institute for Health and Care Excellence), which recommends the Med diet along with exercise and stopping smoking to prevent CVD and reduce the risk of a second heart attack in previous sufferers, and by Diabetes UK and the British Heart Foundation. The Alzheimer's Society also endorses the Med diet [122] and the International Association of Gerontology and Geriatrics recommends the Med diet for early cognitive decline [222]. Although many health bodies involved with heart disease, diabetes and dementia recommend the Med diet, it is recommended along with other "healthy" ways of eating. But the evidence shows that the Med diet is far superior to other diets and this is rarely if ever mentioned.

A Med diet is not often recommended by cancer organisations. However, there is increasing evidence that a Med diet helps reduce the incidence of breast cancer. This diet is also showing promise in preventing breast cancer

---

[122] https://www.alzheimers.org.uk/about-dementia/risk-factors-and-prevention/mediterranean-diet-and-dementia

recurrence, especially when combined with physical activity. This is discussed further below. Improved technologies and earlier diagnosis have greatly increased survival rates for many cancer sufferers, and this has resulted in an ever-greater need to prevent remissions. There is evidence that diet may have a role to play here. For instance, women who switch to a high fibre diet after having had breast cancer reduce their risk of dying prematurely [223]. The Med diet is naturally high in fibre and although studies are still underway to see if the Med diet specifically improves survival in women who have already had breast cancer, its track record in primary prevention of breast cancer makes eating this diet after a diagnosis breast cancer a wise choice [224]. However, it is probably advisable to steer clear of alcohol because of links with breast cancer.

There are increasing calls for dietary assessments and advice to be made a routine part of a visit to the GP [225]. [123] As the diet *par excellence* for preventing a wide range of chronic diseases, a Med diet could play a central role in GP-led prevention programmes. In the UK, the Med diet aligns very well with the objectives of the NHS Health Check programme which aims to reduce heart disease, stroke, type 2 diabetes and kidney disease, and to raise awareness of dementia in the general population. A Med diet could be recommended alongside medical interventions or possibly in some cases even be considered as an alternative. Following an NHS Health Check, cholesterol-lowering statins are the most frequently prescribed drugs (one analysis found that one in thirty three people attending an NHS Health Check were prescribed statins because of a diagnosis of increased risk of CVD [28]). Side effects do however occur in some patients who take statins, including muscle pain, and there is an increased risk of type 2 diabetes. A Med diet offers a side-effects free alternative. Some health authorities have now concluded that a Med diet is a credible alternative to statins for people who are intolerant of these drugs or averse to taking them [226].

So how does the Med diet compare to statins? It is possible to make a direct comparison between statins and the Med diet using an analysis called "number needed to treat" (NNT). The NNT is defined as "an epidemiological measure used in communicating the effectiveness of a health-care

[123] Experts urge evaluation of diet at routine check-ups
https://www.sciencedaily.com/releases/2020/08/200807093752.htm

intervention, typically a treatment with medication." [124] The NNT is the average number of patients who need to be treated to prevent one additional bad outcome. NNT analysis has been carried out for the Lyon heart study and the Predimed study since as randomised control trials these studies are considered sufficiently robust to be able to compare their results with statins. NNT analysis of the Lyon heart study and the Predimed study found that the Med diet outperforms statins for primary and secondary CVD prevention [227]. Using a Med Diet for five years for heart disease prevention, one stroke, heart attack, or death would be prevented for every 61 people (without known heart disease) without any concurrent side effects. For statins given for five years to similar people, one heart attack would be prevented for every 104 people, one stroke for every 154 people and no lives would be saved. One in 100 people would develop diabetes and one in 10 people would suffer muscle damage. This suggests that a Med diet is superior to statins for CVD prevention.

Perhaps the best of both worlds is to integrate a Med diet in medical therapy. An Italian study of over one thousand elderly patients with various forms of CVD (for example patients with angina or those who had already had a heart attack) who were taking statins were found to be far less likely to die from a heart attack or stroke if they were also eating a Med diet [228]. Eating a Med diet also comes with the not inconsiderable additional benefit of concurrently reducing the risk of many other chronic diseases.

Despite these promising indicators, interest in the Med diet by most in the medical profession is at best tepid. The general perception is that it is far easier to convince someone to take a pill than to change his or her eating habits. But with sufficient support dietary change is possible. One-to-one time with a dietitian is one option but may be expensive. However, many new online technologies now offer a way of providing highly motivational individualised support. Maintaining adherence to a dietary change can be a challenge, but so too can be maintaining adherence to drugs - one study found that even in people who had had CVD, less than half were still choosing to take their prescribed statins three years later [229].

Many health bodies do now give fairly general advice on eating healthily to help prevent heart disease, diabetes, dementia and so on. However, the Med

---

[124] http://www.thennt.com

diet is usually given as just another example of how to eat healthily, alongside advice to eat more fruit and vegetables etc. But I believe this does not do justice to the Med diet since the evidence for the Med diet stands head and shoulders above other diets, especially in relation to CVD.

## When is a Med diet not a Med diet?

The Med diet provides a healthy balance of carbohydrates (about half of the calories in the diet), fats (about 35-40% of calories), protein, micronutrients, phytochemicals and fibre. It is this Med diet with *all* its food groups that studies have found is best for protecting against chronic diseases. Low fat and low carbohydrate versions of the Med diet have recently been "invented" but they are not equivalent to the original Med diet and there is very little evidence that they have the same health benefits.

It might seem that at face value a low fat or a low carb Med diets should be beneficial. However, when one macronutrient (ie fat or carbohydrate) is restricted this is usually compensated for by eating more of another macronutrient - that is unless you want to become very hungry! So tinkering with the Med diet means that it is important to consider not only the consequences of reducing one macronutrient but also what that macronutrient will be replaced with.

A low fat version means not only less heart-healthy fat-rich foods such as EVOO, nuts and fatty fish but also the likelihood that the fat will be replaced with refined carbohydrates such as white bread and white rice. It would be unfortunate if this did occur since a high proportion of energy from white bread increases risk factors for type 2 diabetes and heart disease [230]. [125]

A low carb Med diet is also of concern. Low carb Med diets often recommend excluding typical Med carbs such as pasta because of fears that they raise blood sugar. However, both white and whole meal pasta have low glycaemic values [126] and eating whole grains is associated with a reduced risk of type 2 diabetes [216]. This is not to say that all carbs are good, and it should be emphasised that carbs with high glycaemic index values such as white

---

[125] Some studies do not find that refined carbohydrates as a whole increase T2D: but not all refined carbs are the same: pasta has a low GI whereas white bread and rice have high GI values see Neuenschwander et al 2019
[126] https://www.health.harvard.edu/diseases-and-conditions/glycemic-index-and-glycemic-load-for-100-foods. A low GI food has a GI of less than 55.

bread are linked to an increased risk of type 2 diabetes [231]. Whole grains are also an important part of a healthy diet because of their fibre, phytochemicals, vitamin and minerals. Advocates of low carb diets often fail to distinguish between the different types of carbohydrates and excluding all dietary carbs risks throwing out the low glycaemic index baby out with the high glycaemic index bathwater. Not distinguishing between the different types of carbohydrates has led to a huge amount of unnecessary controversy about the role of carbohydrates in diabetes control.

Reducing whole grains also increases the likelihood that fat consumption will go up in order to satisfy appetite. All fats are mixtures of different types of fatty acids, and turning to fat if carbs are restricted risks exceeding recommended levels of saturated fat. This in turn raises blood cholesterol, increasing the risk of CVD. Some Med diets specifically recommend coconut oil but this is exceptionally high in saturated fat and is now considered a risk for CVD [232]. These modified versions may attempt to piggy back on the reputation of the Med diet but distorting the proportions of carbohydrates and fat risks increasing CVD, which is ironic since the *bona fide* Med diet is renowned for reducing the risk of CVD.

Although drastically reducing a food group such as grains invalidates the Med diet, varying the types of foods *within* a food group is perfectly acceptable. There is no need to stick to "Mediterranean" types of fruit and veg. There is, however, one exception to this rule of thumb. And that is that EVOO should always be the cooking oil of choice. EVOO has unique properties and there is increasing evidence that the overall benefits of the Med diet are compromised by using other types of oil. The health benefits of EVOO come both from its main fat, a type of monounsaturated fat called oleic acid, and from its rich variety of phytochemicals. Although replacing EVOO with rapeseed oil provides similar amounts of monounsaturated fat, rapeseed oil does not contain the all-important phytochemicals. [127] These phytochemicals, many unique to EVOO, are crucial for its health benefits. Most are absent even from ordinary olive oil such as "light" versions. One line of evidence (albeit circumstantial) for the unique benefits of EVOO as part of a Med diet comes

[127] Since many scientific studies on the Med diet are carried out in these countries, such as the US and UK, it has been necessary to modify the way adherence to the Med by participants in these studies is estimated. Instead of measuring olive oil the amount of dietary monounsaturated fat is taken into account since this is the main fat in olive oil.

from studies that compare the health benefit of eating Med diets in Mediterranean and non-Mediterranean countries. Studies often find that a Med diet eaten in Mediterranean countries gives greater protection against CVD than when it is eaten in non-Mediterranean countries [233]. [128] This might be explained by the fact that a far higher proportion of people from Mediterranean countries include EVOO as their main cooking oil, whereas people in non-Med countries are more likely to choose another type of oil. It is now established that EVOO has cardiovascular benefits and that this, in part, is due to a phytochemical called hydroxytyrosol. Hydroxytyrosol has been recognised by EFSA (the European Food Safety Authority) to protect against the oxidation of LDL (bad) cholesterol, a key step in the development of CVD.

There is also increasing evidence that EVOO helps protect against breast cancer. The Predimed study mentioned earlier allowed a direct comparison between people eating a Med diet supplemented with EVOO versus a comparable diet not supplemented with EVOO (and instead supplemented with nuts).[129] Women who ate a Med diet supplemented with EVOO reduced their risk of breast cancer by 68% whereas there was no evidence of a protective effect for the women who ate a Med diet supplemented with nuts [234]. So the conclusion is that a Med diet offers optimal protection against breast cancer only when EVOO is part of the Med diet. This is supported by comparing countries with different levels of EVOO consumption. Women from north European countries such as the Netherlands [235], Sweden [236] and the UK [237] where EVOO consumption is typically low did not achieve the same protection against breast cancer from eating a Med diet as that achieved by women from Mediterranean countries such as Spain [234] and Italy [238] where EVOO consumption tends to be higher.

These findings should not be interpreted to mean that it is EVOO alone that is protective against breast cancer, but rather that it is EVOO *in the context of an overall Med diet* that matters. Some other plant-based diets such as the

---

[128] The overall reduced risk of CVD in Med countries is 39% versus 16% reduced risk in non-Med countries. see Rosato V, Temple NJ, La Vecchia C *et al.* (2019) Mediterranean diet and cardiovascular disease: a systematic review and meta-analysis of observational studies. *Eur J Nutr* **58**, 173-191.

[129] Both groups did consume EVOO although levels were three times higher in the MD + EVOO group than the EVOO + nuts group

flexitarian diet are similar to the Med diet. However, they do not specifically recommend EVOO as the main dietary fat and so they will lose the very important benefits that this oil confers. EVOO may be more expensive that other cooking oils but scrimping on EVOO is a false economy.

The Med diet is also severely corrupted by replacing traditional Med dishes with industrial versions. Many of these use inappropriate ingredients and these industrial dishes can no longer be considered Mediterranean. Industrial pizzas use refined flour, little or no EVOO, meager levels of vegetables, and are usually high in salt, saturated fat and calories. Popular commercial Mediterranean dips like hummus and taramasalata may have rapeseed oil rather than EVOO and be high in salt. These types of products have been described as "salt and fat traps" by the organisation Consensus Action on Salt and Health. [130] Artisanal versions may be more acceptable but can be expensive. Homemade is far cheaper and much more dependable.

## The unseen meal

Fully realising a Med diet means far more than just putting meals on plates. The Greek etymological origin for "diet" is "diaita" meaning "a way of life" and the Med diet is better thought of in this broad sense. This is far better way to convey the overall Med diet than the limited meaning we give to the word "diet" today. In its full sense, a Med diet extends to "unseen" factors such as how the food is produced, how the food is cooked, the social context of eating, and even taking a siesta. These and other aspects were recognised by UNESCO when in 2010 it officially designated the Med diet as part of the cultural heritage of the people of the Mediterranean, and as a diet that "provides a sense of belonging and sharing and constitutes for those who live in the Mediterranean basin a marker of identity and a space for sharing and dialogue." Here is part of the UNESCO declaration [131]:

> "The Mediterranean diet constitutes a set of skills, knowledge, practices and traditions ranging from the landscape to the table, including the crops, harvesting, fishing, conservation, processing, preparation and, particularly, consumption of food. The

---

[130] https://www.theguardian.com/society/2016/jul/28/savoury-dips-are-salt-and-fat-traps-warns-health-group

[131] http://www.unesco.org/culture/ich/index.php?lg=en&pg=00011&RL=00394

Mediterranean diet is characterized by a nutritional model that has remained constant over time and space, consisting mainly of olive oil, cereals, fresh or dried fruit and vegetables, a moderate amount of fish, dairy and meat, and many condiments and spices, all accompanied by wine or infusions, always respecting beliefs of each community. However, the Mediterranean diet (from the Greek diaita, or way of life) encompasses more than just food. It promotes social interaction, since communal meals are the cornerstone of social customs and festive events. It has given rise to a considerable body of knowledge, songs, maxims, tales and legends. The system is rooted in respect for the territory and biodiversity, and ensures the conservation and development of traditional activities and crafts linked to fishing and farming in the Mediterranean communities which Soria in Spain, Koroni in Greece, Cilento in Italy and Chefchaouen in Morocco are examples. Women play a particularly vital role in the transmission of expertise, as well as knowledge of rituals, traditional gestures and celebrations, and the safeguarding of techniques."

These culinary and cultural values are not limited to Mediterranean countries and help give the Med diet its global appeal, making it easy to adopt in many other parts of the world. In this age of borderless values, the Med diet can represent the values of many people around the world and not just those living around the shores of the Mediterranean sea.

One of these core values is to demand a diet based on natural foods and not junk foods. Eating by these priorities is really just a way of reacquainting with traditional diets from before the era of junk foods. It may seem a big ask to, say, compare the Med diet with a pre-1950's British diet based as it was on "meat and two veg", but the crucial common factor is that both diets were without junk foods. [132] Building up a diet from a foundation of non-junk foods restores eating to its traditional home. From this historical perspective, a Med diet could arguably be seen as more culturally acceptable to the British than one based on junk foods. The junk food industry may have us believe

---

[132] Spam had appeared in the 1950's https://www.historic-uk.com/CultureUK/Food-in-Britain-in-the-1950s-1960s/

otherwise, and would argue that their products are now part of our food culture. But they are relatively recent imposters out to usurp traditional foods in the name of profit. Adapting to a Med diet would, for most people, mean a far lower adjustment than the huge transition to a diet high in processed foods witnessed between the 1950's and 1980's. By turning the clock back we can move into a future that incorporates far healthier ways of eating.

## Meal patterns through the day

As the UNESCO declaration recognised, sitting down to meals spaced through the day benefits both social cohesion and health. The traditional Cretan diet of the 1960's included eating three meals a day, which, where possible, were eaten with others [239]. Breakfast was a major source of carbohydrates and these would have been needed for the day's exertions ahead. Most protein was eaten at lunch. Physiologically speaking, this may particularly benefit people who have been physically active in the morning (such as would be the case for most Cretan peasants) since optimal muscle building occurs when protein is eaten immediately after exercise [240]. The evening meal for the Cretans consisted mainly of easily digested cooked vegetables.

The Cretan meal pattern is an intriguing one, and one that now finds itself in tune with many recent findings in chronobiology. Chronobiology, as applied to nutrition, examines how what we eat at different times of the day influences how we handle the calories and nutrients. Various internal biological cycles are closely aligned to the 24-hour night-day, sleep-wake cycle. These internal biological clocks form the circadian rhythm. Many physiological processes, including how we respond to what we eat, follow a circadian rhythm. Studies suggest that we are better at metabolising the calories we eat in the morning than those we eat later in the day. This may be because we produce less insulin in the evening and so are less able to regulate blood glucose [241]. One study found that overweight women eating 50% of daily calories at breakfast and 14% at dinner lost over 5 kg more over a 12-week period than women who ate 14% of calories at breakfast and 50% at dinner [242]. This suggests that for weight loss the best time to eat carbs is in the morning. There seems to be veracity in the old saying "eat breakfast like a king, lunch like a prince and dinner like a pauper" (and ditto for queens and princesses). [133] The benefits of eating carbohydrates with a low glycaemic index at breakfast can even extend over several hours by lowering glucose absorption at the subsequent lunchtime meal - an effect known as the "second-meal effect" [243].

Societies that still favour the main meal at midday rather than the evening may well now have the science to justify it, and the Cretan meal pattern is well worth trying. However, it won't be best for everyone since studies have shown that the optimal time for utilising calories varies between people [244]. There is also evidence that we can "train" our clocks to operate at different times of the day [244]. Maintaining a regular eating pattern may be important so that once our biological clock is set, food intake reflects the physiological settings (such as insulin production) that we have created. This will enable the food we consume to be processed in the optimal way by our body.

## Snacks

Advice on not snacking varies widely between countries, but most governments do little to discourage it. France is one exception, and a widely broadcast public health slogan in this country is *Evitez de grignoter entre les repas!* - Don't snack between meals! Perhaps the French authorities assume - probably correctly - that most of the snacks will be unhealthy [245]. Snacks were part of the healthy traditional Cretan Med diet [239]. This might come as a surprise since, even if snacking isn't discouraged by governments, it usually is by public health professionals. However, the mid-morning break of fresh fruit and mid-afternoon break of walnuts or homemade halva enjoyed between meals by Cretan peasants is a far cry from the sugary and fatty offerings most likely to be eaten today.

Although some studies suggest that a healthy snack of fruits or nuts can have a place in a healthy diet, snacking on unhealthy foods as a substitute for regular meals is a particularly bad choice. Well over half of UK people polled for a Harris poll in 2015 said they skip meals and snack, with almost a third

---

[133] https://www.telegraph.co.uk/science/2016/06/22/breakfast-like-a-king-lunch-like-a-prince-and-dine-like-a-pauper/
https://www.nhs.uk/news/food-and-diet/should-we-eat-breakfast-like-a-king-and-dinner-like-a-pauper/
although not all studies support weight loss by eating less in the evening Fong et al Br J Nutr. 2017 Oct;118(8):616-628. doi: 10.1017/S0007114517002550. Epub 2017 Oct 2.

saying they do so daily [246]. Snacking on unhealthy foods like crisps, sweets, chocolates and ice creams is associated with weight gain whereas this is not the case with healthier choices like nuts and yogurt [247]. In one study, a mid-morning snack of almonds caused no overall daily intake of calories in healthy women [248]. [134] This may be because nuts induce satiety and that less is eaten at the next meal. So although there is no consistent evidence that a mid-morning or mid-afternoon break is bad for health, the type of snack food eaten matters. And like eating regular meals through the day, snacking at regular times during the day may also matter. Random snacking may be harmful not only if the snacks are unhealthy but also because of the very randomness of the times they are eaten. [135]

A significant proportion of the junk food industry's products are snacks, and so snacking is a key battleground for this industry, and one vigorously defended. Pepsi Cola is one of the largest snack food companies in the world, owning popular UK snack food brands such as Walker's crisps, Doritos, Nobby's Nuts and Quavers. In 2013 Pepsi Cola funded a review of the health impacts of snacking which came to the conclusion that "for some individuals, including young children, snacking may have a positive rather than negative impact on health and should not be discouraged on a population-wide basis [249]." Many public health workers would strongly disagree with this conclusion. The sports broadcaster Gary Lineker has also come in for criticism because of his adverts for crisps aimed especially at children [250].

Fruit, nuts and seeds are excellent choices for healthy snacks. Dried fruits such as figs and prunes may have lost some of their vitamin C but this is made up for by their excellent levels of antioxidant polyphenols [251]. Roasted chickpeas seasoned with a wide variety of spices are a delicious and healthy snack popular in some Mediterranean countries. They tick all the boxes for their exceptional nutritional value (see ch. 12). Many other pulses and pulse flours are made into snacks, some healthier than others. The NHS website gives recipes for various low calorie snacks [136]. Unfortunately, it is questionable if many people will go to the trouble of preparing these since the

---

[134] It should be pointed out that this study was supported by The Almond Board of California.
[135] https://theconversation.com/circadian-rhythm-liver-gene-helps-body-keep-working-smoothly-after-late-nights-and-midnight-snacks
[136] https://www.nhs.uk/live-well/eat-well/surprising-100-calorie-snacks

Harris poll mentioned earlier found that the main reason why people snacked is because it is "easier".

## Siesta

In some Mediterranean countries, a siesta taken after the midday meal was once almost as much a part of the Med diet as the food itself. That drowsy feeling after lunch is due to more than just a full stomach. The carbs in the meal are an important trigger for inducing the post-lunch feeling of sleepiness since glucose has been shown to switch off a set of brain neurons called orexins that are needed for wakefulness.

Taking a siesta helps the body "rest and digest". And there may be more wide-ranging health benefits as well. Several studies have found that a short siesta of about thirty minutes reduces the risk of CVD and obesity [252; 253]. It is not known why this is so although getting adequate sleep can lower stress and so reduce the risk of CVD, whereas inadequate sleep is known to increase the production of the appetite-boosting hormone grehlin. Longer naps often taken at other times of the day however are linked to increased disease risk and could reflect an underlying chronic disease.

# The Med diet compared to other diets

Once we had no choice: we ate the foods our community could provide. Globalism has changed all that. We are now more or less free to choose a cuisine from anywhere in the world to align with our tastes and moral values. The world has become a global shop for nourishing our bodies and souls. This freedom can be seen as a good thing but with it comes the risk of losing many of the checks and balances that traditionally come from eating similar foods with family and friends. Uprooting these can unleash the persuasive powers of the internet and chat forums. How else to explain Breatharianism, the belief that we can survive on a diet of "the earth's energy"? [137]

The UK's "establishment" dietary guidelines are depicted in the Eatwell Guide. Although these guidelines are fairly similar to the Med diet, there are some important places where these two diets diverge. Firstly, the Eatwell guide recommends using unsaturated fats whereas the Med diet specifically advises olive oil (extra virgin) as the main added fat to use in cooking and raw.

---

[137] https://nypost.com/2017/06/21/breatharian-couple-we-eat-just-not-like-you/

In the Eatwell guide, pulses are classed as a source of protein whereas the Med diet categorises them with fruit and veg highlighting that they are not only a source of protein but also of fibre, vitamins and micronutrients. The Med diet also allows moderate wine consumption whereas alcohol is not included in the Eatwell guide. By trying to fit in with the British way of eating, the Eatwell Guide makes some recommendations that would not be usual in the Med diet. Tinned fruit is deemed to count as one of your five-a-day, whereas it is not mentioned in the Med diet. A recent meta-analysis found that tinned fruit was associated with an *increased* risk of CVD and dying from any cause and so the reliability of advice to recommend tinned fruit has to be questioned [254].

A diet similar to the Med diet, popular over the last few years, is the "flexitarian diet". [138] It is plant-based and, like the Med diet, low in meat. It was ranked equal second overall by a US panel of experts on the Best Diets of 2020. [139] However, it differs from the Med diet in two important ways, namely by not specifically including EVOO or moderate wine consumption - both of which are associated with significant health benefits. Although very similar to a Med diet, the flexitarian diet lacks the massive scientific evidence base of the Med diet, a body of supportive evidence far exceeding that for any other diet.

The popularity of vegetarian and vegan diets is booming. A vegetarian diet excludes fish, meat and products made from them, and a vegan diet also excludes eggs, dairy and honey. [140] The rise in vegetarianism and veganism hasn't occurred evenly between the sexes. A survey by the Vegan Society found almost twice as many vegans were female (63% female versus 37% male). [141] In western societies, more females are also vegetarian. The rise in veganism, in particular, risks leaving many men behind because more men than women prefer meals that include meat. The Med diet does include some meat and so it may prove to be more acceptable to many men than going vegetarian or vegan. A difference in eating preferences between the sexes is an important issue because of its impact on health, but it is one that receives

---

[138] https://www.theguardian.com/environment/2019/jan/19/could-flexitarianism-save-the-planet
[139] https://health.usnews.com/best-diet/best-diets-overall
[140] https://www.vegsoc.org/info-hub/definition/
[141] https://www.plantbasednews.org/opinion/why-arent-more-men-vegan

surprisingly little attention. Encouraging a particular diet is of little value if it discriminates against half the population.

There is no doubt that both vegetarian and vegan diets can be healthy. However, after considering taste, cost and convenience, many people decide these diets are not sufficiently enticing or acceptable. Both diets also suffer a relative lack of variety since meals must be created from a more limited ranges of ingredients (particularly for vegans) and this makes creating tasty and varied dishes challenging for some people and requires more cooking skills. Veganism would also be hard-pressed to be culturally acceptable for the majority of western populations. For instance, according to the trade journal the Farmers Guardian, 98% of UK households buy dairy products, which suggests that a complete ban is unrealistic. [142] Removing all farm animals and fish and switching to veganism would destroy a significant part of the gastronomic, farming, fishing and social culture of many societies. (Chapter 14 discusses the reasons why banning all animals is also unnecessary from an environmental perspective.)

Fulfilling nutritional requirements also requires more care for vegetarians and vegans. It is questionable whether an agriculture system with no animals can provide adequate overall nutrients. A US study concluded that animal-free agriculture would be incapable of supporting the US population's nutritional requirements, especially for calcium, vitamin A, vitamin B12 and the omega-3 fatty acids EPA and DHA (commonly referred to as "fish oils") [255]. As more people adopt vegetarian and vegan diets, appropriate public health information on how to achieve adequate nutrient intake is important. [143] Achieving a nutritionally balanced vegan diet requires a high level of nutritional awareness since most vegans need to take vitamin B12 supplements (since it is not found in plant foods) and many would probably benefit from omega 3 fat supplements too (although many other vegetarians and vegans, by making good diet choices, do survive perfectly well without these). There are also risks of inadequate choline, vitamin D, calcium, iron and zinc. Parents without sufficient nutritional knowledge risk malnourishing their

---

[142] https://www.fwi.co.uk/livestock/dairy/dairy-farmers-reject-vegan-calls-to-switch-to-plant-products
[143] These considerations contributed to why a vegetarian diet was ranked a lowly ninth and vegan an even more disappointing seventeenth in the US Best Diets of 2020 survey out of the thirty five diets considered.

children if they put them on strict vegan diets. In 2019 it was reported that in Sydney, Australia, parents who had put their three-year-old girl on a vegan diet had, according to the judge, left her severely malnourished and they were sentenced to 300 hours community service after they pleaded guilty to failing to provide for their daughter. [144]

Eating a plant-based diet is not necessarily the same as eating a diet of natural foods. Vegetarian and vegan diets are defined by what they exclude and not by what they include. There is no onus on minimising UPFs - unlike in the Med diet. Indeed many vegans may be enticed by vegan versions of processed foods to perk up their diets. Food companies have not been slow to recognise this new market and millennial vegans are heavily targeted with new types of highly processed vegan foods. These are not necessarily healthy, and some are categorised as UPFs that, like other UPFs, contain high levels of sugar, salt, fat and additives. [145] A serving of highly processed plant foods was shown in one study to be no better than a serving of animal foods since the processed plant foods increased the risk of coronary heart disease just as much as the animal foods [256]. We are also on the brink of a massive increase in the consumption of industrially made non-meat burgers. [146] There is an on-going debate about the cancer risk for one leading brand of non-meat burger since the main colouring and savoury flavouring comes from a product called leghaemoglobin. This is similar to the haem in meat, which is a suspected carcinogen (see ch. 12 for more). [147]

A Med diet is based on natural foods and one of the rationales for choosing this diet is that we evolved with natural foods. On the other hand, we did not evolve with processed foods and so these are best avoided. So what about the so-called paleo diet? After all, isn't this a diet that advocates tuning in to our evolutionary past by eating the diet of Paleolithic humans? There are several problems with this diet. Firstly, it is not possible today to replicate the diet from the Paleolithic era. We don't have access to the lean wild meat (which is not just the same as lean meat from domesticated animals) and wild berries.

---

[144] https://www.nytimes.com/2019/08/24/health/vegan-parents-malnourished-baby.html
[145] ww.businessinsider.fr/us/impossible-burger-beyond-burger-nutrition-compared-beef-2019-6
[146] http://www.theedgemarkets.com/article/nestle-plans-vegan-push-nomeat-burger-purple-walnut-milk
[147] https://cspinet.org/news/barebones-fda-review-impossible-burger-soy-leghemoglobin-inadequate-20190903

There is much debate about what Paleolithic people actually ate anyway. And health-wise, this diet raises several concerns. There is now a huge body of evidence that we should be eating far less meat than is advocated in the paleo diet. There are also numerous studies showing that following a paleo diet risks nutrient deficiencies. Cereals and dairy are the main sources of calcium in the UK diet. Because these are excluded from the paleo diet there is an increased risk of calcium deficiencies [257]. Dairy is also the main dietary source of iodine and women on a paleo diet have been found to be at an increased risk of iodine deficiency [258]. It might rank highly with meatarians, but the paleo diet was ranked a lowly twenty-ninth out of thirty-five by the panel of experts who judged the world's best diets in 2020. [148] The paleo diet is best consigned to the Stone Age.

Far more radical diets are also now being debated. An odd alliance of vegans, food industrialists and venture capitalists are proposing that the way to save the planet is with huge vats of fermenting bacteria and by growing animal cells in culture. [149] In their vision, genetically modified bacteria will form the basis of a new generation of processed foods and as a source of various nutrients (such as omega-3 fats). Animal cells will be grown on collagen scaffolds to create meat-like substances. Farmed animals will be banished and meat eaters told to eat "fermed" pastes instead of farmed meats. The food industry is more than happy to oblige with their technological foods, and a few food industrialists stand to achieve powers and profits that could even dwarf those of the current IT giants. It is argued that all this is necessary in order to save the planet because current farming is unsustainable, and because it is destroying vast tracts of land and wrapping the planet in a hot blanket of greenhouse gases emitted by cattle.

Health wise, there is a sense of déjà vu here. There is little reason to believe that this new wave of UPFs will be any different to the current UPFs that have flooded the market and proven in countless studies to represent the nadir of healthy eating. Many of these concerns are similar to those already discussed earlier. Current estimates are that the health risks associated with eating cultured beef cells would be similar to eating beef [259]. And as I discuss

---

[148] https://health.usnews.com/best-diet/best-diets-overall
[149] https://www.theguardian.com/commentisfree/2020/jan/08/lab-grown-food-destroy-farming-save-planet

in chapter 14 on sustainability it is highly debatable whether this new approach is necessary for sustainable food production.

It is clear that the Med diet is far more than just a set of foods and that it is time to move beyond just talking about what we eat to also ask how, when and why we eat. The most progressive eating guidelines have moved away from prescriptive advice such as "five-a-day" - which has done little to increase fruit and vegetable consumption - and towards more holistic advice. Perhaps the most established of these guidelines is the Brazilian system. It gives some excellent advice such as "eat regularly and carefully in appropriate environments and, whenever possible, in company", "shop in places that offer a variety of natural or minimally processed foods" and "plan your time to make food and eating important in your life" [260]. This is a far cry for the Eatwell Guide from the UK. A similar way of holistic thinking has prompted the food writer Gavin Wren to submit a set of "next-generation" dietary guidelines to the UK committee currently considering a new National Food Strategy. [150]

## How close is your diet to a Med diet?

If you are curious to see how closely your current diet is to that of a Med diet, try out the following questionnaire. This has a maximum score of 14 points. A score of seven or more suggests you have good compliance with a Med diet. This scoring system is the one that was used in the original Predimed study and has been adapted for a UK population [261].

---

[150] https://sustainablefoodtrust.org/contributors/gavin-wren/

| | Criterion for 1 point |
|---|---|
| 1. Do you use olive oil as your main fat for cooking? | Yes |
| 2. How much olive oil do you consume per day (including oil used for frying, salads, meals eaten away from home, etc.)? | 4 or more tablespoons |
| 3. How many vegetable servings do you consume per day? (1 serving = 200 g [consider side dishes as half a serving]) | 2 or more (at least 1 portion raw or on salad) |
| 4. How many pieces of fruit (including freshly squeezed fruit juice but not frozen per dried fruit) do you consume per day? | 3 or more |
| 5. How many servings of red meat, hamburgers, or meat products (ham, sausage, etc.) do you consume per day? (1 serving = 100–150 g) | less than 1 |
| 6. How many servings of butter, margarine, or cream do you consume per day? (1 serving = 12 g; 1 tablespoon) | less than 1 |
| 7. How many sugar-sweetened beverages do you drink per day? (1 cup = 100 ml) | less than one cup |
| 8. How much wine do you drink per week? (1 glass = 125 ml) | 7 or more glasses |
| 9. How many servings of pulses do you consume per week? (1 serving = 150 g) (including canned varieties) | 3 or more |
| 10. How many servings of fish or shellfish do you consume per week? (1 serving = 100–150 g of fish or 4–5 pieces or 200 g of shellfish) | 3 or more |
| 11. How many times per week do you consume commercial sweets or pastries (not homemade), such as cakes, cookies, biscuits, or custard? | less than 2 |
| 12. How many servings of nuts (including peanuts) do you consume per week? (1 serving = 30 g) | 3 or more |
| 13. Do you preferentially consume chicken, turkey, or rabbit meat instead of beef, pork, hamburger, or sausage? | Yes = 1 point |
| 14. How many times per week do you consume cooked vegetables, pasta, rice, or other dishes prepared with a sauce of tomato, onion, leek, or garlic sautéed in olive oil (*sofrito*)? | 2 or more = 1 point |

# 10. Core risk states as the triggers for chronic diseases

## Overview

The previous chapter showed that the Med diet can help prevent a remarkably wide range of chronic diseases. One idea for how the Med diet achieves this is that it contains certain foods that help prevent cancer, certain foods that help prevent dementia, and so on. Much like the way different drugs are used to treat different diseases. But the evidence suggests this is unlikely. A more likely explanation is that the Med diet mainly works by suppressing risk states that are common to the very early stages of all these diseases, and hence a Med diet simultaneously prevents many different chronic diseases. There are not different foods each preventing a distinct disease. In this chapter we identify these early core risk states and how changes to them can lead to chronic diseases.

## Common ground between chronic diseases

Chronic diseases are normally considered as distinct entities, each requiring a different treatment. Diabetes is distinct from cancer, which is distinct from CVD, and so on. While it may be true that different treatments are needed for the later stages of these diseases, the picture is quite different for their early stages. Medical research is now unearthing more and more common ground between the early stages of chronic disease development; the perspective that entirely distinct pathways give rise to different chronic diseases is not correct. For instance, some aspects of the early stages of Alzheimer's disease are so similar to type 2 diabetes that Alzheimer's disease has been dubbed "type 3 diabetes".

Just as particle physicists have long sought a theory to unify the forces in nature, so the very early causes of chronic diseases are increasingly being unified. There is no doubt that chronic diseases become increasingly complex and distinct as they develop, and no-one is saying dementia is the same as cancer for instance. But in their very early stages there are a few basic processes that drive the early development of most chronic diseases. Identifying these common early-stage underlying processes opens up huge opportunities in disease prevention. As long ago as 2004, the US associations for diabetes, cancer and cardiovascular disease issued a joint agenda for a common approach to prevent these seemingly distinct diseases [262]. In a few cases, this commonality between diseases is even impacting on treatment: one surprisingly successful recent advance is treating cancer with the diabetes drug metformin.

There is now much evidence that it is the common early stages when a healthy diet intervenes to slow down or even prevent a chronic disease from progressing further. The evidence is mounting that the exceptional benefits of the Med diet relate to its particular effectiveness at intervening during these early stages. This chapter discusses three underlying patho-physiological changes that are root causes of many chronic diseases, diseases that are responsible for fewer healthy years.

## Early stages in chronic diseases

The three patho-physiological changes I will discuss put the body in a heightened "at risk" state for the subsequent development of different diseases. These at risk states don't immediately lead to a full-blown disease since, by definition, chronic diseases develop over many years. Following the "at risk" state is a stage dubbed the "predisease" state.[151] The likelihood of a risk state progressing to the predisease state increases with unhealthy behaviours such as smoking or eating a poor diet or, from having inherited genes that predispose to a disease. Once a predisease state is reached, there is often a high probability of it progressing to a full-blown disease. A good example of a predisease state is "prediabetes", a state characterised by high fasting blood sugar levels and that has a high probability of progressing to the full disease state of type 2 diabetes.

Not all diseases have clearly defined predisease states. For example, stroke does not have a clearly defined "prestroke" stage. Although hypertension

---

[151] The concept of predisease probably has its origins in cancer biology. The term "precancerous" appeared in the medical literature over a century ago, when it was recognized that no sharp line demarcated the histology between benign and malignant tissues.

(high blood pressure) increases the risk of stroke, hypertension is not considered to be "prestroke" since a relatively low proportion of people with hypertension go on to have a stroke, and many people without hypertension may have a stroke. Some examples of prediseases are shown in the table.

**Predisease states and clinical features**

| Disease | Predisease | Example of diagnosis |
|---|---|---|
| Cervical cancer | Cervical intraepithelial neoplasia | Visual |
| Colon cancer | Polyps | Visual |
| Diabetes | Prediabetes | High fasting blood glucose |
| Hypertension | Prehypertension | High blood pressure |
| Alzheimer's disease | Mild cognitive impairment | Memory test |
| CVD | Elevated cholesterol | Blood cholesterol |

Based on this framework of risk states and predisease, the transition from health to disease can be summarised as:

healthy person

↓ *poor diet, smoking, lack of exercise, obesity*

risk state - **disease non-specific/systemic effects in the body**

↓ *genetic / lifestyle factors\**

predisease state - **disease specific/often organ specific**

↓ *genetic / lifestyle factors\**

disease

*Lifestyle factors include obesity, lack of physical activity, smoking, excessive alcohol drinking, sleep patterns, emotional well-being

Identifying risk and predisease states is key to disease prevention. Many predisease states can now be diagnosed and, for some, treatments are available. A particularly common predisease state is elevated cholesterol, and statins are frequently prescribed to help control this.

Unlike predisease states, risk states often go unnoticed. Although a heart attack or cancer diagnosis is usually sudden, dramatic and unexpected, it is simply the maturing of a risk state that has remained undetected for many years, before any personal awareness that something was wrong and before a clinical diagnosis. Healthy diets suppress risk states, and the healthy diet that has prevented a heart attack or cancer is the unsung hero that has been quietly working away to prevent the risk state of a disease from progressing. So what are these risk states and how does understanding them lead to better disease prevention?

## How chronic diseases arise from Core Risk States

In ancient Greece, the physician Hippocrates developed the theory of the Four Humours - the idea that blood, yellow bile, black bile, and phlegm underpin and influence the body and emotions. The new group of risk states in the body that I will discuss can be seen as latter day examples of Hippocrates's humours, but unlike these, the modern versions come with a weighty scientific pedigree. These Core Risk States are harbingers for early disease development and they provide a new lens through which the early development of chronic diseases can be viewed, understood and targeted. The Core Risk States are oxidative stress, chronic low-grade inflammation and insulin resistance. We will now consider each of these.

## Oxidative stress

Oxygen is very much a double-edged sword. Although ubiquitous and essential for life, oxygen readily converts into a group of highly reactive chemicals called free radicals. Free radicals derived from oxygen (they can also derive from nitrogen) are known as Reactive Oxygen Species (ROS). They are present in many environmental pollutants such as car fumes and cigarette smoke [263]. ROS can be very damaging to the body. They attack molecules in the body, particularly the lipids (fats) that surround every cell. Then, vampire-like, the injured lipids themselves become free radicals. This starts a chain

156

reaction with lipid free radicals generating other lipid free radicals. "Radicalised" lipids are the terrorists of the body and can cause extensive tissue damage and cell death. It is not only lipids that can be radicalised, other cellular constituents such as proteins, sugars and DNA can also fall victim to ROS.

Environmental factors are not the only sources of ROS. More surprisingly, ROS are also produced as an unavoidable consequence of normal energy generation by cells. So even living a completely virtuous life does not prevent your body being exposed to ROS. Fortunately, we have an arsenal of antioxidant defences to keep ROS in check. Sometimes, however, the rate at which ROS are produced overwhelms the body's ability to keep them in check. The state when ROS production has outgunned the body's antioxidant defences is called oxidative stress.

Oxidative stress - an excess of ROS - is the first of our Core Risk States. Because ROS are so promiscuous in what they choose to attack, oxidative stress can initiate a wide range of pathological processes. For instance, free radicals from cigarette smoke can attack the DNA of cells in the lung, which may initiate the first step to cancer; they can also damage cells lining blood vessels initiating cardiovascular disease; and they can also damage alveoli in the lungs, which may ultimately result in COPD (chronic obstructive pulmonary disease).

To protect against ROS, we rely not only on our own personal arsenal of antioxidant defences but also on antioxidants found in plant foods such as fruits, vegetables and nuts. These antioxidants include vitamin C and a wide range of phytochemicals. We cannot make these antioxidants ourselves. Presumably they were abundant in the diets of our ancestors and so there was not enough evolutionary selection pressure to deem it necessary to use up precious metabolic energy to manufacture them.

The best strategy to prevent oxidative stress is to prevent excess ROS from being produced. This means having adequate antioxidant defences, both those internally produced in the body and externally obtained from foods. Unfortunately this is often not the case for people who eat a poor diet. Not consuming enough dietary antioxidant phytochemicals increases the risk of disease.

The antioxidant phytochemical lutein can be used to illustrate how important avoiding oxidative stress is for heath. Lutein is a yellow pigment (*luteus* is the Latin for yellow) and is found in particularly high amounts in green leafy vegetable such as kale and spinach. (These vegetables appear green rather than yellow because their very high amounts of chlorophyll mask the yellow lutein.) Lutein is selectively transported into the retina of the eye where it accumulates in a region associated with acute vision known as the macula (in full this region is called the *macula lutea* which translates as yellow spot). The eye is particularly susceptible to light damage. This damage is caused by the energy from light activating free radicals that then damage molecules in the eye by a process called photo-oxidation. Lutein helps protect against this damage.

The eye is an extremely active organ. Neuronal cells in the eye operate at exceptionally high speeds in order to transmit nerve impulses from the eye to the brain. These speeds are made possible by these neuronal cells having very fluid membranes. This fluidity comes from the large amounts of a polyunsaturated fatty acid called DHA (docosahexaenoic acid) in the neuronal membranes. DHA has an irregular structure that prevents molecules of DHA from packing tightly together and so results in a more fluid environment in the neuronal cell membrane. The downside to all this is that DHA is very prone to oxidative damage by free radicals. This is where lutein comes in, by protecting DHA against photo-oxidative damage. Insufficient lutein in the diet is linked to damage to the eye and in particular to an increased risk of age-related macular degeneration (AMD). AMD is the main cause of blindness in western countries. Such is the importance of lutein for the eye that it has evolved specific ways of sucking up lutein from the blood so enabling the eye to accumulate lutein in very high amounts.

There is a second organ in the body that also selectively accumulates lutein: the brain. This is no coincidence. Neuronal cells in the brain and retinal cells in the eye are both derived from the same type of foetal cells. Both the brain and retina are also the two richest regions in the body for DHA and both regions rely on lutein to help protect their DHA from oxidative damage. As with the eye, lutein is also important for the overall health of the brain, and there is increasing evidence that lutein helps prevent cognitive decline.

Hence there are interesting parallels between the eye and the brain. One study found that people with AMD are more likely to have lower cognitive function than normal [264]. It is possible, although not proven, that this could be related to the high reliance of both the eye and the brain for DHA, and so a low dietary intake of lutein could be leading to free radical damage to DHA in both organs. This illustrates that because neuronal cells in the eye and brain have the same foetal origin, they also have similar dietary requirements, and hence that AMD and cognitive decline, two seemingly distinct diseases, are in fact closely related. This may have implications for treatment as well since lutein supplements have been found to both benefit people with AMD and to help cognitive performance in the elderly [265; 266].

Uncontrolled oxidative stress eventually results in ROS and lipid radicals killing cells. The body needs to remove these dead cells and the way it does this is by triggering an inflammatory response. An inflammatory response is part of the body's normal defences to restore healthy tissues. But as we shall see this does not always go according to plan and can lead to chronic low-grade inflammation, the second of the Core Risk States.

## Chronic low-grade inflammation

The word "inflammation" derives from the Latin "inflammo" meaning "I ignite" and alludes to the warm feeling from an infected finger or the burning sensation of an infected throat. The warm feeling is a sign that blood vessels in the region have dilated. This widening of blood vessels creates a super-highway allowing white blood cells from elsewhere in the body to quickly arrive at the scene of infection to deal with invading bacteria. The body is mounting an inflammatory response. Once the marauding bacteria have been dealt with, the immune cells check out and die. This overall process is referred to as an "acute inflammatory response" as it normally lasts only a short period of time. Acute inflammation is tightly regulated and is part of the general housekeeping armoury that the body has evolved to keep healthy.

There is another type of inflammatory response, one that underpins many chronic diseases, and that is of far greater concern for overall health. It can occur in many parts of the body and often goes unnoticed. Here, the stimulus for the inflammatory influx of white blood cells is usually not invading bacteria but tissue damage. Tissues in the body become damaged for many reasons. As we have seen, ROS are one major cause, but there are many others, such as excess alcohol, which damages liver cells, and acid from the stomach refluxing up the oesophagus and damaging cells lining the oesophagus. These damaged tissues send out cries for help in the form of molecules called cytokines. An army of white defensive blood cells responds to cytokines, dutifully arriving at the site of injury. This is an inflammatory response, but in this case it may ultimately lead to serious disease: in blood vessels the eventual outcome may be a heart attack or stroke; in the liver or oesophagus, a cancer may form.

These outcomes appear paradoxical. After all, isn't inflammation meant to be a *defensive* system for the body, not one leading to a life-threatening disease? The problem is that in these situations the inflammation, unlike in the case with bacterial infections, does not always resolve. It is when the inflammation becomes non-resolving or "chronic" in nature that subsequent damaging events can occur. If oxidative stress is the match that ignites many chronic diseases then inflammatory signals circulating around the body are the factors that stoke the flames.

Some people experience chronic inflammation more than others. One of the most significant factors that elevates chronic inflammation in the body is obesity. Adipose (fat) tissue, once considered to be merely an inert depot for excess calories, is now known to pump out inflammatory signals. These signals travel around the body, and can fan the flames of inflammation at sites in the body where white blood cells of the immune system have already accumulated, such as damaged blood vessel walls. Although they are produced at relatively low levels, the inflammatory signals from adipose tissue are continually - chronically - produced. This continual production of low levels of inflammatory signals is known as chronic low-grade inflammation. It is the second of the three Core Risk States.

Chronic low-grade inflammation is a very significant risk state in the body and is probably the main reasons why obesity increases the risk of diseases as diverse as CVD, cancer and dementia. Not all fat stores are equally harmful however. Abdominal obesity (a large waistline) is more dangerous than thigh fat. Fat within the abdominal cavity - *visceral fat* - is stored around a number of important internal organs such as the liver, pancreas and intestines and this is also a significant health risk.

As well as obesity, aging is also a risk factor for chronic low-grade inflammation. Chronic low-grade inflammation linked to aging is known as "inflamm-aging". As the body ages, senescent (dead) cells build up, which trigger an inflammatory response and this is thought to be one of the reasons for inflammaging. Another possible reason is linked to changes in the bacterial population in the gut that occurs with aging [267]. A decrease in "good" bacteria allows more harmful bacteria to flourish. Normally, a layer of mucus protects cells lining the gut (colon) from damage by gut bacteria. But harmful gut bacteria may invade the lining of the colon and trigger a chronic inflammatory response [268].

Increased inflammation with age is thought to be one of the main reasons why many chronic disorders usually occur in later life. Age-related chronic disorders linked to inflammaging include atherosclerosis, type 2 diabetes, Alzheimer's disease and osteoporosis. Inflammaging is also incriminated in muscle wasting or sarcopenia (sarx = muscle, penia = lack of) [269; 270]. This is because inflammaging increases inflammatory factors that can trigger the breakdown of muscle tissue [270]. The fat in muscular areas is not affected, and so signs of sarcopenia can be masked in obese individuals. Obese people with low muscle mass are at particular risk of mobility and disability problems [270].

Reduced inflammaging is now being linked to successful aging in very old people who experience very little disease. This may be because of their innate ability to produce higher than normal levels of factors that counter inflammaging. For elderly people without such a good innate anti-inflammatory defence system, strategies that reduce inflammaging may lower disease burden and increase healthspan and overall life expectancy.

Chronic low-grade inflammation is clearly an important factor that drives many chronic diseases and blocking inflammatory signals has been found to be an effective way of reducing CVD. This was demonstrated for a drug that very specifically blocks an inflammatory signal called interleukin-1. This drug was found to dramatically reduce the likelihood of a second heart attack or stroke in high-risk patients [271]. [152] Also, although statins were designed to reduce cholesterol levels, there is some evidence that statins have anti-inflammatory activity and this may be an important way they lower the risk of CVD [272].

Inflammatory mediators produced during chronic low-grade inflammation can induce a state of resistance in the body to respond to insulin. Insulin resistance is the third of our Core Risk States.

---

[152] https://www.theguardian.com/science/2017/aug/27/anti-inflammatory-drugs-may-lower-heart-attack-risk-study-finds

# Insulin resistance

During the digestion of carbohydrates from a meal, glucose is released into the bloodstream. The rise in glucose in the blood triggers the release of insulin from the pancreas. The insulin is produced to allow cells to take up glucose from the blood: it is the key that opens the door on a cell to allow glucose in. Muscle cells and other organs use glucose to generate energy and any left over glucose is taken up by adipose tissue and converted into fat for storage. Blood glucose levels then fall, the insulin is no longer needed and so no more is produced. Sometimes this normal rise and fall no longer operates. This can result in insulin taking on a completely different, more sinister role, and one linked to driving many chronic diseases.

The crucial switch that triggers this less desirable role arises when muscle and fat cells change so that they no longer respond to insulin. They are no longer responding to the key that allows the cells to open their door to glucose and so these cells can no longer take up glucose from the blood. The cells are said to be insulin resistant. Cells in the pancreas sense that glucose levels in the blood are remaining high and so the insulin-producing cells in the pancreas try and compensate by producing more insulin. If there is still no response, the pancreas carries on producing insulin. The normal rise and fall of insulin is lost. The consequence is both high levels of glucose in the blood (hyperglycaemia) and high levels of insulin (hyperinsulinaemia).

There are various causes of insulin resistance. Continually elevated levels of blood sugar - caused for example by eating a very sugary diet - can result in continually elevated levels of insulin. This can eventually desensitises cells to insulin, resulting in insulin resistance. Paradoxically, too much dietary sugar is leading to cells being starved of glucose.

Another major culprit is obesity. Some of the inflammatory signals produced by adipose tissue can block cells from responding to insulin. If insulin is the key that opens doors on cells to allow glucose in, then inflammatory signals are the locksmiths that change the locks preventing insulin from working. Inflammaging also increases the likelihood for insulin resistance. Hence various situations that cause chronic low-grade inflammation can ultimately then lead to insulin resistance.

This shows that the three Core Risk States are related as follows:

oxidative stress → chronic low grade inflammation → insulin resistance

## Why insulin can be dangerous

Hyperglycaemia and hyperinsulinaemia are hugely important predisease states. A person with elevated blood glucose is said to have prediabetes. According to one report, a staggering one in three adults in the UK now has this condition – a figure that has tripled since 2003 [273]. A review of a large number of studies found that being prediabetic increases the risk, albeit to a small extent, for many different cancers [274]. Hyperglycaemia also increases free radicals in the body that damage blood vessels [275]. A simple strategy that may reduce the risk of this damage is to stick to three meals a day. The tradition of three meals a day allows time between meals for antioxidants to repair oxidative damage. With snacking on sugary foods there may be less of a reprieve, and with the damaged blood vessels comes an increased likelihood of a heart attack or stroke [276; 277].

Although detecting and treating prediabetes has huge implications for public health, most people don't even know they are living with this pre-disease state and so take no remedial action. In the UK, an NHS Health Check will detect prediabetes, enabling patients to reverse it by adopting a healthier lifestyle.

Hyperinsulinaemia is of equal if not even greater concern. As mentioned earlier, obesity can lead to insulin resistance and the body tries to compensate for the failure to respond to insulin by producing more insulin, which results in hyperinsulinaemia. Because of the high prevalence of obesity, hyperinsulinaemia is very common in western society. A chronically elevated level of insulin has widespread pathological effects in the body. This particularly relates to cancer. Although some cells such as muscle cells can become insulin resistant others known as epithelial cells do not develop this resistance. Insulin can act like a fertiliser for these epithelial cells, keeping them alive for longer and increasing their chances of dividing. This effect will be greatly enhanced when insulin levels remain chronically high. A high rate of cell division in epithelial cells greatly increases the likelihood that some of the cells will become altered and change into cancerous cells. Epithelial cells are found all over the body. For example they line "tubes" in the body such as in the gastrointestinal tract, in the respiratory system and in the breast. Epithelial cells are the main cell type that forms cancers. Consequently, hyperinsulinaemia is associated with an increased risk of many different types of cancer.

## Why obese people can have different health risks

In his 1988 Banting Lecture, the American endocrinologist Professor Gerald Reaven described "a cluster of risk factors for diabetes and cardiovascular disease". He named this cluster of factors "Syndrome X" [278]. He used the term "syndrome" rather than "disease" because to be positively diagnosed a person must have a cluster of (usually three or more) pathological changes that exceed defined levels. These changes are a large waist circumference, high blood fats, high blood pressure, high fasting blood glucose, and low HDL (good) cholesterol.

Although syndrome X represents a collection of risk factors, Reaven realised that there was a fundamental pathological change underlying this condition. This is insulin resistance. Being insulin resistance causes many pathological metabolic changes in the body, and it is for this reason that syndrome X is now usually called metabolic syndrome.

Although few people have heard of it, metabolic syndrome is an extremely common condition. It is age-related. Up to a third of middle-aged people in more developed countries have metabolic syndrome, and this increases to almost two thirds in those over 70 [279]. Metabolic syndrome frequently evolves to type 2 diabetes, CVD or various types of cancer and its high prevalence means that metabolic syndrome is the driving force for chronic disease in huge numbers of people.

As mentioned a moment ago, obesity creates a state of chronic inflammation in the body, which may then lead to insulin resistance. Hence it is not surprising that obesity is a risk factor for metabolic syndrome. But the sequence of obesity leading to chronic inflammation leading to insulin resistance and then metabolic syndrome is not inevitable. For some people this sequence appears to stop at obesity since they do not go on to develop the further pathological changes that define metabolic syndrome. People who are obese but have no signs of metabolic syndrome are said to be metabolically healthy obese (MHO). Just as there are many people with metabolic syndrome, so too the number who are MHO is very high with one analysis categorising 7–28% of European women and 2–19% of European men as MHO [(280)].

There is currently much debate about whether the state of being MHO really exists - in other words that it is possible to be obese and yet not have an increased risk for obesity-related diseases such as CVD. This is sometimes referred to as being "fat and fit". It can be quite difficult to decide if an obese person is not being affected by their weight since obesity can cause very many pathological changes. Measuring all of these would be necessary before being able to conclude that an obese person is not being adversely affected by their weight. One important change rarely measured is a thickening of and build up of calcium in the arteries. If this change goes undetected, an obese person could still be categorised as metabolically healthy, even when this is not really the case[(281)]. Current evidence suggests that an obese person having none of the standard markers of metabolic ill health has a reduced risk for CVD compared to a person with metabolic syndrome, but that they are not at as low a risk as someone who is of normal weight and metabolically healthy. [153] In other words, there is still some increased risk of ill-health in a person who is defined as MHO.

Even allowing for this slightly increased disease risk, we can accept that there are a significant number of people who are obese but still relatively metabolically healthy. This gives rise to an important question: why are some obese people relatively metabolically healthy? In fact, this situation is not always stable, and many obese people who start out as metabolically healthy eventually develop the normal adverse metabolic changes associated with obesity [(283)]. So the next question to ask is what causes the switch from being obese but metabolically healthy (ie MHO) to being metabolically unhealthy? One explanation relates to diet. Diet is likely to be an important factor that influences the metabolic health of an obese person. Many studies have found that obese people eating a traditional Mediterranean-style diet are more likely to retain metabolic health. For instance, obese women in Lebanon who followed their traditional diet were almost twice as likely to retain metabolic

---

[153] For example, a meta-analysis of prospective cohort studies found MHO individuals to have approximately four times increased risk (relative risk (RR) = 4.03, 95% confidence interval (CI) 2.66–6.09) and MUO approximately nine times increased risk of developing T2DM (RR = 8.93, 95% CI 6.86–11.62), compared to MHNormalWeight -see 282. Bell JA, Kivimaki M, Hamer M (2014) Metabolically healthy obesity and risk of incident type 2 diabetes: a meta-analysis of prospective cohort studies. *Obes Rev* **15**, 504-515.

health than similarly overweight women who ate a diet of fast foods [284]. Other studies have also shown that a Med diet can counteract the adverse effects of abdominal obesity [285]. So the important overall conclusion is that not all obese people are alike, and not all obese people are at the same risk of obesity-related disorders.

## How the Core Risk States drive cancer

A simple view of cancer is that it is caused by a carcinogen. This implies that avoiding exposure to carcinogens removes cancer risk. This direct cause and effect rationale of identifying and removing carcinogens from the environment has saved many lives. Not smoking is the single most important way of reducing exposure to carcinogens. Avoiding occupational carcinogens such as asbestos and greater awareness of environmental carcinogens such as uv rays from the sun and pollutants in the air has been of great benefit in reducing cancer risk.

But the way a cancer develops - the process of carcinogenesis - is far more complex causes than this, and carcinogenesis cannot simply be pinned down to being caused by a single carcinogen. A more sophisticated view of carcinogenesis is as a two-step process. A carcinogen is the initial trigger that damages (mutates) the DNA of a cell, but for carcinogenesis to progress other agents called tumour promoters are also needed. [154] Tumour promoters create an environment that drives the carcinogenic process forward. It is tumour promoters that largely determine whether or not a cell with mutated DNA matures into a full-blown tumour, and eventually - usually after many years - for it to be sufficiently aggressive and invasive to be called a cancer. [155] If initiators are the on-switch then tumour promoters are the volume control. Without turning up the volume there is no music; without tumour promoters there is no cancer. All three Core Risk States are strongly implicated in carcinogenesis. Oxidative stress can act as a tumour initiator by causing mutations in DNA, and inflammatory mediators and insulin can act as tumour promoters. Hence the Core Risk States are a useful framework for understanding and helping prevent cancer.

---

[154] The body has various defence mechanisms to repair the mutated DNA, but these are not always successful.
[155] A fundamental step in the transition from a solid tumour to a cancer is when it acquires the ability to become invasive.

Links between inflammation and cancer have been known since the time of the Roman Empire. In the second century AD, the physician Galen observed that cancers can arise from inflammatory lesions, but, as he noted, they can be differentiated from them because "they are blacker in colour than inflammations and are not at all hot" (a reference to black bile one of the original four humours) [286]. A rather more recent study from 2016 found that Finnish men with the highest levels of markers of inflammation in their blood were 47% more likely to get cancer and 48% more likely to die from cancer [287].

Because adipose tissue is a major source of tumour-promoting inflammatory mediators it is not surprising that obesity increases the risk of some types of cancer. There is a particularly increased risk of cancers of the breast, colorectum, kidney, pancreas, endometrium and oesophagus [288].

Insulin can also be described as a tumour promoter because of its ability to stimulate cell growth. Adipose tissue doesn't itself produce insulin, but leads to an increase in insulin production in a more roundabout way. The adipose tissue produces inflammatory mediators, these then cause insulin resistance in some organs, and the body then tries to compensate for these organs failing to respond to insulin by producing more. This elevated insulin state in the body is hyperinsulinaemia.

A very important question is whether it is obesity itself that increases cancer risk or whether it the insulin resistance caused by the obesity. A prospective study conducted in the US provided clinical evidence that it is insulin resistance that is a cancer risk factor and that this can be independent of obesity [289]. They demonstrated this by showing that people who had insulin resistance but were of normal weight were over twice as likely to develop cancer as people who were of normal weight and not insulin resistant. So the conclusion is that although many cancers are referred to as "obesity-related" it is the underlying metabolic changes such as inflammatory mediators and insulin resistance caused by obesity that are the real cause, and not obesity *per se*. [156]

Even though new approaches to cancer prevention are desperately needed, the association between cancer risk with chronic low-grade inflammation and

---

[156] see also: Obesity, Inflammation, and Cancer  annurev-pathol-012615-044359

insulin resistance receives relatively little attention in cancer prevention programmes. Instead, government policies mostly tackle carcinogens. It is true that these policies have been very successful in reducing the incidence of some types of cancer. Anti-smoking campaigns are now starting to reap their reward as seen by the fall in the incidence of lung cancer in men (although not yet in women), and many previously permitted chemicals, such as some pesticides, are now banned because they are suspected carcinogens. But despite these actions, more and more people in the UK are still being diagnosed with cancer. In 2008 just over 300,000 people were diagnosed with cancer in the UK and this is predicted to rise to almost 400,000 by 2030. In some high-income countries, cancer is already the main cause of death in middle-aged people. [157] Cancer is soon expected to overtake CVD as the number one cause of death.

It is the failure to identify and target the main risk factors for some of the most deadly cancers that is mostly to blame for these worrying statistics. The effectiveness of targeting risk factors to tackle chronic diseases is exemplified by the success in reducing the incidence of CVD in developed countries. For cancer, there is a strong argument that government prevention campaigns that previously focused on carcinogens now need to put far more resources into tackling tumour promoters. I believe we now have our eye on the wrong ball. I will illustrate why I think this is the case by discussing two cancers with worryingly high incidences, which are still rising: those of the breast and oesophagus.

## Breast cancer

The good news about breast cancer is that survival rates have been steadily improving. This is mainly because of earlier detection and improved treatments. The not so good news is the continual increase since the 1970's in the number of UK women getting this disease (see Figure).

---

[157] https://www.bbc.com/news/health-49558223

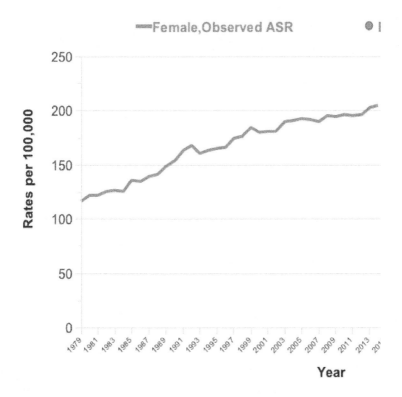

**Female, Observed ASR** ● I

**Incidence Rates of Breast Cancer in UK Females** [158]

As the next Figure shows, this rise varies markedly between age groups. Figures from Cancer Research UK show that since the early 1990's incidence rates in the 25-49's have increased by 17%, by 14% in the 50-64's, by 70% in the 65-69's, by 32% in the 70-79's and by 22% in the 80 plus. Breast cancer rates in the under-50's are now at record highs. [159]

---

[158] Cancer Research UK https://www.cancerresearchuk.org/health-professional/cancer-statistics/statistics-by-cancer-type/breast-cancer/incidence-invasive#heading-Five (accessed Sept/2020)

[159] https://www.nhs.uk/news/cancer/breast-cancer-rates-in-under-50s-at-record-high/

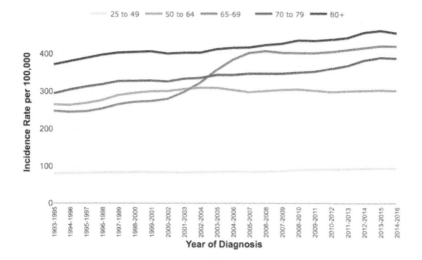

**Breast Cancer Incidence Rates by Age in Females in UK** [160]

The precise reasons for these worrying increases are unclear. Many factors could play a part such as improved screening (and so detecting more women with breast cancer), having children later, women living longer (since risk increases with age), increasing rates of obesity and various lifestyle factor such as alcohol consumption and low levels of physical activity.

But these risk factors are not as clearly linked to breast cancer as, say, the link between smoking and lung cancer. For instance, if obesity were a major risk factor for breast cancer it would be expected that the prevalence of breast cancer in UK women from lower socio-economic groups would be higher since their prevalence of obesity is higher (see ch. 3). But breast cancer prevalence is actually lower in women from lower socio-economic groups (see Figure below).[161] This suggests that multiple factors interact in breast cancer risk. Although obesity is a risk factor it is not the dominant one.

---

[160] (Cancer Research UK https://www.cancerresearchuk.org/health-professional/cancer-statistics/statistics-by-cancer-type/breast-cancer/incidence-invasive#heading-Two (accessed Sept/2020))

[161] This is the opposite of most other cancers where there is an association between lower socio-economic class and increased risk of cancer.

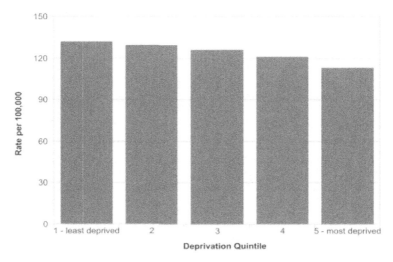

**Incidence if Breast Cancer by Level of Deprivation in UK Females** [162]

If obesity *per se* isn't the dominant risk factor for obesity then perhaps more important is the elevated level of insulin that results from obesity. There is increasing evidence that this may be the case. In one study, the risk of breast cancer in a large group of postmenopausal women from the US was measured according to the women's weight and insulin status. It was found that the women who were obese but with normal insulin levels were not at increased risk of breast cancer [(290)]. But the women with elevated insulin levels - even if they were of normal weight - were at almost twice the risk of breast cancer. This suggests that elevated insulin levels are a more important risk factor for breast cancer than obesity *per se*.

Elevated insulin levels are an indication that the body has experienced a preceding period of insulin resistance. This is because when the body becomes insulin resistant the pancreas has tried to compensate for the lack of a response to the insulin by producing more insulin. This period of over-producing insulin may have persisted for many years. These are many years when the body is at increased cancer risk. Type 2 diabetes is also usually preceded by many years of elevated insulin levels (which often goes often undetected) and this is probably a reason why being diabetic increases the risk

---

[162] https://www.cancerresearchuk.org/health-professional/cancer-statistics/statistics-by-cancer-type/breast-cancer/incidence-invasive#heading-Six (accessed Sept 2020)

(by about 20%) of breast cancer in postmenopausal women. Again this is independent of obesity [291].

Being diagnosed as obese *and* insulin resistant carries a higher risk of breast cancer than having just one of these risk factors [292]. One reason for this could be that as well as elevating insulin levels, obesity can also increase chronic inflammation, and chronic inflammation is also known to be a risk factor for breast cancer risk [291].[163] So both elevated insulin and increased chronic inflammation resulting from obesity can drive breast cancer.

Insulin increases breast cancer risk by acting as a tumour promoter - that is, it stimulates the growth and survival of cells. But insulin does not operate alone: it has two major partners in crime. The first is a closely related miscreant called IGF1 - insulin-like growth factor. As its name implies, IGF1 mimics many of the actions of insulin by stimulating cell growth and cell survival. The second miscreant is oestrogen. Insulin, IGF1 and oestrogen can all interact to increase the risk of breast cancer. And - even more importantly - is that the interaction between oestrogen and insulin, and the interaction between oestrogen and IGF1, are synergistic. In other words, when oestrogen interacts with either insulin or IGF1 the adverse effects are greater than sum of these molecules acting alone.

One reason why insulin, IGF1 and oestrogen make cells in the breast more likely to become cancerous is because of the way they stimulate breast cells to divide more quickly and to survive longer. An increased rate of cell division is, on its own, not sufficient to cause a cancer: rapidly dividing cells may accumulate into a mass forming a benign tumour, but this tumour will not be invasive (the trademark sign of a cancer). But every so often one of the rapidly dividing breast cells is likely to fail to faithfully replicate its DNA and so the next generation of this cell (the "daughter" cell) carries a mutation. [164] It is when this mutated daughter cell divides further that a cancer can develop. What this means is that a breast cancer can arise without the need for an environmental carcinogen to cause the initial mutation since all the factors

---

[163] Also, obesity and type 2 diabetes, or perhaps the associated inflammation, promote oestrogen-independent breast cancer particularly in premenopausal women Rose DP, Gracheck PJ, Vona-Davis L (2015) The Interactions of Obesity, Inflammation and Insulin Resistance in Breast Cancer. *Cancers (Basel)* **7**, 2147-2168

[164] Cells can repair damage when they fail to replicate faithfully but this ability decreases when cells are dividing more rapidly

driving the development of the cancer - oestrogen, insulin and IGF1 - are produced by the body itself. This is unlike in more familiar scenarios such as lung cancer where it is usually environmental carcinogens - such as cigarette smoke - that start the process of carcinogenesis.

As well as interacting at the cellular level, insulin and oestrogen also interact at the whole body level because insulin increases the production of oestrogen by the body. Oestrogen is generally regarded as the most important risk factor for oestrogen-responsive breast cancers (known as ER-positive cancers) in postmenopausal women. [165] Insulin increases oestrogen production in adipose tissue and this might be particularly important as a risk factor for breast cancer in obese postmenopausal women [291].

From these discussions it is clear that obesity, insulin (and the related IGF1) and oestrogen all interact to drive breast cancer. So how much do these interactions explain the link between obesity and breast cancer? The authors of one important study analysed the blood levels of insulin and estradiol - which is equivalent to oestrogen - in 835 postmenopausal women with breast cancer. They concluded that "our data indicate that hyperinsulinaemia and high endogenous estradiol [oestrogen] levels are independent risk factors for postmenopausal breast cancer and largely explain the association between obesity and the risk of breast cancer in postmenopausal women [293]." [166] Since every extra 5 kg of weight gained over normal increases the risk of breast cancer by 6% in postmenopausal women in European and North American countries this conclusion deserves serious attention and greater action. [294]

The benefits of physical activity for preventing breast cancer

This brief discussion of this very active area of research suggests that inflammation, insulin and oestrogen are all strongly implicated in breast cancer risk. Some studies have also found that high circulating insulin increases the chances of breast cancer recurring in survivors of breast cancer [291]. Hence any action that lowers these risk factors may help reduce the risk of breast cancer. Physical activity is one such action. This is because physical activity makes the body more sensitive to insulin. When the body is more sensitive to insulin it does not need to produce so much insulin in order to

---

[165] ER is the abbreviation for estrogen receptor

[166] By contrast, there is not reliable evidence that obesity increases the risk of breast cancer in premenopausal women.

respond to it. Hence insulin levels fall. Physical activity also lowers inflammation in the body. These effects probably help explain why physical activity, especially when it is fairly vigorous, has been found to reduce breast cancer risk (in both premenopausal and postmenopausal women) [294]. Physical activity also reduces the likelihood of breast cancer recurring in women who have already had breast cancer [295]. One meta-analysis calculated a 38% decreased risk of women dying from a recurrence of breast cancer if they had high levels of physical activity [296]. There is also observational evidence that women being treated for diabetes with the insulin-lowering drug metformin, have a reduced risk of developing breast cancer. This further supports a central role for insulin as a driving force for breast cancer. A randomised control trial of metformin to prevent obesity-associated breast cancer is currently underway [297].

Diets that modulate inflammation may also be important in influencing breast cancer risk. A meta-analysis found that diets that increase inflammation in the body increases the risk of breast cancer risk by on average 14% [298]. And another review concluded that diet-induced chronic inflammation in breast adipose tissue "produces a local microenvironment that, regardless of ER status, is conducive to increased tumor cell proliferation and metastatic capacity" [291]. The Med diet is an excellent anti-inflammatory diet that also lowers the risk of insulin resistance and this diet has been found to reduce the risk of breast cancer. This is discussed more in the see next chapter. We now turn our attention to a second very serious cancer, oesophageal cancer.

## Oesophageal cancer

After swallowing food, the rippling oesophagus cajoles and massages the food downwards towards the stomach. Once in this acid bath, backflow back up the oesophagus is normally prevented by a sphincter muscle closing tight. But things don't always go to plan, and sometimes acid does flow back into the oesophagus. Most people experience this acid reflux occasionally, and a brief episode is not likely to do any harm. But acid continually refluxing from the stomach damages cells lining the lower part of the oesophagus. The cells respond to this damage by changing their morphology (shape) becoming more like cells that line the intestine rather than cells lining the oesophagus. This change in cell morphology is called Barrett's oesophagus. It affects about 1-2% of the adult population in western countries, and is more common in

174

men than in women (by about 2-4 times in the UK [(299)]).

Barrett's oesophagus will be diagnosed in about 8% of people who go for an endoscopy for acid reflux. It is estimated that in the UK between 400,000 and one million people have Barrett's oesophagus. Although not a danger in itself, Barrett's oesophagus can progress to a particularly aggressive cancer called adenocarcinoma of the oesophagus, also called oesophageal adenocarcinoma (OAC). [167] Around 3-13% of people with Barrett's oesophagus in the UK will develop OAC in their lifetime and the risk of OAC is more than 11 times higher in people with Barrett's oesophagus than in the general population. [168] Only about 50% of people diagnosed with OAC survive a year. Knowing if you have Barrett's oesophagus means that it can be checked at intervals to make sure it is not changing into OAC. Unfortunately, only about 10% of people with Barrett's oesophagus know it and for most it goes undiagnosed. [169]

In the western world, the prevalence of OAC has increased six fold in the last two decades, an increase that is more rapid than for any other cancer [(300)]. The UK has the highest incidence of OAC in the world [(301)]. This very worrying statistic receives very little publicity and rather than launching a campaign to highlight the dangers of acid reflux, it seems to have been quietly sidelined.

OAC is about four times more common in men than women. Both UK men and women top their league tables. Rates for men in the UK are five times higher than in France, twelve times higher than Italy and eighteen times higher than Greece [(301)]. This international variability strongly suggests that lifestyle factors play a key role in this cancer. But it is unclear what these are. The incidence of Barrett's oesophagus is not much higher in the UK than many other countries, and neither smoking nor obesity seem likely explanations [(302)]. Obesity is a factor, but it is unlikely to be the main one since obesity rates in different countries do not correlate with the different incidences of OAC. Also, whereas obesity rates have risen similarly in men

---

[167] There is also a second type of oesophageal cancer called squamous cell carcinoma, which is more strongly linked with smoking and is more common in South East Asia.
[168] https://www.cancerresearchuk.org/health-professional/cancer-statistics/statistics-by-cancer-type/oesophageal-cancer/risk-factors#heading-Five
[169] https://www.medtronic.com/uk-en/patients/conditions/reflux-disease/what-is-barretts.html

and women, the prevalence of OAC is far higher in men than women. There is, however, abundant evidence that inflammation is a key driver for OAC.

Inflammation

Refluxing acid is a toxic and deadly brew. It can damage DNA and so act as a carcinogen [303]. It also causes chronic inflammation in the oesophagus, a condition known as oesophagitis. A person with oesophagitis is four-times more likely to develop OAC. Having oesophagitis and Barrett's oesophagus increases the risk of OAC thirty fold [304]. It is clear that inflammation is a key driver in the development of OAC.

The most direct way of tackling this inflammation medically is by stopping acid reflux. This is routinely achieved with drugs called proton pump inhibitors such as omeprazole, and these are highly effective in lowering the risk of OAC. There is also evidence that aspirin - the most commonly used anti-inflammatory drug - is beneficial. A randomised controlled trial involving over 20,000 patients with Barrett's oesophagus evaluated a combination of aspirin and a proton pump inhibitor. The study found that this combination significantly reduced progression to OAC [305]. There is also some evidence that hyperinsulinaemia drives the development of OAC [306]. The importance of inflammation, and possibly hyperinsulinaemia too, suggests that diets that reduce these Core Risk States are interesting targets for preventing OAC. This is discussed in the next chapter.

# Cardiovascular disease

Until recently, there was little debate that a raised level of cholesterol in the blood - or more specifically of cholesterol-containing particles called LDL-cholesterol - increases the risks of a heart attack and stroke. LDL-cholesterol is raised by dietary saturated fat and this is why dietary guidelines recommend an upper limit of saturated fat consumption (11% of energy in the UK). But the idea that saturated fat is a risk factor for CVD is now being challenged. This has resulted in much media attention along the lines of "butter is back". So how can these two opposing views about whether or not saturated fat is a risk factor for CVD be reconciled? The role of oxidative stress and inflammation in CVD may provide an answer.

A heart attack or stroke is preceded by a disease process called atherosclerosis. Atherosclerosis starts with damage to the cells, called endothelial cells, which line the inside of arteries. For instance, chemicals in cigarette smoke can cause damage to endothelial cells. The damaged endothelial cells become "sticky" to white blood cells in the blood stream and these blood cells adhere to the damaged area of the artery wall. This area also becomes more permeable and particles of LDL-cholesterol can pass from the blood into the artery wall. Here the LDL-cholesterol particles are "eaten" by a type of white blood cell called macrophages ("macrophage" means "big eater"). These macrophages take on a whitish appearance (because of the cholesterol inside them) and they are now called foam cells. The foam cells, engorged with LDL-cholesterol, accumulate and form the "fatty streak" - an area of damage on the wall of a blood vessel. Other types of cells then become involved and the fatty streak enlarges and eventually, after many years, a "plaque", known as an atheroma, is formed. Inflammatory white blood cells are key players in this process and this is why atherosclerosis is now seen as an inflammatory reaction. Eventually a blood clot or thrombus may form on the atheroma and this can block the blood flow in the artery. Cutting off the blood supply to the heart can cause a heart attack, or to the brain, a stroke.

This sequence of events clearly implicates LDL-cholesterol early on in atherosclerosis, and suggests that the higher the concentration of cholesterol in the blood the greater will be the risk of atherosclerosis. But there is one crucial extra detail. Macrophages have a very limited appetite for normal LDL-cholesterol; they quickly become replete and stop engulfing it. By contrast, macrophages have an insatiable appetite for LDL-cholesterol that has been oxidised - it is the salt that makes their cholesterol meal so much more appetising. This is key. If the LDL-cholesterol does not become oxidised then very little is taken up and atherosclerosis is far less likely to develop. If the LDL-cholesterol becomes oxidised, the macrophages engulf it in an uncontrolled way greatly speeding up atherosclerosis and with it the risk of a heart attack. This sequence of events is summarised below:

LDL ➜ Oxidised LDL ➜ Fatty streak (inflammation) ➜ Atherosclerosis ➜ Heart attack/Stroke

It seems reasonable to assume that the more LDL-cholesterol there is in the blood then the more likely it is to be oxidised. So blood cholesterol levels are a risk factor for atherosclerosis. But more important during the early stages of atherosclerosis is the amount of LDL-cholesterol that becomes oxidised at the developing fatty streak in the artery wall. This implies that preventing LDL-cholesterol oxidation is key. Laboratory studies with cells and animal models clearly demonstrate the importance of oxidised-LDL in the formation of an atheroma (atherogenesis) [307]. Also, some clinical studies have found that people with higher levels of oxidised cholesterol are at increased risk of CVD [308].

However, the role of oxidised LDL-cholesterol in CVD is far from being universally accepted. One of the main thorns in the side of the oxidised-LDL hypothesis is that clinical trials with antioxidant vitamins, such as vitamins E and C, have not been found to reduce cardiovascular events. One possible explanation for this is that the antioxidants are given after the oxidised LDL has already initiated the disease process. Oxidised LDL cholesterol is involved in formation of the fatty streak, an event that occurs very early on in atherosclerosis, a process that itself develops over decades. Giving antioxidants to middle aged people may be too late. The antioxidants may close the door on oxidised LDL cholesterol but the horse of atheroma formation may already have bolted.

In sharp contrast to the disappointing results with antioxidants in preventing CVD, the Med diet is pre-eminent in reducing cardiovascular events such as a heart attack - even in middle aged people. The Med diet is rich in antioxidants and these may help with early stages of atherosclerosis. This diet also has many other arrows in its anti-atherosclerosis quiver, such as anti-inflammatory foods, that may also help tackle CVD. Anti-inflammatory substances may be more able to prevent the later stages of atherosclerosis and so be of more benefit to middle aged people who have already passed the early oxidative stage of atherosclerosis. This is discussed in the next chapter.

## Brain health, Alzheimer's disease and insulin resistance

Even though the link between a healthy diet and a healthy body is clear enough, our brain is seen as somehow different, obeying different and more obscure rules, and so the possibility that diet could play an important role in mental health receives little attention. But the link between mind and body has long been recognised. As the Buddha is reputed to have said: "To keep the body in good health is a duty... otherwise we shall not be able to keep our mind strong and clear". This link is illustrated by the increased risk of dementia in people with cardiovascular disease and diabetes. This also suggests that the three Core Risk States may play an important role in brain

178

health. And as we shall see, there is considerable evidence that this is the case.

The brain is particularly susceptible to oxidative stress. Although only 2% of the body's weight, the brain consumes about 20% of the oxygen needed by a person at rest. The brain has relatively low levels of antioxidant defences and so it is highly vulnerable to oxidative attack by reactive oxygen species (ROS), oxygen's hyperactive cousins. Less antioxidant defences are produced as we age and this increases the likelihood of oxidative stress. A major target for attack by ROS is the polyunsaturated fat DHA, which is found in high amounts in the brain and which is essential for neurones to function correctly. As well as damaging DHA and other important molecules in the brain, oxidative stress also triggers inflammation. This inflammation in the brain - neuroinflammation - is an important pathological change that drives many brain disorders.

It is not primarily the neurones that cause neuroinflammation in the brain but rather cells that form part of the immune and inflammatory systems called microglia and astrocytes [309]. These cells normally support and nourish neurones but during neuroinflammation they become over-activate and can turn on the neurones and kill them. Dying neurones increase the level of oxidative stress in the brain. This then sets up a vicious cycle whereby oxidative stress causes neuroinflammation, which then causes more oxidative stress. This creates a non-resolving - ie chronic - type of inflammation. Death of neurones resulting from neuroinflammation is linked to Alzheimer's disease and other brain disorders. In Alzheimer's disease - an incurable condition and the most common cause of dementia - a progressive increase in memory lapses affects the performance of everyday tasks. Progressive decline not only affects cognitive function: Alzheimer's disease and other dementias are now the leading cause of death in women in the UK and second for men.

Just as chronic low-grade inflammation causes insulin resistance in the body (see above), so neuroinflammation in the brain can lead to insulin resistance there too. Insulin resistance in the brain - and the resulting inability of cells to take up glucose - is key to understanding the pathology of Alzheimer's disease. Glucose is the preferred energy source for the brain. It was long thought that glucose uptake in the brain was insulin-independent (unlike skeletal muscle which needs insulin to take in glucose for fuel). But it is now known that, although not totally dependent on it, insulin influences glucose uptake by the brain, particularly during periods of high activity [310]. Hence insulin resistance in the brain means that the parts of the brain that need insulin in order to take up glucose can no longer do so.

Because of the parallels between chronic low-grade inflammation in the body causing insulin resistance that leads to type 2 diabetes, with neuroinflammation in the brain causing insulin resistance that leads to Alzheimer's disease, some researchers have dubbed Alzheimer's disease "type 3 diabetes"[311]. There are also more apparent links between the risks of these two diseases since people with type 2 diabetes have a two to three fold increased risk of Alzheimer's disease. One study that followed 824 elderly Catholic priests and nuns for nine years found that being diabetic greatly increased their likelihood of going on to develop Alzheimer's disease. In the study, two-thirds of those who went on to develop Alzheimer's disease were subsequently found to be diabetic even though only 15% of the priests and nuns were diagnosed with diabetes at the start of the study [312]. The underlying explanation is likely to be that the conditions that caused insulin resistance in the body leading to type 2 diabetes also caused insulin resistance in the brain leading to Alzheimer's disease.

Only certain regions of the brain need insulin in order to take in glucose. If these brain cells cannot respond to insulin because of insulin resistance, they will not be able to take in adequate amounts of glucose for fuel and so they will "starve" and die. The hippocampus is one such region. The hippocampus is involved in memory and this explains why memory loss is one of the main symptoms of Alzheimer's disease. Insulin and its cousin IGF1 are also needed for brain cells simply to survive. Brain cells are not strong swimmers and are unable to navigate the sea of life unsupported. Rather they need the buoyancy aids of insulin and IGF1 to stay afloat. Without these survival factors, brain cells will drown and die, laying to waste essential parts of the brain. [170]

Insulin resistance leaves glucose fuel in the brain unused. This spare glucose in the blood stream can attach to - glycate - various proteins. These glycated proteins are called advanced glycation endproducts (AGEs) and they accumulate in people with Alzheimer's disease. AGEs cause damage by

---

[170] This is not limited to brain cells. All cells need survival factors in order not to die. Cells that cannot respond to survival factors will die (by a process called apoptosis). Dying is the default position for cells and is thought to have evolved to prevent uncontrolled cell growth leading to cancer.

stimulating oxidative stress. And so the circle is complete, with AGEs - the endproducts of insulin resistance - initiating oxidative stress all over again.

The risk of insulin resistance increases with age. This is probably because of increased inflammaging, which can cause insulin resistance. This increase in insulin resistance with age, and consequent build-up in AGEs, helps explain why old age is the main risk factor for Alzheimer's disease. AGEs cause oxidative stress and brain damage after binding to receptors called RAGEs ("Receptors for AGEs") on the surface of cells. Dylan Thomas expressed rage in his poignant poem to his dying father: "Do not go gentle into that good night, Old age should burn and rave at close of day; *Rage, rage against the dying of the light.*" In the case of Alzheimer's diseases, it is the RAGEs that are the problem. We should indeed rage against Alzheimer's disease and not succumb to the consequences of RAGEs. The next chapter shows that a Mediterranean-style diet is highly effective at suppressing the three Core Risk States, and that this goes a long way to explaining why this diet is so effective at not only preventing Alzheimer's disease, but other chronic diseases.

# 11. Suppressing Core Risk States with a Med diet

## Overview

This chapter shows that by suppressing the Core Risk States of oxidative stress, chronic low-grade inflammation and insulin resistance, the Med diet can substantially reduce the risk of many different chronic diseases. Ultra-processed foods (UPFs) by contrast promote these risk states and so increase the risk of many chronic diseases. So UPFs can be seen as the complete antithesis of a Med diet. From the perspective of the three Core Risk States, eating fewer UPFs is just as important as eating a healthy Med diet.

## The inflammatory risk state and diet

### Pro- and anti-inflammatory foods and nutrients

The extent to which different foods and diets stimulate inflammation in the body can be assessed by measuring changes in the levels of "inflammatory biomarkers" in the blood. These biomarkers increase when inflammation increases. Hence, the higher the level of an inflammatory biomarker the greater the inflammatory effect of a food or diet. [171] By measuring inflammatory biomarkers it has been possible to show that many nutrients and foods in a typical western diet are pro-inflammatory whereas many of those in a healthy diet are anti-inflammatory (see Table).

Since inflammation is linked to chronic diseases, foods that alter inflammation can influence the risk of many seemingly unrelated chronic diseases. For instance, red and processed meats increase inflammation and this increase in

---

[171] Biomarkers for inflammation are measured in blood samples and include white blood cells and a protein called CRP. There are now companies that measure biomarkers of inflammation, mainly because they are used to monitor inflammatory conditions such as rheumatoid arthritis. 313. Liu CH, Abrams ND, Carrick DM *et al.* (2017) Biomarkers of chronic inflammation in disease development and prevention: challenges and opportunities. *Nat Immunol* 18, 1175-1180.

inflammation may help explain why these meats can increase the risk of colorectal cancer, CVD and type 2 diabetes [314]. It is possible that people already with increased inflammatory stress, due for example to a poor diet, diabetes or irritable bowel syndrome, may be particularly susceptible to meat's harmful effects by making their inflammation worse. The inflammation associated with having diabetes may contribute to why diabetic people are a third more likely to get colon cancer than the rest of the population [315].

**Foods and nutrients that are pro-inflammatory or anti-inflammatory**

| Pro-inflammatory | Anti-inflammatory |
|---|---|
| Excess calorie intake | Calorie restriction |
| Saturated fats | Monounsaturated fats |
| Trans fats, oxidised fats | Olive oil |
| High ratio of omega-6 to omega-3 fats | Fish oils |
| Low fibre intake | High fibre intake |
| High fructose, glucose, refined grains | Fruits, vegetables, whole grains, herbs, nuts |
| Domesticated meat | Wild meat, fish |
| Salt | Chocolate, tea |
| High alcohol consumption | Moderate alcohol |

On the other side of the coin are beneficial anti-inflammatory foods. In the case of type 2 diabetes, not only do pro-inflammatory foods increase the risk of type 2 diabetes, some anti-inflammatory foods decrease the risk. Whole grains help protect against type 2 diabetes. High blood glucose increases inflammation, which is a risk factor for diabetes. Whole grains are anti-inflammatory and so lowering the inflammatory effects of high blood glucose may be an important part of how whole grains protect against type 2 diabetes [316; 317]. It is usually considered that the whole grains reduce the risk of diabetes simply by helping control blood glucose levels but this may be only a partial explanation.

Forty-five foods and nutrients have been ranked in a league table according to how pro- or anti-inflammatory they are. This was achieved by measuring the extent to which the foods and nutrients changed inflammatory biomarkers in people. For example, saturated fat causes a big rise in inflammatory biomarkers and is ranked as highly inflammatory, whereas the spice turmeric does not cause a rise in inflammatory biomarkers and is ranked as highly anti-inflammatory. By measuring how much of these forty-five foods and nutrients a person eats, it is possible to determine how inflammatory their diet is. This is their Dietary Inflammatory Index (DII) [318]. Since most people consume more than just the forty-five foods and nutrients included in the DII, and some they may not eat at all, the DII is modified to suit the population being studied.

The DII is very useful to see if there is an association between a person's DII and disease risk, and then to see if reducing their DII can reduce their disease risk. Many studies have now shown that the DII of a person's diet does indeed influence their risk of disease and disability. In one study of elderly people, those with a lower DII reported being able to lead a more rewarding old age because of their improved mental and physical function and greater capacity to participate in various social activities [319; 320; 321]. In an analysis of forty-four studies involving over a million people, people with the highest DII score had a 58% increased cancer risk compared with those in the group with the lowest DII scores [322]. This is convincing evidence that an inflammatory diet increases cancer risk. Choosing a diet based on its anti-inflammatory ranking, rather than a diet simply based on its foods, could help prevent some of the most feared diseases. I will illustrate this by showing how important an anti-inflammatory diet is for preventing oesophageal adenocarcinoma.

## Inflammation and Oesophageal Adenocarcinoma

As I mentioned in the previous chapter, oesophageal adenocarcinoma (OAC) is the most rapidly increasing cancer in the western world. Cells lining the oesophagus are quite unusual because they are directly exposed to any carcinogens in the diet (a similar example is cells in the lungs that are directly exposed to carcinogens in cigarette smoke). Cells in most other organs in the body are only exposed to dietary carcinogens after they have been absorbed across the gut, metabolised by the liver and then released back into the blood stream. So, perhaps not surprisingly, the oesophagus is particularly sensitive to diet.

There is a particularly strong association between a pro-inflammatory diet and OAC and several studies suggest that a pro-inflammatory diet harms the oesophagus. In a Swedish study, patients were three and half times more likely to be diagnosed with OAC if they had eaten a diet high in inflammatory foods [323]. Because OAC, like most other cancers, develops over many years, people in this study were asked to recall their diet from twenty years previously since it was assumed that their diet at this time was likely to have influenced the early stages in the development of their cancer. Recalling a dietary habit from such a long time ago is clearly problematic and a limitation of this study. Requiring less of a memory feat, patients from Northern Ireland and the Republic of Ireland were asked to recall their diets from five years ago and their DII was calculated. Patients who had eaten a diet with the highest DII were about twice as likely to have developed the precancerous condition Barrett's oesophagus or full-blown OAC [324].

Inflammation is the most clearly established risk factor for driving the progression of precancerous oesophageal cells to cancer. A person with an inflamed oesophagus (oesophagitis) is four times more likely to develop cancer, and this rises to thirty times more likely if they already have Barrett's oesophagus [304]. So can reducing inflammation - by diet or any other means - reduce the likelihood of this progression? An important source of inflammation for many people is abdominal fat. Compared to other cancers, there is a particularly strong association between abdominal obesity and the risk of developing Barrett's oesophagus and OAC [325; 326]. Although many studies support the view that obesity-related chronic inflammation drives oesophageal adenocarcinoma, unfortunately there is no good evidence that losing weight will then reduce a person's risk of Barrett's oesophagus from progressing [327].

Although weight loss does not reduce the progression of Barrett's oesophagus, the anti-inflammatory drug aspirin does [305]. This suggests that inhibiting inflammation is beneficial. Even though it is not yet known if eating anti-inflammatory foods slows Barrett's oesophagus from progressing, there are some tentative indications that this may be the case. Turmeric is a well-known anti-inflammatory spice. Its presumed main active constituent is a substance called curcumin. Curcumin (rather than the spice itself) has been

186

shown in a small clinical study to reduce inflammation in the damaged area of the oesophagus in patients with Barrett's oesophagus [328; 329]. Curcumin has also been shown in lab studies to kill oesophageal cancer cells [330]. These studies were with purified curcumin rather than the spice turmeric and clinical trials are needed to see if curcumin or turmeric are of real benefit in preventing Barrett's oesophagus from progressing.

Curcumin is given as a tablet. However curcumin is not very well absorbed across the gut and it is also rapidly broken down in the body. So a better option may be to take the spice turmeric. Turmeric is cheap and easy to buy. It is not very soluble in water and so taking the powder dissolved in a teaspoon of olive oil may help the medicine go down. It is possible that turmeric dissolved in olive oil may be able to act directly on damaged cells in the upper gut - rather like cough medicine.

Other dietary anti-inflammatory substances may also help in the fight against OAC. The omega-3 fatty acids EPA and DHA are converted in the body into anti-inflammatory substances. A small-scale clinical study evaluated the effects of giving a daily dose of 3.6 grams of EPA and DHA (about the same as in 300 grams of oily fish) to obese people with Barrett's oesophagus. When measured six months later, the participants receiving the omega-3 fatty acids had significantly less inflamed oesophagi [331]. However, the study was not carried out for long enough to see if this translated into fewer cancers.

As always, an overall healthy lifestyle is the way to go, and a study that encouraged people to be physically active, eat a lot of fruit and avoid processed meat halved their risk of developing Barrett's oesophagus [84]. At present, dietary advice to avoid strongly pro-inflammatory foods is not part of the recommendations given to patients with Barrett's oesophagus in the UK. [172] I believe this is a serious missed opportunity for helping the up to a million in the UK with Barrett's oesophagus avoid getting a cancer with a particularly poor prognosis.

So what about the Med diet? Some Mediterranean countries have remarkably low rates of OAC compared to the UK. In Greek men, OAC is eighteen times lower than for UK men [301]. This variation cannot be explained by known risk factors for this cancer such as obesity or smoking. It is not known

---

[172] https://www.nice.org.uk/guidance/cg184/ifp/chapter/if-you-have-barretts-oesophagus

if it is eating a Med diet that reduces the risk of OAC in Mediterranean countries. Some studies of North Europeans found no evidence that when they ate a Med diet it reduced their risk of OAC [332; 333]. However, there is an important caveat here since most people from Northern Europe do not consume much EVOO and there is evidence that a Med diet that excludes EVOO has reduced anti-cancer benefits (see ch. 12). EVOO has very potent anti-inflammatory properties that could make it particularly useful against OAC [334]. Until a study is done with the traditional Med diet that includes EVOO it is not possible to establish if a Med diet reduces the risk of OAC.

## The anti-inflammatory Med diet

Eating a Med diet is perhaps the best of all diets for lowering chronic low-grade inflammation [335]. A Med diet also reduces inflammation brought on by aging - so-called inflammaging - and this could help explain how the Med diet extends life expectancy [336]. Since inflammation is a key stage in the development of CVD, inhibiting inflammation may explain how the many anti-inflammatory foods and nutrients in the Med diet work to reduce the risk of CVD [337; 338]. A study from Italy concluded that it was an anti-inflammatory effect, and not the lowering of cholesterol, that was responsible for the cardiovascular benefits seen in patients taking statins and eating a Med diet [339].

The Med diet is not only high in anti-inflammatory foods, it is also low in pro-inflammatory foods. Using the DII system for measuring inflammation, the Med diet achieved a score of +4 indicating a highly anti-inflammatory diet [340]. This was the precise converse for a fast food diet, which had a highly pro-inflammatory score of -4. So from an inflammation perspective, a fast food diet is the antithesis of the Med diet. From a practical perspective it suggests that a fast food diet can negate the anti-inflammatory benefits of a Med diet. If the western diet transforms the body into a parched landscape ready to ignite with the smallest inflammatory spark, then the Med diet is the welcome anti-inflammatory shower.

## Does evolution explain why some foods are more inflammatory than others?

It is probably more than just chance why natural foods are mostly anti-inflammatory whereas foods typical of the western diet are mostly pro-inflammatory. The way our immune system evolved may provide the explanation. The immune system is designed to recognise friend from foe. Most environmental viruses and bacteria, for instance, are recognised as foe. Our foods also come from the environment but clearly we must recognise them as friend and not as foe. So over thousands of years, our immune system has evolved to accept and benefit from the natural foods eaten by our ancestors.

This is not the case with UPFs in the western diet. Evolutionarily speaking our immune system has had very little time to evolve to accept the current western diet. The inflammatory response is one part of the immune system, and as mentioned earlier, most junk and industrially processed foods trigger a pro-inflammatory response. So the body, by mounting an inflammatory response to junk and industrially processed foods, is saying *this western diet is foreign and I am trying to reject it.* We did not evolve to eat these foods and so they cause an inflammatory immune response. Ill-adapted to these foods, we become ill. This argument leads to the provocative proposition that through evolution we have become inextricably bound to a diet of natural foods and that this is an inviolable reason why we should minimise consumption of UPFs.

We can support this proposition by considering dietary fats. During early human evolution, the relative amounts of the different types of fats in the diet were quite different to those in the modern western diet. Meat was an important source of fats for our ancestors, but compared to the meat from the domesticated animals we eat today, the wild meat in the diet of early humans was low in saturated fat and high in unsaturated fat. The problem now with some nutrients in the western diet such as saturated fat may simply be the relative amounts compared to the levels that humans were used to from the time when our immune system was evolving. So why are some saturated fats pro-inflammatory and so more of a disease risk than unsaturated fats?

To answer this question we need to consider the immune system in a little more detail. There are two parts: the innate immune system which mounts a general and rapid response to foes, and the adaptive immune system which produces more specifically targeted antibodies. The innate immune system evolved to recognise bacteria from the saturated fatty acids on their surfaces.

[173] When bacteria are detected, the innate immune system mounts an inflammatory response in order to remove them. Unfortunately one of the saturated fatty acids on the surface of bacteria, called palmitic acid, is present in high amounts in many junk foods and in the western diet. High levels of palmitic acid in the diet may be enough to confuse the innate immune system into thinking that the dietary palmitic acid is actually invading bacteria. And so it mounts an inflammatory response [341; 342]. In other words, junk foods are treated like an infection. And like an infection, junk foods trigger fever. This link between junk foods and a pro-inflammatory response has led one researcher to declare that fast foods trigger "fast food fever" [341].

Another group of ingredients of concern in UPFs are trans fats. Trans fats are strongly linked to an increased risk of CVD and although levels in foods in western countries have decreased recently through government initiatives, they still crop up in some foods that contain partially hydrogenated vegetable oils and in fast foods. [174] Levels in fast foods vary considerably, but in the UK some doner kebabs and fish and chips have been found with particularly high amounts [171]. [175] Trans fats are pro-inflammatory. Industrially produced trans fats cause vascular inflammation in blood vessels, which is a risk factor for CVD [343]. Industrial trans fats also raise LDL cholesterol. The raised levels of LDL cholesterol can trigger an inflammatory response in the body which adds further to the risk of cardiovascular disease and having a heart attack or stroke [344].

Industrial trans fats are completely foreign to the human body and this may be why we attempt to reject them by mounting an inflammatory response [345; 346]. But not all trans fats are the same. As well as industrial trans fats, trans fats are also produced naturally by bacteria in the stomach of ruminants (cattle and sheep). These trans fats end up in meat and dairy products. However, unlike industrially produced trans fats, similar levels of these naturally produced trans fats do not seem to increase the risk for CVD and they do not cause vascular inflammation [343; 347]. It is generally agreed that unlike industrial

---

[173] These saturated fatty acids are part of a cell surface molecule on bacteria called LPS (lipopolysaccharide).
[174] These foods include hard margarines, some fried products, and some manufactured bakery products (biscuits, pastries and cakes). https://inews.co.uk/news/health/trans-fats-ban-avoid/
[175] https://www.telegraph.co.uk/news/2018/05/14/countries-urged-wipe-killer-trans-fats-foods/

trans fats, normal dietary levels of trans fats from ruminants do not pose a health problem. Indeed, some trans fats found in dairy produce may even be beneficial [348]. So quality matters as well as quantity, and even closely related molecules - one from nature and one from industry - can have quite different effects on the immune system.

One surprisingly anti-inflammatory part of the Med diet is alcohol when it is consumed in moderate amount as red wine. Again, evolution may provide an explanation for why this is the case. The archaeological evidence for alcohol consumption (as wine) only dates back to about 7000 years ago in Iran. This is far too short a time period for our immune system to have evolved to benefit from it. So how did our immune system evolve to recognise alcohol as friend and not as foe? One suggestion is that exposure to dietary sources of ethanol increased in hominids 10 million years ago during early stages of hominid evolution when they were adapting to a terrestrial lifestyle from a previous life in trees [349]. Fruit falling to the forest floor would quickly start fermenting and hominids evolved to benefit from the resulting alcohol by learning to metabolise what is quite a calorific food source. Just as is recommended today, the alcohol would have been consumed with - or, rather, in - a solid food! Moderate alcohol consumption, particularly red wine, is linked to benefits against chronic diseases such as CVD and Alzheimer's disease and this has been linked to antioxidants in the wine with anti-inflammatory properties [350].

## Why natural foods contain antioxidants

Unprocessed natural foods are naturally rich in antioxidants. But why is this? Again, evolution provides an answer. It is easy to forget in this age of packaged foods that virtually all natural foods (fruits, vegetables, fish and so on) were once living organisms or at least a part of one (salt being a rare exception). All living organisms must confront the challenges of daily life. One of those challenges is oxygen because of its ability to change into dangerous free radicals called reactive oxygen species. As we saw in chapter 10, organisms have evolved to produce a range of antioxidants to protect themselves against these free radicals.

Unsaturated fats are particularly prone to oxidation and so food plants rich in unsaturated fats such as nuts and olives evolved to produce high levels of protective antioxidants. Antioxidants will reduce the oxidative stress in the body. Oxidative stress can trigger inflammation and this may explain why nuts and EVOO with their high levels of antioxidants are such important anti-inflammatory foods in the Med diet. Nuts wrap their lipids in a protective blanket of antioxidants - the brown skin around the nut. The main nuts in Mediterranean countries such as almonds, walnuts and hazelnuts are eaten with their skins on. Consuming a nut without its skin or consuming a nut oil puts more of a burden on our body to prevent the nut fats from being oxidised and this increases the risk of the nut fats triggering a dangerous chain reaction of lipid oxidation.

So by consuming a natural food - an ex-organism - we are consuming that organism's arsenal of defensive antioxidants. By eating minimally processed natural foods we are benefitting from the millions of years of evolutionary R&D that went into developing stable organisms-cum-foods where oxidation is kept in check. Processing foods often unbalances the nutrient mix by separating oxidation-prone fats from their antioxidants. Although manufacturers of processed foods are obliged to add back sufficient antioxidants to their products to prevent the foods going rancid, some synthetic antioxidants have come under scrutiny because of possible side effects [351].

When beneficial fats are removed from their antioxidant milieu they can be quickly converted into lipid peroxides by the process of lipid peroxidation. Lipid peroxides are harmful substances. The omega-3 fatty acids found in fish oils (EPA and DHA) are particularly prone to lipid peroxidation. We detect these oxidised lipids in rancid fish by their smell. However it is less likely that an oxidised omega-3 fat in a supplement will be noticed. This is not a minor issue since one review found that the majority of omega-3 supplements being sold are oxidised. The dangers of consuming oxidised omega-3 fats aren't fully resolved, but some studies have found that people taking oxidised omega-3 fats have increased inflammation and oxidative stress. This means that a supplement which is supposed to protect against CVD may actually be having the opposite effect [193]. When farm animals such as pigs are fed unsaturated fats to boost their growth they are often given a side order of antioxidants to prevent lipid oxidation [352]. If it's good enough for pigs, then it should be at least as important for people to know that when they are consuming omega-3 fats that these fats are not going to change into potentially dangerous lipid peroxides, which may be a particular danger for people who eat a diet low in antioxidants.

## After a meal

The risk of damage to the body from inflammation and oxidative stress is not uniform through the day. A particularly critical time is the few hours after a meal. During this so-called post-prandial period both oxidative and inflammatory stress rise dramatically, triggered by increased concentrations in the blood of newly acquired glucose and fats [353]. Uncontrolled, postprandial oxidative stress and inflammation increase the risk for many chronic diseases and so it is essential for the body to activate adequate antioxidant defences at this time [354]. Obese people and diabetics have a more pronounced postprandial inflammatory response, and so for them counteracting this response is particularly important [355].

A Med diet has been shown to significantly reduce postprandial oxidative stress in the elderly [356]. Antioxidants eaten as part of a Med diet will counter postprandial oxidative and inflammatory stress at the most important time of all: as it occurs. This is far better than taking an antioxidant supplement at a time divorced from when the damage is being done. EVOO appears to be particularly beneficial in reducing postprandial oxidative stress compared to other cooking oils. In one study, volunteers given mashed potatoes and EVOO were far less likely to develop postprandial oxidative and inflammatory stress than if they were given mashed potatoes with either refined olive oil or corn oil [357]. Eating more slowly is another strategy shown to prevent postprandial damage. In healthy people, postprandial vascular dysfunction was less when a meal was consumed in small portions over a longer period of time compared to when it was consumed more rapidly [358].

Another activity that increases antioxidants in the body and so helps counter postprandial oxidative stress is sleep. The sleep hormone melatonin has potent antioxidant and anti-inflammatory properties and an intriguing possibility is that triggering melatonin production with a postprandial siesta may be an effective way of reducing oxidative damage to the brain, and so of reducing the risk of dementia [359]. Melatonin is not restricted to the brain, and so other parts of the body also benefit from its anti-inflammatory and antioxidant actions. A siesta is associated with a lower risk of CVD and the rise of melatonin during the siesta could possibly have a role in this since it has been shown to protect against atherosclerosis [360].

# Insulin resistance

Insulin resistance is a state when the body becomes desensitised to insulin and is one of the three Core Risk States discussed in the previous chapter. Insulin resistance can arise from eating too many carbs. Excess carbs cause the body to produce too much insulin, and the body eventually responds to the excess insulin by becoming less sensitive to it - much as we become desensitised to background noise. Hence a low carb diet should reduce the risk of insulin resistance developing and so reduce the risk of the many diseases associated with insulin resistance. There is some evidence for this. For instance, a diet low in sugars is associated with a reduced risk of coronary heart disease (CHD) [89], and a large scale study that included people from 18 countries called the PURE study found that a low carb diet increased longevity [361].

But there is a problem with this simple correlation between a low carb diet and health benefits. The problem is that some very long-lived peoples have diets high in refined carbohydrates - such as the Okinawans who eat white rice as a staple. It is clear we must dig a bit deeper to find an explanation for this apparent paradox.

One possibility is that health benefits relate more to the quality of the carbohydrates. Refined cereals raise blood sugar levels far more than their whole grain equivalents. Instant porridge raises blood sugar half as much again as a more traditional version [362]. But again this cannot explain the long lives of the Okinawans since refined rice has amongst the highest capacity of any food to raise blood sugars, in other words it has a high glycaemic index [362].

Perhaps more important than the quality of the carbohydrates is how they are consumed in the context of the overall diet. One important influence on blood sugars is dietary fibre. A study conducted by highly respected researchers from the Harvard School of Public Health examined if a high-fibre cereal could influence the risk of type 2 diabetes in men and women who were eating a diet with a high glycaemic index. They found that the men and women had a 59% increased risk of type 2 diabetes if they ate a high glycaemic index (GI) diet (compared to a lower GI diet) but only a 19% higher risk if they consumed a lot of high-fibre cereals as well as the high GI diet [363]. High-fibre cereals have also been shown to mitigate the potentially harmful effects of a sugary diet for CHD [80]. It is thought that dietary fibre achieves this by slowing sugar absorption into the body. These studies show that it is important to consider the overall diet when evaluating the potential risks of sugary foods.

It is not only other foods in a diet that make a difference to the risks of a high sugar diet. The types of people who consume it matter too. Fit, active, lean people are highly responsive to insulin and can readily handle a rise in blood glucose. People who are insulin resistant, however, cannot take up the glucose from a sugary meal into their muscles. Instead the glucose languishes in the blood and is converted into fat. This leads to a rise in fats in the blood which increases the risk of CHD [92] and the risk of putting on weight [362].

Being overweight or obese doubles the risk of CHD from eating a high carbohydrate diet and this is probably because of insulin resistance and so not being able to adequately handle blood sugars [89]. Studies are finding that people with type 2 diabetes benefit far more from a low carbohydrate diet than fit and lean people [94]. So the important conclusion is that people respond differently to a carbohydrate-rich diet depending on whether or not they are insulin resistant: there is a far greater need for people who are insulin resistant such as diabetics and the overweight to reduce their carbohydrates.

There is far less sense in going on a low carb diet if you are lean and fit. This is because this diet can lead to other dietary problems. Low carb diets usually advise against eating grains. However, grains are the main source of fibre in the western diet, and so avoiding grains increases the risk of not getting enough fibre. To avoid going hungry, the lack of carbs will be compensated with eating something else, most likely fat. But eating more fatty foods will increase saturated fat consumption (since all dietary sources of fat are a mix of saturated and unsaturated fat). If the diet isn't carefully chosen, this may increase the risk of CHD and other diseases.

## Brain disorders and insulin resistance

There are many reasons why sitting down to a good meal can raise the spirits. One of the more surprising ones could be the mealtime surge in insulin. In 1924, Dr David Cowie and colleagues from the University of Michigan Hospital observed that their child patients with type 1 diabetes - a condition where no insulin is produced - had marked symptoms of depression and that "the most noticeable reaction from the use of insulin was the clearing of the depression" [364]. More recent studies have shown that intranasal insulin

195

treatment improves mood and lowers stress even in healthy people [365]. In fact, insulin was one of the first drugs used to treat severe psychiatric disorders [310].

Insulin may be enhancing mood by promoting glucose uptake in the hippocampus - one of the main areas of the brain involved in mood regulation. Glucose is the brain's preferred energy source. It was thought for a long time that uptake of glucose by the brain did not require insulin (unlike other organs in the body). [176] However, it is now known that a few regions in the brain including the hippocampus do need insulin for optimal glucose uptake.

Regions of the brain that require insulin for glucose uptake will suffer if they become insulin resistant and so are unable to take up glucose. This has a major impact on another of the hippocampus's actions, namely its role in learning and memory. The hippocampus is one of the brain regions that becomes insulin resistant in Alzheimer's disease. So the inability of the hippocampus to use glucose as an energy source helps explain why memory loss is one of the key features of this disease. An inability to use glucose is now seen by many researchers as the "defining metabolic signature of Alzheimer's disease" [366].

Insulin resistance in the hippocampus is receiving intense interest as a possible root cause of Alzheimer's disease. Deprived of their energy supply, hippocampal neurones "curl up" to try and defend themselves. They do this by retracting their dendrites and axons, the parts of their neurones that connect them with other neurones. The loss of these communicating connections (synapses) reduces cognitive function. Eventually the isolated and starving neurones in the hippocampus die, which leads to further mental deterioration.

Since insulin resistant hippocampal cells are unable to take up glucose from the blood, blood sugar levels around the cells will rise. This is also a problem. High blood sugar levels are toxic to neurones and cause increased atrophy in the hippocampus [367]. This is because the excess glucose binds to proteins forming toxic compounds called AGEs (advanced glycation endproducts) that

---

[176] The brain is only 2% of total body mass, but uses 50% of the glucose in the body. Gibas, K. J. Neurochemistry International 110 (2017) 57-68

kill hippocampal neurones. So hippocampal neurones die both from insufficient glucose inside the cells and excess glucose outside. Glucose starvation is an early event and has probably already occurred by the time patients have the pre-disease state for Alzheimer's disease called mild cognitive impairment.

One of the major defining pathological features seen in the brains of patients with more advanced Alzheimer's disease is the build up of insoluble plaques. These are made of a protein called amyloid beta. Amyloid beta builds up in the brains of Alzheimer's disease patients not because their brains are producing more of this protein but because less is broken down. Amyloid beta is normally broken down by the same enzyme that breaks down insulin. Patients with Alzheimer's disease frequently have hyperinsulinaemia and one idea is that the enzyme responsible for breaking down amyloid beta is so busy trying to break down the insulin that it has no time to break down the amyloid beta. Hence this may help explain why the beta amyloid accumulates [366]. As plaques build up, further changes in the brain occur and with it the development of full-blown Alzheimer's disease.

As mentioned earlier, continually high blood sugar results in continually high amounts of insulin being produced. Cells desensitise to insulin and this can lead to the cells no longer being able to respond to the insulin despite the high levels. High insulin levels are now recognised as a major risk factor for Alzheimer's disease [366]. But excess sugar in the diet isn't the only cause of insulin resistance in the brain. As we have seen in the previous chapter, inflammatory signals produced because of low-grade chronic inflammation in the body can also cause insulin resistance.

**Brain disorders and inflammation**

Inflammation in the brain can increase for various reasons such as aging (inflammaging) or because of a build up in the brain of AGEs, which causes inflammation of neurones - neuroinflammation. Because inflammaging and neuroinflammation increase with age, this explains why age is the single most important risk factor for Alzheimer's disease. Aging is in effect *AGEing*. Obesity also increases inflammation. However, currently there is no clear evidence for a link between obesity and Alzheimer's disease. An important study of over one million women (the so-called Million Women study) found that although obesity during midlife was associated with dementia over the long term, this was dementia caused by *vascular disease* and not dementia caused by Alzheimer's disease [368].

There is some evidence that a pro-inflammatory diet can adversely affect cognitive function. This was shown in a long running study set up in 1985 that has been examining factors that influence the health of British civil servants. This so-called Whitehall II study identified a pattern of eating in some of the civil servants that included meat, processed meat, an "English breakfast", and low intake of whole grains. This dietary pattern increased inflammatory markers and the civil servants who ate this inflammatory diet had a far greater cognitive decline over a ten-year period [369]. (This study did not look specifically at Alzheimer's disease.)

Studies that look at the role of diet in brain health often consider overall diets rather than individual nutrients. This seems reasonable since the brain needs many different nutrients to function properly. For instance, deficiencies in B vitamins and omega-3 fats are linked to cognitive problems and dementia. The hippocampus is particularly sensitive to diets that increase inflammation and oxidative stress. In one study, 60 to 64 year-old healthy Australians eating a western diet high in sugar and fat were found to have smaller hippocampi [370]. One reason why their hippocampi may have shrunk is because the hippocampus is one of the few areas in the brain where new neurones continue to be produced during adulthood in order to sustain the hippocampus. For new neurones to grow (by a process called neurogenesis) a nerve growth factor called BDNF (brain-derived neurotrophic factor) is needed. Unhealthy foods in the western diet reduce the production of BDNF and so the hippocampus is not able to grow properly.

Although a healthy brain has complex nutritional requirements, diet isn't everything. The complex pathological changes that occur even in early stages of cognitive decline suggest that approaches that encompass more than just diet are needed to maintain good cognitive health. A Californian study used a multi-pronged approach with impressive results. Patients, most of whom had mild cognitive impairment, were put on a low glycaemic diet, rich in micronutrients and omega-3 fats. They also received relaxation therapy and were asked to increase their sleep and physical activity [371]. At the start of the study, six of the ten participants were no longer able to work because of their mental impairment. After the intervention there were major improvements. All six participants who had stopped working were well enough to return to work. Of the other participants, only one experienced no improvement in cognitive function, probably because this person already had advanced Alzheimer's disease at the start of the study. Importantly, the participants maintained or even improved their cognitive function for at least the next two and a half years.

This study, impressive though it was, was not a properly controlled study since it lacked a control group and was not conducted under controlled conditions. Fortunately, a multipronged approach has now been evaluated in several randomised control trials (RCT). In one RCT from Finland, cognitive decline in elderly people at risk of poor mental health because of their lifestyle and general health was reduced when they were given a healthy diet that followed national dietary recommendations, they exercised regularly, received cognitive training, and were monitored for their vascular health [372; 373].

It is now clear from the Finnish and similar studies that a healthy lifestyle is good for cognitive health. It is not possible to know precisely which are the most beneficial changes. But based on the huge body of research around this area, it is likely that reversing or bypassing insulin resistance is important. (A second important factor is improved blood supply to the brain.)

As mentioned earlier, low levels of dietary antioxidants increase oxidative stress in the brain. Oxidative stress increases the risk of neuroinflammation, which in turn can cause insulin resistance, starving the brain of glucose. As might be predicted from this sequence of events, anti-inflammatory diets are associated with improved memory [374; 375; 376]. So dietary factors that suppress the Core Risk States are beneficial for the brain and dietary factors that promote the Core Risk States are harmful for the brain, just as they are in other parts of the body.

Beneficial and harmful nutrients are usually considered separately, but one study looked at how these opposing forces might interact within a single diet. In a group of elderly Swedes it was shown that a high level of compliance with foods typical of a healthy diet - vegetables, fruit, cereals and legumes, whole grains, rice/pasta, fish, low fat dairy, poultry, and water - counteracted the adverse effects on cognitive decline of eating foods associated with a less healthy western diet - more frequent consumption of red/processed meat, saturated/trans-fat, refined grains, sugar, beer, and spirits [377]. The more healthy diet is sometimes referred to as a "prudent diet" and eating this diet is indeed a wise decision.

It is not known how a healthy diet can oppose the adverse effects on cognitive decline of a western diet. However it is tempting to speculate that this could relate to differences between the inflammatory natures of these two diets. A healthy Med diet has an anti-inflammatory score of +4 and this just happens to be the opposite of the pro-inflammatory score of -4 that has been calculated for a western diet. So a tempting explanation for the opposing effect of a prudent diet on a western diet in the Swedish study is that anti-inflammatory foods in the prudent diet counter pro-inflammatory foods in the western diet.

## The Med diet and dementia

The Med diet has received a huge amount of attention as a way of delaying cognitive decline [378]. Its impressive benefits were summed up in a recent review: "there is general consensus that greater adherence to a Med diet is associated with better cognitive performance, slower rates of cognitive decline, a reduced risk of developing mild cognitive impairment and Alzheimer's disease and a reduced risk of progressing from mild cognitive impairment to Alzheimer's disease" [379]. The evidence that a Med diet can slow down or even reverse mild cognitive impairment is hugely important since there are no medications currently recommended for mild cognitive impairment. It is important to emphasise though that there is little evidence that later stages of Alzheimer's disease are reversible by a Med diet.

As for other diseases, it is likely that many nutrients in the Med diet work together synergistically to counteract risk factors for Alzheimer's disease. The Med diet is particularly nutrient-rich and its favourable composition sets it apart even from other healthy diets. A Med diet provides high levels of many vitamins and minerals, it has a low glycaemic index, and it provides especially high levels of many different anti-inflammatory and antioxidant nutrients. These include carotenoids and phenolics found in many plant foods such as fruits, vegetables and nuts, omega-3 fatty acids found at especially high levels in oily fish, moderate alcohol, dairy produce from goats and sheep milk and EVOO. Many of these foods are discussed more in ch. 12 but a couple warrant further mention here since they may be particularly important for preventing cognitive decline. These are dairy products from goat and sheep milk, and EVOO.

## Can eating goat's cheese reduce your risk of Alzheimer's disease?

A rise in insulin resistance is common as we age. This can result in a decline in the ability of the brain to use glucose and a gradual decline in cognitive function. Without any glucose, neurones in the brain will die, leading to cognitive decline and an increased risk of Alzheimer's disease. This process can start many years before there are any clinically detectable changes in cognitive function. Being able to continually monitor and correct this silent deterioration would be a major advance towards delaying the onset of Alzheimer's disease [380].

One way to compensate for a loss in the ability of the brain to use glucose is to provide the brain with an alternative energy supply, especially for those regions in the brain such as the hippocampus that develop insulin resistance. Most tissues in the body use fatty acids when glucose is in short supply, but the brain cannot use these. There is only one significant alternative energy source to glucose for the brain and that is a group of substances called ketones. Ketones are the main energy source used by the brain during fasting and can provide about 60-80% of the brain's energy needs when glucose is not available [381]. There is increasing evidence that strategies that increase ketones in the blood benefit cognitive performance.

We do not consume ketones directly from the diet. Rather they are produced in the body from fats. A group of fats called medium chain fatty acids (MCFAs) are readily converted by the body into ketones. The word "chain" refers to the number of carbon atoms linked together in a linear fashion in a fatty acid. MCFAs have an even number of between six and twelve carbons linked together in a chain.[177]

MCFAs made up in formulations have been found to benefit cognitive function in people with mild cognitive impairment. In one study, a group of elderly patients with mild cognitive impairment were given a drink containing MCFAs for six months. Scans showed that there was increased use of ketones in the patients' brains, and cognitive function such as memory and language use improved significantly [381]. These ketogenic drinks offer great hope for people with mild cognitive impairment and even possibly with early Alzheimer's disease. However, these are people who have already developed

---

[177] There are three categories of fatty acids: short chain, medium and long.

brain damage due to glucose deprivation. A more desirable strategy is to prevent the brain damage in the first place. Another limitation of MCFA drinks is that they are not suitable for the general population since they can cause gastrointestinal side effects. Diet, on the other hand, is a more acceptable way to consume high levels of MCFAs.

Diets designed to increase ketones in the blood - so-called ketogenic diets - often improve cognitive performance [380]. Since ketones are derived from fats, one way to increase ketones in the body is with a high fat diet. In these high fat diets, about 70% of the total energy comes from fats. However, these diets are nutritionally unbalanced, not least because of the high levels of saturated fat, and so again are not recommended for everyday use. Another way to increase ketones is by prolonged fasting since carbohydrate stores (glycogen) are used up first during fasting and the body then switches to burning fat, which generates ketones. But fasting is not a very welcome option for most people either. A third approach is to use a regular diet and supplement it with MCFAs. This was done in the multipronged Californian study mentioned earlier by including MCFAs in the patients' diets.

A Med diet is another way to consume above average amounts of ketones. This is because a *traditional* Med diet includes dairy produce from the milk of sheep and goats rather than from cows. [178] As a proportion of all types of fatty acids, the amount of MCFA in sheep and goat milk is about twice that in cow's milk. This special feature of goat and sheep milk was acknowledged by naming some MCFAs after the scientific name for the goat, *Capra*. In increasing chain length of carbon atoms, these MCFAs are called caproic acid (six carbons in the chain), caprylic acid (eight) and capric acid (ten). Although there are no scientific studies that show whether MCFAs in a traditional Med diet that uses dairy from goat and sheep milk is a superior way of tackling cognitive function, it is worth looking at some of the circumstantial evidence that suggests this is a possibility.

The first line of evidence is to consider the type of MCFA. There are four MCFAs, the three with goaty names (caproic acid, caprylic acid and capric acid) and a fourth called lauric acid. Lauric acid is the largest MCFA with 12 carbons. Studies have found that caprylic acid (eight carbons) is far better at

---

[178] Traditionally these would have been mostly fermented dairy products, namely yogurt and cheese.

being converted in the body into ketones than the larger MCFAs capric and lauric acids [382]. The smallest MCFA, caproic acid (only six carbons) is probably better still but there are fewer studies with this. [179] These details matter because about 4 - 9% of the fats in goat's milk are the high ketone-generating MCFAs (six and eight carbons) [383]. By comparison coconut oil - which has received a lot of interest as a source of ketones for preventing Alzheimer's disease - consists of only about 1.5% of these fats [384].

The amount of sugary foods in the diet also influences ketones. This is because a sugary diet raises blood insulin, and insulin suppresses ketone production. A Med diet is low in sugars and relatively high in fat. These two factors together make it likely that a person eating a Med diet will efficiently convert MCFAs to ketones.

As well as acting as an alternative energy source to glucose, ketones have another trick up their sleeve: they are anti-inflammatory and reduce neuro-inflammation in neuronal cells [385]. These dual functions of ketones - as alternative energy sources for the brain and as anti-inflammatory substances - offer considerable promise in helping to protect the brain to delay dementia.

Although the overall level of MCFAs even in a traditional Med diet is not high compared to giving MCFA supplements, the dietary approach does provide a way of supplying ketones on a constant basis that may help out the brain before any damage due to glucose deprivation or neuroinflammation is done. At the moment, including sheep and goat milk dairy products is rarely if ever mentioned when recommending the Med diet. This may be squandering a potentially important health benefit of the more traditional Med diet.

**Extra Virgin Olive Oil and dementia**

Some clinical studies with the Med diet have found it does not reduce cognitive decline or the onset of Alzheimer's disease. This would seem to rather undermine confidence in recommending this diet for preventing Alzheimer's disease. But rather than dismissing the Med diet, there are other possible explanations. One is how the Med diet is defined in the study. A person can still be classed as adhering to a Med diet even when they are not consuming olive oil. (This is permitted so as to enable studies on a "Med diet"

---

[179] https://ketosource.co/caprylic-acid-c8/

in countries where olive oil is not routinely consumed.) This olive oil-less Med diet frequently shows less benefit against cognitive decline, and so this suggests that olive oil is a very important part of a brain-protecting Med diet [386]. Experimental studies with neuronal cell cultures and animals show that EVOO contains potent phytochemicals that protect against neuro-inflammation and the toxic effects of amyloid-beta [387; 388]. Two of the most important of these phytochemicals, hydroxytyrosol and oleuropein, are almost completely absent from any other food. [180] Although no clinical trials have yet evaluated these phytochemicals from EVOO on cognitive function, the experimental studies suggest that if EVOO is absent from a Med diet, then its cognitive benefits may be compromised.

Despite the considerable evidence for a protective effect of a Med diet against Alzheimer's disease, there are currently only modest recommendations to eat a Med diet from organisations such as the Alzheimer's Society [181], and the world isn't exactly scrambling to recommend the Med diet for brain health. There is no indication, for example, of dementia care homes prioritising a Med diet for their clients. GP's prefer to prescribe drugs to their patients and many have reservations about diet. However, this perspective is worth challenging since confidence in the therapeutic benefit of currently available drugs for treating Alzheimer's disease is showing signs of waning. In 2018, France removed drugs for treating Alzheimer's disease from its list of recommended ways to manage Alzheimer's disease patients [389]. In a way, it's a shame that the Med diet wasn't "invented" by a drug company as a means to help prevent or delay Alzheimer's. If it were, it would in my opinion probably be one of the most widely marketed and prescribed drugs in the world.

## The Med diet and mood

The idea of mood foods has been around a long time without ever conclusively proving that diet has a significant effect on mood. One of the main problems is that being depressed can influence a person's food choices, since when they are depressed they may change their diet and eat more "comfort foods". This means that it is the mood influencing the food whereas nutritionists want to establish if food is influencing a person's mood.

---

[180] Small amounts of hydroxytyrosol are found in wine
[181] https://www.alzheimers.org.uk/about-dementia/risk-factors-and-prevention/mediterranean-diet-and-dementia

Observational studies which simply compare a person's existing diet with their mood have very limited ability to distinguish between these two possibilities and interpreting these studies can lead to the possibility of "reverse causality" (see ch. 5) and mistakenly concluding that the food is influencing the mood whereas in fact the mood is influencing the food.

The way round this problem is with an RCT. These studies assign one group to a test diet (the Med diet) and the second group to a "control" diet and then see how their moods change over the following few months. Several recent RCTs have shown promising results with participants assigned to the Med diet arm of the study showing less depression than the participants eating the control diet [390; 391]. It is worth mentioning that studies with supplements such as vitamins are mostly ineffective in reducing depression [392]

So how is a Med diet reducing depression? One idea relates to glucose regulation. A diet high in refined sugars can lead to poor glucose regulation, which periodically deprives the brain of glucose. This in turn triggers hormonal changes leading to adverse effects on mood [393]. Because a Med diet has an overall low glycaemic index it helps prevent these fluctuations in blood glucose and their adverse effect on mood. A second idea is that inflammation is important. [182] Increased inflammation is linked to mood disorders in some people and so the powerful anti-inflammatory Med diet could also benefit mood by damping down inflammation in the brain. By contrast, a western diet is pro-inflammatory because of its high calories and high levels of saturated fat and, it has been suggested, this could be linked to adverse effects on mood [393].

## Insulin, diet and cancer

We saw in the last chapter how elevated insulin - hyperinsulinaemia - increases the risk for some cancers. The reason is not because of insulin's role in regulating blood sugar levels, but rather because of its role as a growth factor. Since a sugary diet is the main cause of hyperinsulinaemia, this raises the possibility that people who eat a sugary diet have an increased risk of some cancers. A meta-analysis that looked into this found that postmenopausal women eating a diet high in sugary carbohydrates had a 28% increased risk of

---

[182] https://www.theguardian.com/commentisfree/2020/jan/19/inflammation-depression-mind-body

breast cancer (hormone receptor–negative tumours) [394]. Although hyperinsulinaemia is a likely explanation for this association between a sugary diet and breast cancer risk, this study did not specifically measure insulin. Another possible contributory factor could be that a sugary diet is raising chronic inflammation.

It is not only insulin itself that increases cancer risk. Insulin also increases levels of the related growth factor IGF-1. Both insulin and IGF1 stimulate the division of many types of cells in the body, and in addition to breast cancer, the risks of several other types of cancer, including colorectal, endometrial and prostate, are also slightly increased when people eat a sugary diet [395]. However, the risks of a sugary diet and of insulin resistance on cancer are generally small, and disentangling their importance from many other aspects of diet and lifestyle is complicated. This has led to many conflicting conclusions about just how important elevated levels of insulin are as a risk factor for cancer. Hence this area of cancer risk has been mostly ignored by organisations that give advice on cancer prevention.

However, epidemiological studies should be seen as only one part of the overall picture, especially when the epidemiological studies are difficult to interpret. Studies on cancer cells grown in culture and studies in animal models strengthen the argument that elevated levels of insulin/IGF1 are likely to increase breast cancer risk, and other cancers. I believe it is likely that the rise in sugar consumption that has occurred over the last decades and the resulting disruption of insulin regulation could be making a far greater contribution to the rising incidence in breast cancer than is currently appreciated.

## Diabetes and the Med diet

Many healthy diets reduce the risk of type 2 diabetes [396]. The Med diet is amongst the most effective of these, not only for preventing it but also for managing people already with this condition. A recent meta-analysis of meta-analyses concluded that "Current evidence indicates that the Mediterranean diet is effective in improving both glycaemic control and cardiovascular risk factors in people with type 2 diabetes, and should therefore be considered in the overall strategy for management of people with diabetes" [397]. The Med diet also reduces the risk of healthy people developing type 2 diabetes. In one meta-analysis, higher adherence to the Med diet was associated with a 23%

reduced risk of developing type 2 diabetes [215].

It is unlikely that there is just one mechanism to explain this. The Med diet is not particularly low in carbohydrates, but it is low in foods that cause a rapid rise in blood glucose (ie foods with a high glycaemic index). Equally importantly, the Med diet contains high levels of nutrients and foods that prevent or control hyperglycaemia. Dietary fibre delays gastric emptying rate, which slows down digestion and glucose absorption and reduces plasma insulin levels. Dietary fibre (mainly bran) also contains a lot of magnesium and magnesium is known to help maintain insulin sensitivity [215]. Other foods present in the Med diet such as vegetables, nuts and legumes are also rich in magnesium. Moderate alcohol consumption has been associated with enhanced insulin sensitivity and preventing type 2 diabetes [398]. The Med diet is also associated with weight control, which is another important aspect in preventing type 2 diabetes. A person with diabetes will typically have experienced a period, often many years, of hyperinsulinaemia before they are diagnosed. This may explain why having type 2 diabetes increases the risk of some cancers (colorectal, breast, endometrium, liver, pancreas, and bladder) [399].

## Beyond the three Core Risk States

The Core Risk States - oxidative stress, chronic inflammation and insulin resistance - are only early steps towards disease and many other changes occur before a cancer is diagnosed or a heart attack strikes. Some of these changes are caused by so-called "risk genes" where a person inherits a predisposition to a particular disease. This helps explain why one person with chronic inflammation will go on to develop cancer whereas another may get heart disease.

The pathological changes that need to accumulate before a disease is clinically diagnosed are sometimes referred to as liabilities. A disease becomes clinically diagnosable after a certain number of liabilities have accumulated and a threshold passed - rather like being banned from driving after accumulating a certain number of points on a driving licence. For example, a genetic predisposition, together with exposure to a carcinogen and chronic inflammation, may be sufficient liabilities for cancer to develop.

This idea of liabilities implies that the trick to not getting cancer is to tackle the liabilities as they arise and to avoid passing beyond the threshold number needed for full-blown cancer to develop. One way to achieve this is to increase your capacity to reverse liabilities - like going on a driving safety course to avoid points being added to your licence after a speeding offence. Consider cancer. A carcinogen causes a genetic change in a cell that "initiates" the cancer process. This is a first liability. We are continually exposed to carcinogens - such as from cooked meat and other foods and environmental pollutants - but fortunately this rarely leads to cancer. This is because the body can detoxify carcinogens and also even repair small amounts of damage to DNA caused by carcinogens. As long as these defensive abilities of the body to neutralise the carcinogen are not overwhelmed, cancer will not develop. This may be why small amounts of meat are safer even though only one genetic change from a single carcinogen molecule is required to initiate cancer. It is worth noting that this capacity to reverse carcinogens is only possible below a certain threshold dose of the carcinogen since excess exposure can overwhelm the defence mechanisms [400]. (In virally transmitted diseases there is the similar concept of "viral load" - beyond a certain amount of virus the immune system is overwhelmed and this leads to the viral disease.)

Building up defence mechanisms to reverse liabilities is building up resilience in the body. Resilience can be considered as a way of building up an arsenal of defence mechanisms that tackle liabilities so that the threshold to disease is not breached. Resilience raises the bar so that more liabilities are needed to reach the threshold. Many phytochemicals build up resilience in the body to cancer by increasing the capacity of the body to neutralise carcinogens. One of the best-known examples is a phytochemical called sulphoraphane found in broccoli. Sulphoraphane induces various enzymes in the body including antioxidant enzymes that can detoxify carcinogens.

Increasing resilience is a fundamental goal for maintaining good health. Human biology is full of examples of homeostatic mechanisms that explain the self-regulation of the body. The extent to which these processes operate successfully can vary widely between people depending on their level of fitness, diet and genes. Fit, active, lean people have high resilience and so can handle liabilities that pose a risk for unfit, inactive, overweight people. For instance, a sugary diet is better tolerated in fit healthy people because of their greater capacity than less fit people to process glucose.

We are now entering the era of "personalised nutrition" which will take these differences between individuals into account when making dietary recommendations. However current epidemiological research is only just starting to discriminate between different people when interpreting nutritional epidemiological studies and making recommendations. Most current nutrition advice is still based on population-wide recommendations. But what is good for the goose may not always be good for the gander.

## Reducing disease liabilities with physical activity

Being fit, active and lean is one of the most effective ways to keep liabilities in check. Physical activity and diet are usually considered as separate parts of a healthy lifestyle. But in fact they both influence many of the same processes in the body. So in order to fully understand a person's disease risk, it is necessary to consider their level of physical activity.

The time and effort needed to burn calories makes exercise a pretty challenging way to lose weight. It takes only a few minutes to eat a slice of pepperoni pizza. But to burn off these 198 calories would take 45 minutes swimming, for example. [183] Burning off calories with exercise is even more challenging for many overweight and obese people. It would of course be more effective to not eat the pizza in the first place, but the promise from junk food manufacturers that a bit of exercise will cancel out the calories can be hard to resist.

And yet there are very important reasons why exercise or another form of physical activity is good for health. Not so much to burn calories, but rather to help prevent chronic low-grade inflammation and insulin resistance [401]. Physical activity helps keep inflammation and insulin levels under control and the result is that the risk of many chronic diseases tumbles. This is a big part of why physical activity reduces the risk of many chronic diseases such as breast cancer, colon cancer, diabetes, ischemic heart disease and stroke, as well as the recurrence of breast and other cancers in cancer survivors [401; 402; 403; 404; 405].

You probably noticed that the diseases that physical activity protects against are essentially the same as the diseases a healthy diet protects against. This hints at the intriguing possibility that at a fundamental level both a healthy

---

[183] https://www.theguardian.com/lifeandstyle/2010/sep/19/exercise-dieting-public-health
https://www.vox.com/2018/1/3/16845438/exercise-weight-loss-myth-burn-calories

diet and physical activity are working in very similar ways. This is of huge importance for how we view a healthy diet.

## Identifying the master switches for the three Core Risk States and for health

Unearthing the links between physical activity, diet and risk states begins to expose the true master switches for health. One of these master switches is an enzyme called AMPK [406]. As we shall see, AMPK is central to both why physical activity is beneficial, and how many phytochemicals work to promote health.

AMPK's main role in a cell is to ensure that the cell maintains adequate energy reserves. Glucose is the main source of these energy reserves and so after exercise, when energy supplies in muscle cells have been depleted, more glucose needs to be taken in. This is achieved by making the muscle cells more responsive to insulin. It is AMPK that is switched on by exercise and that is able to make cells more insulin responsive. In other words AMPK improves insulin sensitivity, which is the same as saying it reduces insulin resistance. AMPK also reduces inflammation. The ability of physical activity to switch on AMPK which in turn reduces insulin resistance and inflammation is far more influential on health than burning a few calories [134].

So how does exercise switch on AMPK? AMPK monitors the main energy currency in cells, a molecule called ATP. It does this indirectly by monitoring the molecule that ATP is changed into when ATP is used for energy. This is a molecule called AMP.[184] AMPK is switched on when it detects an increase in levels of AMP since this is a sign that ATP is being used up. [185] AMPK then switches on processes in cells to restore adequate levels of ATP. This it does by increasing insulin sensitivity (which then facilitates more glucose uptake). This sequence of events is depicted below:

---

[184] ATP and AMP are abbreviations for adenosine triphosphate and adenosine monophosphate respectively
[185] AMPK is short for AMP-dependent kinase.

Glucose is taken up by cells and used to produce ATP

 *physical activity*

ATP is converted into AMP, and the rise in AMP activates AMPK

AMPK increases insulin sensitivity

## Coming full circle with the Med diet

It is not only physical activity that activates AMPK. Some pharmaceutical agents also do so. One of the most interesting of these is metformin. Metformin is best known as a widely prescribed drug for treating type 2 diabetes, and this drug is also now being used to enhance cancer treatment. Clues that metformin might be having fundamental effects in the body came from a study conducted on obese diabetics in the UK in the late 1990's. This study found that metformin reduced all-cause mortality [407], a finding that has subsequently been confirmed in other studies. Hence, even though it is probably going too far to call metformin and its mediator AMPK panaceas, they do nonetheless provide important clues on how to manage the risk states for many chronic diseases.

Because of side-effects, metformin is only available as a prescription drug. But if you are eating a Med diet then it is likely you are also eating phytochemicals that activate AMPK. Amongst a wide range of phytochemicals in the Med diet that activate AMPK are resveratrol in red wine, quercetin found in onions and other vegetables, and a chemical found in green tea called EGCG. Structurally these phytochemicals are all quite different and so it is not immediately obvious what they have in common that enables them to all switch on AMPK. The answer is probably that they can all poison a cell's ability to manufacture ATP in its mitochondria. [186] By depleting a cell of its ATP, these phytochemicals then trigger the cell to switch on AMPK in order to produce more ATP [134]. And at the same time the body profits from all the other benefits that AMPK confers such as increased insulin sensitivity.

There is more. In chapter 6 we saw that plants produce more phytochemicals under conditions of environmental stress and it has been hypothesised that

---

[186] They are toxins of mitochondria - the organelles in cells where ATP is made.

these stress-induced phytochemicals trigger resilience in humans. This cross-talk between plants and humans is dubbed "xenohormesis". Xenohormesis is considered to increase our resilience to disease at times of environmental stress. Maybe a milder version of xenohormesis occurs all the time in people eating a diet rich in phytochemicals and who take regular exercise. Activating AMPK may be one of the underlying mechanisms to explain the increased resilience that comes from exercise and eating a Med diet. A common criticism of phytochemicals is that their concentrations in the body are too low for them to have any physiological effect. But if each phytochemical is simply acting as a mitochondrial poison then added together they may have a cumulative effect due to their gradual build up in mitochondria which eventually triggers AMPK.

As well as activating AMPK, many phytochemicals found in the Med diet activate other "master switches" that switch on anti-oxidant and anti-inflammatory responses [408]. [187] These effects can also occur at low concentrations of phytochemicals whereas at higher concentrations the phytochemicals can be toxic. This is being true to the underlying principle of hormesis, namely that there are benefits at low doses but adverse effects at higher doses - "that which does not kill us makes us stronger". This shows that more is not always better and suggests that supplements providing very high amounts of phytochemicals are not necessarily a good thing.

The ability of AMPK to respond to signals declines with aging and this is probably an important reason why age is the main risk factor for many chronic diseases [409]. Hence there is now much interest in phytochemicals that activate AMPK as lifespan and healthspan extenders - or "gerosuppressants" as they have been branded [410]. However there is no need to take these phytochemicals as supplements. The evidence suggests that moderate physical activity and a diet high in phytochemicals are good ways to ensure that AMPK remains active during aging and to ensure that you achieve your maximum healthspan [406; 411]. AMPK is the quintessential healthspan extender [407].

If these discussions all sound rather theoretical, let's consider the case of Bill. Bill is a 70-year-old retired executive with a history of heart diseases and type 2 diabetes who has recently been diagnosed with mild cognitive impairment.

---

[187] These include sirt1 and nrf2.

Bill wants to improve his memory and blood sugar levels by changing his lifestyle. He was prescribed a ketogenic diet, which is low in glucose and so activates AMPK, and a 10-week high intensity interval training programme. By the fourth week of the intervention Bill's fasting insulin was down and his HbA1c levels (a marker for type 2 diabetes) had returned to normal. His memory had improved significantly when measured by established techniques. This is a real case study and although it only involved a single patient, the authors of the study commented, "restoring dysregulated mitochondrial function via AMPK pathway activation through a ketogenic protocol offers promising trends for future neurological and metabolic research" [412]. For patients such as Bill and the millions of others who want to lower their risk of dementia, nutrition and exercise offer one of the greatest hopes.

We have come a long way in these discussions from a simple view of disease prevention as suppressing what I have dubbed the three Core Risk States, but these discussions reveal deep, evolutionary conserved processes. Organisms - and humans are no exception - have remarkable abilities to maintain health through self-righting homeostatic mechanisms. This provides the capacity to adapt to new challenges. The ability to do this is a sign of resilience [413], and the master processes triggered by a healthy diet and physical activity are key allies in maintaining resilience and preventing a descent into frailty and ill health. I hope I have convinced you of the benefits of adopting a Med diet. We are now ready to get down to the practicalities of how to adopt this diet.

# 12. The food groups in the Med diet

# Fruit and Vegetables

## Carrot or stick?

A child eating a raw carrot stick is a popular image in campaigns to encourage children to eat more fruit and veg. To me this image seems misplaced and conveys far more stick than carrot. A carrot stick is not particularly tasty; it is hard and not very digestible. This is the opposite of the many tasty Med dishes in which carrots crop up, often along with onions and celery (such as in a French *mirepoix* or Italian *soffritto*) as the base of a stew or soup. Carrots tick many boxes: they are cheap, locally produced in the UK, easily available, nutritious and store well. It is not *moussaka* that the Greeks consider as their national dish but a simple white bean soup with carrots and other veg called *fasolada*.

Mouthwatering vegetable casseroles cooked in EVOO are served daily in traditional Med cuisine, often finished with a sprinkling of cheese such as parmesan which greatly lifts the taste and adds protein. Lack of imaginative ways with veg - unadorned and boiled to tastelessness - is probably a major reason why the UK ranked a lowly fifteenth out of nineteen European countries in a league table of fruit and veg consumption. [414] Although most people in the UK are familiar with the five-a-day campaign for fruit and veg, successive governments have failed to reverse the low consumption, which has stayed stubbornly below target levels for the last decade. [188] In England only 31% of adults eat five-a-day and this figure falls to 24% in Wales and 20% in Scotland. [189] It has been estimated that over 42,000 premature deaths would be prevented if the five-a-day target were achieved across the UK. This

---

[188]https://www.nutrition.org.uk/nutritioninthenews/newreports/ndnstrends.html?__cf_chl_js chl_tk__ F&V consumption in UK see Food Statistics Pocket Book 2015
[189] These figures come from NDNS for England, National Wales Survey and Scottish Health Survey as reported in Peas Please Progress Report 2018

is far more lives saved than would be achieved by reducing salt or saturated fat consumption. [190]

In the UK, people from higher socio-economic groups eat up to one and a half more portions of fruit and veg per day more than those in the lowest group [415]. The perceived cost of fresh fruit and veg is often given as a reason why less well off people eat less fruit and veg and this is also extrapolated as a major reason why on average they are less healthy [416]. [191] But this is only part of the picture since inexpensive fruit and veg cost no more than the less healthy eating options that many choose instead. The reasons are broader, and include time constraints on cooking, lack of cooking skills, and the cultural reprogramming of diets by the food industry to encourage the consumption of junk food. These complex interrelated reasons explain why public health initiatives to encourage greater consumption of fresh fruit and veg are so challenging.

There is little doubt that eating more fruit and veg reduces the risk of many chronic diseases. The evidence has been classed as "convincing" for cardiovascular diseases and as "likely" (a notch below the "convincing" category) for cancer [417]. The WCRF/AICR has scrutinised the role of specific classes of fruits and vegetables in cancer risk. They found a wide range of protective benefits and their conclusions are summarised in the Table.

---

[190] McColl K, Lobstein T. (2015) Nutrient Profiling: Changing the food of Britain. London: Coronary Prevention Group and World Obesity Federation. Daily salt intake reduced from average 9g to 6g 20,200 lives saved. Saturated fat intake reduced by 2.3% of energy 3,500 lives saved

[191] By contrast, it has been argued that smoking and alcohol abuse do not present strong cases to explain social discrepancies since both are falling while mortality is rising 416. Hiam L, Dorling D (2018) Government's misplaced prevention agenda. *BMJ* **363**, k5134..

**The types of cancer fruit and veg protect against** [418]

| Level of evidence | Type of fruit and veg | Type of cancer |
|---|---|---|
| Strong | Non-starchy veg and fruit | Aero-digestive |
| Limited | Non starchy veg | Mouth, pharynx, larynx, oesophagus (adenocarcinoma and squamous cell carcinoma), lung, breast (ER negative) |
| | Fruit | Oesophagus (squamous cell carcinoma, lung |
| | Citrus fruit | Stomach |
| | Non starchy veg and fruit | Bladder |
| | Foods containing carotenoids | Lung, breast |
| | Foods containing beta-carotene | Lung |
| | Foods containing vitamin C | Lung, colorectal |
| | Foods containing isoflavones | Lung |

A large scale study from the EPIC trial found convincing evidence that even a modest increase in fruit and vegetable intake could help to prevent type 2 diabetes, regardless of whether the increase is among people with initially low or high intake [419]. Another large review estimated that the risk of dying prematurely is reduced by 5% for each extra serving of fruit and vegetables [420]. The authors of this review suggested that protective mechanisms against CVD could include the high levels of antioxidants in fruits and vegetables preventing the oxidation of cholesterol, and high levels of magnesium and potassium, which lower blood pressure. The benefits in this study were maximal with five servings a day but some studies suggest that even more servings may bring even greater health benefits. In the EPIC study, which followed more than 450,000 Europeans for 13 years, participants who ate more than seven portions of fruit and veg per day (a portion is equivalent to

80 grams) had a 15% lower risk of death from heart disease and stroke, 27% for respiratory diseases such as flu, pneumonia and COPD and 40% for diseases of the digestive system such as liver disease compared with participants who consumed less than three portions per day [421].

Some of the most convincing evidence why eating fruit and veg is so healthy is because they reduce the Core Risk States. I will illustrate this with that unassuming vegetable the onion.

## Know your onions

Preparing a savoury Med dish from scratch more often than not starts with peeling an onion. Even though they start so many dishes, onions are usually regarded as lowly pace setters that are expected to anonymously melt away to just leave behind a lingering savoury note so that the star ingredient(s) in the dish can then take centre stage. The onion's presence in the dish is forgotten. Which is a shame, since onions not only add taste, they also have wide-ranging although little appreciated health benefits.

Onions suppress the three Core Risk States in various ways. We can first consider how onions regulate glucose levels and so reduce the risk of insulin resistance. Clinical studies have shown that diabetics given diets supplemented with onions have significantly reduced blood glucose levels [422]. This can be demonstrated by simply seeing how onions reduce glucose uptake in people. A PhD student of mine recruited twenty sturdy undergraduates to study this. The students were asked to first swallow a glucose solution so that their blood sugar levels could be measured. As expected, blood glucose levels rose over the first half hour and then fell away again over the next few hours. The students were then asked to swallow a solution of onions before swallowing the glucose solution again. The amount of glucose in the blood was halved compared to when the students had swallowed only the glucose solution. This demonstrates that onions have a powerful effect on blocking glucose uptake [203].

There are various substances in onion that may be reducing the glucose absorption. One is a polysaccharide called inulin. Inulin slows the emptying of the stomach into the duodenum and small intestine and so glucose (along with other foodstuffs) is absorbed less quickly [112]. Inulin has been found to reduce fasting blood glucose levels in diabetics [423]. Good control of blood glucose helps prevent insulin resistance developing which will have a wide range of benefits as was discussed in chapters 10 and 11. Inulin is a molecule that signals its presence in onions by developing sweetness when onions are fried for long time. This sweetness is due to individual fructose molecules breaking off from the long fructose chain that makes up the inulin molecule. So inulin provides both sweetness to the tongue and takes away excess sweetness from the blood. [192]

Inulin also helps tackle chronic inflammation, another of the three Core Risk States. Inulin is a type of soluble fibre. This means that our digestive system is unable to break it down, and so it reaches the colon intact where it acts as a prebiotic providing nourishment for billions of colonic bacteria. This nourishment keeps the bacteria content. It also stimulates colon cells to produce a protective mucus lining to prevent harm from the gut bacteria. But if there is not enough dietary inulin then less protective mucus is produced, and so some of the gut bacteria can invade into the colon cells and trigger low-grade chronic inflammation. This damaging response was demonstrated when mice were fed a diet low in fibre and this damage was prevented by providing the mice with inulin in their diet.[193]

Glucose molecules are normally absorbed across the intestinal wall by a specific transporter. This transporter will also transport other molecules in the diet that contain a molecule of glucose as part of their structure. If there are a lot of these "part-glucose" molecules then these can outcompete glucose itself for binding to the transporter. This will reduce the amount of glucose absorbed. One of these part-glucose molecules comprises glucose attached to a phytochemical called quercetin. These quercetin-glucose couplings called quercetin glucosides are found in particularly high amounts in onions. So eating a meal rich in onions leads to glucose transporters in the gut busily binding quercetin glucosides which means less free glucose is absorbed across the gut wall.

This brief description shows that even such a seemingly humble vegetable as the onion can still be a rich treasure trove of beneficial compounds. Onions are the second most commonly consumed vegetable after tomatoes, and so it is definitely worth knowing your onions.

---

[192] A good website for inulin: https://draxe.com/inulin/
[193] Fiber Is Good for You. Now Scientists May Know Why.
https://www.nytimes.com/2018/01/01/science/food-fiber-microbiome-inflammation.html

Onions aren't the only food able to reduce glucose absorption. Clinical studies have shown that apples and coffee do so too, and, like onions, they contain phytochemicals able to block glucose transporters lining the gut wall [424]. In fact, few vegetables have unique health benefits despite the media hype that often draws attention to a specific benefit of a particular vegetable. Beetroots, for instance, attract a lot of attention because of their high levels of blood pressure-lowering nitrates. But many other vegetable such as spinach and rocket also contain high levels of nitrates [425].

A lot of the glucose we consume comes from eating starchy foods. These are broken down in the gut to glucose. Because they cause a rapid rise in blood sugar levels, starchy diets are linked to an increased risk of type 2 diabetes [426]. Many fruits and vegetables contain phytochemicals that reduce this starch digestion. In one study, supplementing a diet containing starchy bread with polyphenol-rich dried strawberries, blackberries, blackcurrants and green tea reduced glucose levels in the blood by a quarter and insulin levels by half [111]. It is thought that the polyphenols were both blocking starch breakdown and glucose absorption across the gut wall into the blood stream and that the fibre (which is high in dried fruits) was reducing glucose uptake from the gut. This is another illustration of why it is a mistake to just consider one food outside the context of the other foods with which it is eaten. Anti-glycaemic (glucose lowering) foods need to be in the gut at the same time as starchy foods in order to effectively reduce blood glucose levels. This suggests that to realise the anti-glycaemic benefits from berries, it is better to eat them at the end of a starchy meal rather than at a time separate from the meal.

## Shopping

Shopping the Mediterranean way starts with the tastiest, freshest, best value, seasonal fruit and veg and the cook then usually fits the recipe around these. A Mediterranean cook is less likely to go out searching for unusual, expensive produce for a newly discovered recipe. [194] It is not necessary to buy only typical "Mediterranean" veg such as aubergines and peppers. Local produce is equally acceptable. Resources that provide many different enticing recipes for even commonplace veg such as cabbages or carrots are a great asset. The internet is a good source, as are the more comprehensive cookery books that

---

[194] In the UK a useful website for advice on eating seasonable veg is http://eatseasonably.co.uk

have stood the test of time such as The Silver Spoon for Italian cuisine and Vefa's Kitchen for Greek cuisine (for more cookery books see ch. 13).

## Variety

Choosing a variety of colours - "eat a rainbow" as they say - by including both green leafy vegetables (cabbage, lettuce etc) and red, orange and yellow root veg (such as beetroot, carrots and parsnips) ensures that you consume all classes of phytochemicals, from red and yellow carotenoids to blue and purple anthocyanins. There is good evidence that eating a diverse range of veg promotes health; it's not just how much you eat that matters. In one study, smokers who ate the greatest variety of veg were 27% less likely to contract lung cancer than smokers with a diet low in variety, and this beneficial effect was independent of the actual amount of vegetables consumed [427].

## Varieties

Driven by demands from supermarkets, farmers often cultivate varieties - cultivars - with the best shelf life, uniformity and yield. But these cultivars may not necessarily be best for phytochemicals. Phytochemical levels vary enormously between cultivars, and so a simple way to boost health from vegetables without eating more is by being choosy about the cultivar you buy. Phytochemicals give fruit and vegetables their taste and so a tastier variety often equates with higher levels of phytochemicals. An iceberg lettuce has 32 times less antioxidants than a *cos* lettuce and an enormous 690 times less than a *lollo rosso* lettuce [428].

Bitterness is one taste consumers often avoid and this has led to a boom in the sale of bland varieties and "baby veg" with low levels of bitter compounds. But this comes at the cost of health-promoting bitter compounds. Rather than avoiding bitterness altogether, balancing bitterness with sweetness results in a far tastier food - marmalade is made with bitter Seville oranges balanced for sweetness rather than from sweet dessert oranges, and a rocket salad with a sweetened dressing is a far tastier and healthier option than salad leaves where the bitterness has been bred out.

A well-stocked salad bowl makes a tempting display, but only if the fruit is sweet and juicy, not bitter and hard. Not all fruits continue to ripen after they have been picked. Those that do are called "climacteric" and include apples, avocados, bananas, figs, mangoes, papayas, peaches, pears and tomatoes. [195] Fresh fruit is the ultimate convenience food to eat with breakfast cereals, as a healthy snack, and is the customary way to round off a Med meal, rather than a sweet dessert. Bananas - the UK's favourite fruit - are rich in potassium, which is good for helping lower blood pressure, but they have only low levels of many of the vitamins and phytochemicals found in other fruits. So if your preference is for bananas, why not try chopping up a banana with another fruit such as grapes, an apple or an orange – or go the whole hog and use that banana as the starting point for a fruit salad sweetened with honey…

## Organic

Because the Med diet is plant-based and veg-centric, choosing quality fruit and veg is particularly important. Increasing numbers of people choose organic hoping it will be more nutritious and not have the pesticide residues found in conventionally grown produce. So is there good evidence for this?

### Toxic compounds

Agricultural practices mean that small amounts of potentially toxic compounds find their way into many conventionally grown plant foods. One of the less well-known toxic compounds is the metal cadmium. Cadmium is present in rocks mined for the phosphate fertilisers that are then used to grow crops. Cereals in particular have been found to have high residues of cadmium - on average 48% higher levels than organically grown produce. Cadmium is toxic to the kidneys and accumulates in the body since we have no way of excreting it. It is one of only a few metals (the others being mercury and lead) that the European Commission has set maximum recommended levels for in foods. Cadmium induces oxidative stress throughout the body and is linked to an increased risk of a wide range of chronic diseases from breast cancer to CVD [429]. However, it is currently up to individuals to decide about the health risks from cadmium since this is not regulated by law.

The possible cancer risk from pesticide residues in conventionally grown crops is much debated. A couple of studies found a lower incidence of non-Hodgkin lymphoma in people consuming organic foods [430; 431] and one of these studies also found a lower incidence of post-menopausal breast cancer

---

[195] https://www.knowablemagazine.org/article/living-world/2017/getting-it-ripe

(430). But it is difficult with these studies to completely disentangle the possible influence of other lifestyle factors (confounders) since people who eat organic also tend to lead healthier lives in general.

The possible cancer risk from eating conventionally grown fruit and veg needs to be considered in context. It should not be used as an argument to eat less fruit and veg, since the benefits of eating fruit and veg far outweigh any possible increased cancer risks. A study from the US estimated that approximately 20,000 cancer cases per year could be prevented by increasing fruit and vegetable consumption, while only 10 cancer cases per year might be caused by the added pesticide consumption[432].

This may still not ally the fears for many individuals. So is the extra cost of organic fruit and veg worth it? Studies usually find that pesticide residues in organic crops are lower than in conventionally grown crops. In one large international study, pesticide residues were found to be four times lower in organic crops [433]. It may come as a surprise that *any* pesticides are found in organic crops. The authors of the study suggested this may have been because the organic crops containing pesticides (about 11% of all the organic crops) had been cross-contaminated from neighbouring conventional fields, or that there was fraudulent labeling.

Various countries produce league tables showing the likelihood of pesticide residues being present in conventionally grown produce. In the UK, the Pesticide Action Network provides very useful information. [196] According to their tables, almost all citrus fruit and oats for instance have pesticide residues. But this information taken out of context is not very helpful. It is of little concern if the pesticides are on a part of the food that is usually discarded (such as the skin of an orange). Also, simply stating that residues were detected does not say if these exceed permitted levels. For the quarter ending September 2018, the UK Expert Committee on Pesticide Residues in Foods reported that of 21 foods examined (including 16 fruit and veg), pesticide residues were above the maximum permitted level in 8% of the food samples [434]. The majority of these foods were specialty beans from developing countries. High levels of the chemical chlorate were detected in various frozen veg. The main dietary source of chlorate is chlorinated drinking water.

---

[196] http://www.pan-uk.org/our-food/best-and-worst-foods-for-pesticide-residues-uk/

Chlorate can reduce iodine uptake but the EFSA does not consider it likely to be hazardous. [197]

There is still no consensus on whether or not permitted pesticide levels in foods are harmful to health. Drawing conclusions can be challenging. This can be illustrated by considering the herbicide glyphosate. Glyphosate is the most widely used herbicide (weedkiller) in the world and is used by farmers and gardeners in products such as Roundup. In 2015, the International Agency for Research on Cancer (IARC) classified glyphosate as a probable human carcinogen, but this decision was criticised. [198] A meta-analysis concluded that there is "compelling evidence" that workers directly exposed to glyphosate are at increased risk of non-Hodgkin lymphoma [435] and France has now banned gardeners and professionals from using one form of glyphosate with other glyphosate products set to follow. [199]

Most people do not use glyphosate themselves and for them the more pertinent concern is whether or not levels of glyphosate found in food - so-called "residues" - are dangerous. There is unequivocal evidence that glyphosate residues are indeed found in foods and this looks set to increase. Use of glyphosate is increasing in many countries because of the introduction of genetically modified (GM) foods such as soya and rapeseed. These are engineered to be glyphosate resistant and so fields can be sprayed destroying weeds but sparing the crop. A less well-known use for glyphosate is to spray normal (ie non-GM) grains and pulses a few weeks before harvesting them. This kills the crop since these crops are sensitive to glyphosate. This is done in order to cause a faster and more uniform final ripening of the crop. As a bonus it also clears the ground of weeds that may contaminate the harvest of the crop. Spraying so close to harvest has the downside for consumers of significantly increasing the levels of glyphosate residues in the crop food [436]. Glyphosate also has environmental impacts and these are considered in chapter 14. Overall, there are complex issues on the pros and cons of glyphosate which means that the debate on its use continues.

---

[197] https://www.efsa.europa.eu/en/press/news/150624a
[198] https://www.theguardian.com/business/2019/feb/14/weed-killing-products-increase cancer-risk-of-cancer
[199] Barbara Casassus French court bans sale of controversial weedkiller Nature 24 Jan 2019 https://www.nature.com/articles/d41586-019-00259-x

A couple of pesticides (malathion and diazinon) were also classified by the International Agency for Research on Cancer in 2015 as probable carcinogens, and there are concerns about occupational exposure to these agents.

Overall, for most pesticides, there is no strong evidence that the legal limits of pesticide residues in foods pose a health risk to the public. However, determining these limits is not an exact science. Multiple factors interact over many years to cause cancers and so it is perhaps not surprising that it is unclear how pesticide residues in foods contribute to this potpourri of risk factors. This is complicated even more by the many different pesticides consumed in a normal diet. A related concern is the possibility that the dangers of pesticides arise from the continual low dose exposure to a cocktail of interacting pesticides. There is evidence that chronic moderate exposure to a cocktail of pesticides may increase the risk of Parkinson disease and have hormonal effects in the body [437; 438]. Based on the precautionary principle, rather than on definitive research, a strong case can now be made to minimise occupational exposure during spraying and for consumers. [200] Governments are now using this principle as the basis for banning certain pesticides.

<u>Is organic richer in nutrients?</u>

As with uncertainties over pesticide residues, there is no consensus between experts whether or not organically grown vegetables are healthier. On the whole, studies *do* find that organic crops contain more phytochemicals. One comprehensive review concluded that a person eating organically grown fruits, vegetables and grains would increase their intake of antioxidant polyphenols by between 20% and 40% [433]. What is still lacking, though, are long-term studies that measure *health* outcomes such as heart disease or cancer. The difficulty with conducting these studies is trying to isolate the contribution of eating the organic foods from all the other potentially confounding factors in the person's diet and lifestyle. Again the precautionary principle is a useful guide, and based on fewer pesticide residues and higher levels of antioxidants, buying organic can be recommended. However, buying organic fruits and vegetables is prohibitive for some. If this is the case then prioritising organic produce where the skins are eaten, such as apples and

---

[200] A useful website on how to avoid exposure to glyphosate is at
https://www.mygenefood.com/why-glyphosate-is-dangerous-and-how-to-avoid-eating-it/

potatoes, makes sense since the skins of fruits and vegetables are often highest in phytochemicals and also most likely to have pesticide residues.

The composition of organic fruit and veg is influenced by many aspects of how they are grown. Plants must adapt to their environment since they are literally rooted to the spot. For instance, when plants are crowded together their growth is stunted. Growing conditions also influence nutrient composition, although this is less obvious at first glance. Plants adapt in order to make the most of where they are, much as we might adapt to our own circumstances. As Drs Ingrouille and Eddie summed up in their book Plants: Diversity and Evolution: "Growth in plants is somewhat analogous to behaviour in humans." [201]

Organically grown crops are less pampered with pesticides than their conventionally grown counterparts. This "neglect" results in organically grown plants becoming more stressed, and this behaviour change is expressed by the plant producing more phytochemicals [135] (see ch. 6). Many of these are defensive phytochemicals since organic crops are not able to rely on synthetic pesticides to protect themselves; so instead they produce their own. Organic farmers are also more likely to choose cultivars with a higher capacity to produce defensive phytochemicals and this may benefit our health as well as that of the plant. These scenarios make it likely that organically grown fruit and veg will have higher levels of phytochemicals.

Since they are not fed synthetic fertilisers containing nitrogen and phosphorus, organically grown crops are also distinguished from conventionally grown produce by not having such easy access to soil nutrients. This can also result on greater accumulation of phytochemicals. Conventionally grown crops suck up nitrogen from the soil, which is then combined with carbon compounds to produce complex molecules needed for growth. The carbon compounds are mostly sugars made by fixing carbon dioxide from the atmosphere by photosynthesis. Organically grown crops form similar amounts of carbon compounds by photosynthesis. But because they often have a harder time getting nitrogen, they may build up excess carbon compounds - since they cannot switch off photosynthesis. Most plants have only limited ways of excreting the excess carbon and so instead channel

---

[201] Ingrouille, M and Eddie, B (2008) Plants: Diversity and Evolution. CUP

some into producing phytochemicals. Phytochemicals are effectively acting as carbon stores.

These examples illustrate that it is not so much labeling a crop plant as "organic" or not that is the real determinant of how nutritious it is - at least in terms of phytochemical content, but rather how the plant grows. After all, a plant is responding to its environment not to a label it has been given. So it is not surprising that growth conditions may sometimes result in conventionally grown crops having better nutritional value. In one study, non-organic grapes had higher levels of purple antioxidant pigments called anthocyanins than grapes grown organically. This was attributed to a combination of the very hot summer and spraying with pesticides, which, the authors of the study suggested, acted together as more important stressors for phytochemical production than growing the vines organically [439].

There is a huge increase in demand for organic produce across Europe, and governments are incentivising farmers to grow more organic produce to satisfy this demand.[202] Health concerns is one reason why people choose organic. However, the strongest rationale to choose organic is to help protect the environment and this is discussed in chapter 14.

## Cooking

Veg dishes as the main courser have more of an image problem than a steak or coq au vin. For most omnivores, it is the meat in a meal that conjures up the most eating pleasure. Veg dishes are simply not deemed worthy to sit centre-stage. Some of this can be traced back to childhood. Studies have found that parents putting pressure on children to eat healthy foods like veg and avoid unhealthy foods can backfire and reduce a preference for healthy foods and increase the preference for unhealthy foods [440]. The childhood order to "eat your greens" lingers in the ears of many a veg-denier.

Psychologists from Stanford University have suggested that changing the mindset that healthy foods are not tasty foods could be an effective way of increasing veg consumption. They found that labeling vegetables in a university cafeteria with indulgent descriptors like "twisted citrus-glazed carrots" was a better way to get people to choose the dish than describing it as

---

[202] https://ec.europa.eu/agriculture/organic/eu-policy/data-statistics_en

healthy [(441)]. Ultimately, however, fancy labels are unlikely to be enough of a sleight-of-hand to increase consumption. To achieve this requires a genuine desire to want to eat more veg.

It is its many clever ways with veg that gives the Med diet a head start, even for omnivores. Key to eating more veg is to use EVOO either for cooking or for sprinkling over raw veg. The oil solubilises and liberates fat-soluble phytochemicals, including flavoursome phytochemicals, that enhance taste and it makes it easier for our body to absorb them. Tomatoes and herbs are frequently added to vegetables as flavour enhancers. The traditional Cretan Med diet included salads several times a week and salads still form an important part of the Med diet. In the large EPIC study mentioned earlier, health benefits were even more pronounced for raw vegetables than cooked ones especially for protection from cancers [(421)]. Eating vegetables raw preserves heat-sensitive vitamins, and salad dressings of olive oil, vinegar, marjoram and other herbs or spices greatly increase antioxidants in the dish [(442)].

## Food preparation

The time needed to prepare fresh veg is a barrier for some when deciding whether or not to include them in a meal. Although pre-chopped fresh vegetables are one option, these are relatively expensive, they can lose nutritional value and they may have been chemically treated - this can even be the case when there is nothing on the label to signify this. [203] Ready prepared frozen veg may be a better option. Investing in a good chopping board and knife and knowing how to use it makes preparing your own veg so much easier. Jamie Oliver's videos on how to chop key ingredients such onions and garlic can be very motivating.

The 19th century Irish-American Augustus Saint-Gaudens said of garlic "What garlic is to food, insanity is to art." Fortunately the health benefits of garlic are now more widely appreciated. It is the very act of chopping garlic that creates much of its healthiness. An intact bulb of garlic has very little smell compared to a clove that has been chopped. Chopping or crushing garlic starts chemical reactions that generate a diverse range of very healthy

---

[203] https://www.mashed.com/151312/the-real-reason-you-should-never-buy-pre-cut-fruit-and-vegetables/

sulphurous compounds. [204] One of these is a compound called allicin, and it is allicin that is mainly responsible for garlic's characteristic sulphurous odour. Allicin develops over time, something well known to cooks who leave foods containing garlic overnight in the fridge, which can taste more 'garlicky' the following day. Allicin is thought to have antibacterial activity in the stomach and this may help protect against stomach ulcers since these are caused by the bacterium *Helicobacter pylori*.

Allicin is not very stable and is rapidly converted into a range of other sulphur-containing compounds. Allowing time for these to form can increase the health benefits of garlic. In one study, waiting ten minutes after crushing garlic before cooking with it greatly increased the ability of the garlic to prevent platelets sticking together [443]. This is an important action that reduces the risk of CVD.

Some other sulphur compounds in garlic called sulphides have anti-cancer activity. Heating garlic has been found to reduce this anticancer properties and, as for CVD, allowing the chopped garlic to stand for a few minutes before cooking helps retain anticancer benefits [444; 445]. Some of the sulphides from garlic get taken up by red blood cells and are converted into hydrogen sulphide (best known to school boys as "bad egg gas"). Hydrogen sulphide reduces blood pressure by dilating blood vessels, which lowers the pressure within them. A lower blood pressure reduces the risk of strokes.

Because allicin and some of the other sulphur compounds are not very stable to heat, Mediterranean foods that include raw garlic as an ingredient may be particularly beneficial. The health benefits of sauces made using raw garlic, like Catalan *allioli* (raw garlic mashed with salt and olive oil), French *aiolli* (with added egg yolks made into a mayonnaise) and Greek *skordalia* (with potatoes), may be as powerful as their flavours. Garlic breath may not be popular with those around you but it may be doing you good. One study found that raw garlic eaten two or more times per week decreased the risk of lung cancer by 44%, and the researchers speculated that this may have been because the volatile oil from raw garlic (which includes allicin) is largely excreted in the lungs and hence may be able to exert a beneficial effect there [446].

---

[204] Chopping breaks down structural barriers in garlic cells allowing an enzyme called alliinase to come into contact with a molecule called alliin which it then converts into allicin.

Crushing generates more damage to the garlic than chopping it and may produce more bioactive compounds. Crushing garlic is preferred in some recipes especially in Spanish cuisine. Adding garlic towards the end of the cooking time will also preserve more of the important heat sensitive sulphur compounds.

Members of the cabbage family (brassicas) are, like garlic, well known for their sulphur compounds. And like garlic, the chemical reactions that produce these compounds are initiated by chopping. Some of the sulphur compounds help protect against cancer, and a number of epidemiological studies have shown a relationship between above average intake of Brassicas and a reduction in cancer. Brassicas are chopped to a lesser extent than garlic but chewing may also initiate the production of these substances.

## Cooking for taste and health

Raw and cooked veg bring different things to the table and so a combination is probably best. Many people avoid vegetables because of perceived bitterness, so making them a little sweeter can make them far more satisfying. Roasting root veg such as parsnips brings out their natural sweetness. Other veg such as carrots and cauliflower benefit from a small sprinkling of sugar and then cooked or fried in olive oil to caramelise the sugars. Stews that include tinned tomatoes also usually benefit from a pinch of sugar. Although too much sugar is never a good thing, the fibre and phytochemicals in veg are likely to reduce the amount of sugar absorbed by the body.

The way veg are cooked can have as big an impact on health as how much of them you eat [3; 442]. Loss of vitamin C is perhaps the best-known example of nutrient loss due to cooking. Claims that potatoes are a good source of vitamin C need to be tempered by the fact that much of the vitamin C is destroyed during cooking - and eating raw potatoes is not an option. Some other vitamins including A, B1 (thiamine) and B9 (folate or folic acid) are also lost at high temperatures. By contrast, many micronutrients and phytochemicals (polyphenols, carotenoids and glucosinolates) are relatively stable at high temperatures.

An interesting example of a chemical reaction involving a carotenoid occurs when shrimps and lobster are boiled. Heating separates the carotenoid astaxanthin in the carapace from a protein, which then changes the colour of the shellfish from blue-green to a pinkish-red. Liberating carotenoids in an active form may also be important for the health benefits of carotenoids in fruit and veg. In the plant world, tomatoes, bell peppers and many leafy green vegetables are excellent sources of carotenoids. However, carotenoids often occur in vegetables in less-readily available forms. In green leafy veg the carotenoids are bound to proteins inside chloroplasts - the cell's photosynthetic unit. In many other veg, they occur in semi-crystalline forms. Protein bound and crystalline forms of carotenoids are harder for the body to absorb than when the carotenoids are free. Cooking has the benefit of breaking down plant cell walls and helping release the trapped carotenoids. This enables the carotenoids to be more easily absorbed - increasing their so-called "bioavailability". A good example of this is chopping and stewing tomatoes with olive oil, actions that help solubilise the main, and fat-soluble, carotenoid in tomatoes called lycopene. Studies suggest that olive oil is better than other oils at increasing carotenoid absorption. Enhancing the bioavailability of lycopene may help explain the observational studies which suggest that cooked tomatoes are better at protecting against prostate cancer than eating raw tomatoes. In one study of Greek men, eating cooked tomatoes (most likely cooked in olive oil) was associated with a 91% reduced risk of prostate cancer whereas this protection dropped to 55% for men eating raw tomatoes [447].

A base of onions, garlic and tomato lightly fried in EVOO called *sofrito* is the starting point for numerous stews in Spanish cooking. [205] As well as carotenoids, this base contains many phenolic and sulphur compounds (as discussed above). Many of these phytochemicals are released into the cooking oil and then readily absorbed by the body. This sauce is considered a key component of the Spanish Med diet [448]. *Sofrito* was included as one of the beneficial components in the Med diet in the Predimed study (see ch. 9) since eating this base on a regular basis provides an excellent source of many healthful phytochemicals linked to reducing cancer and protecting against CVD.

Boiling veg

Varying amounts of water-soluble nutrients leach from veg into their cooking water. A very visible example is purple pigments called betalains that colour

---

[205] Not to be confused with Italian *soffritto* which is a mixture of slowly cooked carrots, onions and celery.

the water when beetroots are boiled. The loss of healthy nutrients due to leaching may be substantial with up to 90% of anti-cancer glucosinolates from brassicas (cabbages, broccoli etc) ending up in the cooking water. Many water-soluble vitamins (vitamin C and the B vitamin family) also leach into cooking water. Not throwing away cooking water may be one of the ways that makes the Med diet so nutrient rich. In Mediterranean cooking, making a sauce using the cooking liquid from cooked brassicas ensures no loss of the beneficial glucosinolates and vitamins. Left over cooking water from vegetables is excellent as the stock for making risottos, and eating a risotto once or twice a week is an excellent way of eliminating this waste. Soups, stews and "stewps" (very thick soups) are very popular in Med cuisine, and since the liquid is consumed, there will be no loss of water-soluble nutrients. Even when vegetables are simply boiled in water, as is the case with very bitter vegetables to reduce bitterness, the leftover water was traditionally drunk by the Mediterranean cook rather than being thrown out! Another common technique is to cook vegetables in a small amount of water with added olive oil. The olive oil will dissolve some of the phytochemicals left in the saucepan that may otherwise be lost.

## No Waste

According to the waste reduction organisation WRAP, a third of all fresh veg and salads purchased by UK households is wasted [449]. Potatoes are by far the most commonly thrown away veg, followed by carrots, lettuce and onions. The main reason why so much food is thrown away is because it is not used in time. However, root veg like carrots, onions and potatoes are storage organs and given the correct cool conditions will store for many weeks. One culprit is "best before dates" which often don't reflect the actual storage potential of root veg if they are stored correctly. [206] By contrast, leaf veg are not produced by the plant to be stored and they can start losing their nutrients as soon as they are harvested. Frozen veg retain nutrients for far longer, and veg like peas that are often frozen within a few hours of harvesting can be more nutritious than fresh alternatives.

Because the Med diet is so focused on veg there should never be any risk of waste. Med cuisine has very many recipes for the same veg ranging from

---

[206] https://www.theguardian.com/science/2018/may/25/times-up-for-best-before-dates-in-move-to-tackle-food-waste

simple soups to sophisticated stews. Similar combinations of veg are also often used in different Med cuisines and so there is no likelihood of becoming bored with a leftover veg that has already been used in a previous recipe. For instance, most Med countries have a vegetable stew that includes various combinations of aubergines, peppers, tomatoes and courgettes. They are all good reheated the next day or served cold and include

- ratatouille - the classic French combination - can accompany chicken and is also good served with eggs poached on the top

- briami - a Greek stew with potatoes rather than aubergines and with the addition of cinnamon
- caponata - a very tasty Italian sweet and sour dish with celery rather than courgettes
- escalivada - Spanish grilled veg; simple and versatile

# Grains

## History

About 10,000 years ago in the Eastern Mediterranean region known as the Levant early humans had the groundbreaking idea of cultivating various grasses for their seeds. These seeds we now call "grains" or "cereals". They are relatively easy to cultivate and have good yields. The first grains to be cultivated were early varieties of wheat and barley, and today wheat, rice, corn (maize), barley, oats, and rye are a staple food for billions of people around the world. [207]

## Health benefits of whole grains

In ancient times, grains in western countries were mainly eaten as porridge-like gruel, made famous when Dickens's Oliver Twist asked his workhouse supervisor for more. Gruel's reputation as the food of workhouses and prisons was cemented and has never really recovered. Describing something as "gruelling" is hardly a positive association for a food. And today, whole grains do not rank highly on most people's choice of healthy foods compared to say eating more fruit and veg or less meat. Eating them is indeed often seen as gruelling; which is a great shame.

With this pedigree it is not surprising that milled and refined grain products became so desirable. But with this transformation has come the loss of much of the natural goodness of the whole grain. In the landmark international Global Burden of Disease Study published in 2017, an inadequate intake of whole grains was the number one dietary risk factor for death and disability, ahead even of high salt consumption or low fruit and veg [450].

Many studies have confirmed the benefits of eating whole grains. For instance, one study that analysed over two million people concluded that eating whole grains reduces death from any cause by 17%, CVD by 25% and cancer by 10% [451]. These conclusions were backed up by a large meta-analysis published in 2019 by a team of New Zealand nutritionists who found that people who ate a lot of whole grains were reducing their risk of coronary

---

[207] A highly informative article on the history of wheat is at
https://sustainablefoodtrust.org/articles/a-brief-history-of-wheat/?

heart disease, stroke, type 2 diabetes and colorectal cancer by between 15% and 30% [452].

For grains, the issue is not so much one of quantity, as it is, say, for red meat or fruit and veg. Rather it is one of quality: eating the wrong types and replacing whole grains with refined grains. This is why eating more whole grains is one of the main dietary recommendations in UK and many other national dietary guidelines.

So the question arises as to why so many of the health benefits of whole grains are lost when the grain is refined. The three Core Risk States provide a useful framework for understanding the health benefits of whole grains and why refining out beneficial substances reduces protection against oxidative stress and inflammation and increases insulin resistance.

# Nutritional consequences of milling, refining and fermenting

Few natural foods have lost as much of their nutritional value at the hands of food processors as grains. The breakfast "cereals" we sit down to eat have lost much of both their original physical structure (food matrix) and nutrient content and are altered beyond all recognition. Natural whole grains consist of an outer bran layer, an inner germ - the embryo, which will grow into the new plant, and the endosperm - a starchy mass that nourishes the embryo (see ch. 8 for a figure of a whole grain). All three parts must be retained for a food to be called "wholegrain". Even when milled into flour, a food can still be called "wholegrain" as long as all three parts of the whole grain are retained in their original proportions. This flour is called wholemeal flour and is made into bread, pasta etc. All of the nutrients in whole grains are retained in wholemeal flour. Some examples of wholegrain foods are:

- wholegrain breads
- wholegrain breakfast cereals (for example, muesli and porridge)
- popcorn
- wholegrain rice
- cooked grains (for example, wheat, millet and roasted buckwheat)
- bulgur

Refining grains removes the bran and germ. The brown whole grain is replaced with a white, mainly starchy product. Some examples of refined foods and foods made with refined flour are:

- white breads, sweet rolls
- noodles, pasta
- cakes, biscuits, viennoiseries
- muffins
- refined grain breakfast cereals
- white rice
- pancakes, waffles
- pizza

## Milling: flours versus grains

Although milling a whole grain into flour does not affect the overall nutrient composition there is one important change. And that is loss of the intact physical structure, or matrix, of the whole grain. Loss of the matrix makes nutrients in the grain more accessible to digestive enzymes. As well as enhancing the absorption of some beneficial nutrients, this also has significant negative health effects. One of these is on the rate of digestion of starch. In the intact whole grain, the outer bran layer acts as a protective shield reducing the ability of digestive enzymes called amylases to penetrate through to the inner endosperm and break down the starch located there into glucose. So in the gut, glucose is absorbed relatively slowly from intact whole grains. When grains are milled to produce wholemeal flour the protective shield is lost and this allows digestive enzymes to rapidly break down the starch to glucose and so cause a rapid rise in blood glucose.

The extent to which a food raises blood glucose levels is expressed by its glycaemic index (GI). The more a food raises blood glucose levels, the higher its GI value. Since an intact matrix is needed for the low GI of wholegrain foods, milled flours have higher GI values than the intact grains from which they are derived. The matrix is degraded in wholemeal flour and this explains why the GI of wholemeal flour is little different to white or brown bread. Wholemeal bread is still far healthier than white bread, though, because it retains many nutrients that are lost in white bread (see below).

**Glycaemic index of some grains** [208]

| FOOD | Glycaemic index (glucose = 100) |
|---|---|
| White wheat bread* | 75 ± 2 |
| Whole wheat/whole meal bread | 74 ± 2 |
| Specialty grain bread | 53 ± 2 |
| Unleavened wheat bread | 70 ± 5 |
| Spaghetti, white | 49 ± 2 |
| Spaghetti, whole meal | 48 ± 5 |
| White rice, boiled* | 73 ± 4 |
| Brown rice, boiled* | 68 ± 4 |
| Couscous | 65 ± 4 |

* Different types of rice vary enormously in their GI values with some having GI values classed as low [209]

Pasta is a little different. Both white and brown pastas have relatively low GI values (see Table). This is because the starch in the pasta - whether brown or white - coils when it cools making it less easy for digestive enzymes to break it down to glucose. This starch is called resistant starch and is classed as a form of dietary fibre since it reaches the colon intact where it can be broken down by bacteria. Although both white and brown pasta have similar quite low GI values, brown pasta is still preferable since, like wholemeal bread, it retains the micronutrients of the whole grain.

The advantages of consuming intact whole grains were demonstrated in a study with patients with type 2 diabetes. One group of patients ate a diet that

[208] https://www.health.harvard.edu/diseases-and-conditions/glycemic-index-and-glycemic-load-for-100-foods
[209] (Foster-Powell et al Am J Clin Nutr 2002;76:5–56)

included ground up grains and the other group ate the same diet except that their grains were left intact. The diabetics eating the diet that included ground grains had higher levels of blood glucose because of the higher GI of this diet. An important finding in this study was that the diabetics eating the ground grains also had much higher levels of risk markers for CVD compared to the group eating the diet containing the intact grains [453]. CVD is a risk factor for people with type 2 diabetes, and this study suggests that diabetics who choose whole grains over refined grains can lower their risk of CVD.

Whole grains have another important difference from their milled counterparts, namely their effect on appetite. Whole grains give a greater feeling of fullness (satiety) than milled grains. In one study, eating whole grain buckwheat was shown to raise a signal in the body for satiety far more than when eating pancakes made from buckwheat flour [454]. Since feeling full is the most basic way of regulating appetite and so not putting on excess calories, eating whole grains is a good strategy to help lose weight.

## Refining

Refined grains have had their bran and germ layers removed and most of what remains is the starchy endosperm. Many people prefer refined grains since they are more digestible and quicker to cook than whole grains. Refining grains also benefits manufacturers and retailers since it extends shelf life by removing unsaturated fats that easily go rancid. But refining is throwing out the embryonic baby germ of the grain with the bathwater, since it is the germ, along with the bran, where most of the goodness is stored. The germ is rich in the omega-3 fat ALA and the bran contains most of the fibre. Both bran and germ are also excellent sources of vitamins (especially B vitamins and vitamin E), minerals, phytochemicals and protein. Because of the loss of these important nutrients, refining compromises nutritional value to a far greater extent than milling.

In the 1950s, Bread and Flour Regulations in the UK were made law in order to enforce the mandatory fortification of white and brown flour with calcium, iron, and the B vitamins niacin and thiamine lost during milling. Cereal manufacturers also sometimes add other micronutrients. The list of micronutrients on the side of a cereal box may look impressive. But it is still a pretty feeble attempt to recreate the original nutrient content of the wholegrain since it excludes many of the dozens of vitamins, minerals and phytochemicals, and importantly the fibre, that were present in the germ and bran [243]. Even though iron is added back, there are major concerns about the usefulness of this since the type of iron added to flour and to cereal products is poorly absorbed by the body [166].

It matters that the nutrients added back to refined cereals by manufacturers are only a fraction of those in the original grain. Although regulatory authorities seem quite happy to ignore these other nutrients, it is highly probable that many have important health benefits. The cancer prevention associations the WCRF and AICR highlighted some of these in a joint report published in 2018, saying: "Whole grains provide various nutrients including vitamin E, selenium, copper, zinc, and bioactive non-nutrient compounds such as lignans, phytoestrogens and phenolic compounds as well as dietary fibre. Many of these compounds which are mainly found in the bran and germ of the grain, have plausible anti-carcinogenic properties" [418]. Fibre is the main food for gut bacteria, which the bacteria convert into a fatty acid called butyrate. This has anti-inflammatory properties, and this may help explain why fibre reduces the risk of CVD. Butyrate also inhibits the growth of colon cells and this is thought to be important for reducing the risk of colon cancer. In addition to these protective anticancer nutrients, grains are also a major source of cholesterol-lowering phytosterols, which may help protect against CVD. Adding back a few vitamins and minerals to refined grains fails badly in trying to reproduce the complex synergistic interactions that occur between different components in the whole grain.

<u>Fibre</u>

The relative amounts of soluble and insoluble fibre in whole grains differ from those in vegetables. In most whole grains, including wheat, rye, barley and oats, most of the fibre is of the insoluble type, although oats and barley do contain some soluble fibre. Soluble fibre is the type more commonly found in vegetables. Most of the fibre in whole grains is located in the bran layer. A large meta-analysis by nutritionists from New Zealand found that the dietary fibre from cereals had a similar spectrum of health benefits as the whole grains from which it was derived, reducing the risk for coronary heart disease, type 2 diabetes and several cancers including breast, colorectal and oesophagus [452]. This suggests that the fibre in whole grains is very important for the health benefits. Their analysis found that the more fibre a person consumed the greater the health benefits. A large study from the UK's authorative Scientific Advisory Committee on Nutrition that looked specifically at fibre intake from whole grains also concluded that it reduces the risk of CVD, type 2 diabetes, colorectal cancer and heart disease [455].

Micronutrients and phytochemicals

It is not only the fibre in whole grains that matters. There is also evidence that the phytochemicals are important. Wholegrain foods are the main dietary source of a phytochemical called ferulic acid. In one study, there was a significant reduction in markers of inflammation in overweight and obese people who ate whole grains for four weeks and this was linked to the ferulic acid in the whole grains [456]. Ferulic acid is a potent antioxidant and it may also make a significant contribution to the protective effects of whole grains against colorectal cancer [457]. Wholegrain foods also contain a group of phytochemicals called alkylresorcinols that protect against colorectal cancer. This was shown in the highly respected EPIC study [418]. There is now good evidence that ferulic acid, alkylresorcinols and possibly other phytochemicals contribute to the protective effect of whole grains against type 2 diabetes [458].

These findings matter since white bread contains only a fraction of the protective antioxidants such as ferulic acid found in wholegrain bread [459]. For alkylresorcinols the situation is particularly bad since they are completely absent from white flour. In fact, the presence of alkylresorcinols in a person's blood is used as a marker that they are eating whole grains [460]. These and other important phytochemicals are never added back as supplements to white bread and this highlights the inadequacy of current policies aimed at restoring the nutritional value of refined cereals.

The micronutrients and phytochemicals in whole grains are an important source of nutrients for our gut bacteria. Some micronutrients and phytochemicals (including ferulic acid) are tightly bound to fibre in an inactive form. The fibre chaperones these nutrients intact through the digestive system to the colon where they are released in an active form by bacteria that reside there [461]. As well as benefitting the colon, these newly released nutrients can be absorbed from the colon into the body. This makes the colon a second important place, along with the small intestine, where nutrients from our diet are absorbed into the body. There is an important difference between these two sites of absorption. Nutrients absorbed from the small intestine immediately drain into the liver where they are scrutinised by the vast metabolic army of liver enzymes before they are allowed into the rest of the body. This does not happen with nutrients absorbed across the colon and instead these nutrients can immediately enter the blood stream and circulate around the body. It is fibre that enables this to occur by preventing some nutrients being absorbed in the small intestine. The health implications for this are only slowly being unraveled.

The protective effect of whole grains against colorectal cancer has usually been attributed to its high dietary fibre content. But the recent research mentioned above suggests that phytochemicals such as ferulic acid found in whole grains may also reduce the risk of colorectal cancer. This has important implications for how we choose our dietary fibre. Many people substitute processed bran products for whole grains in the hope that this is a like-for-like substitution. But many of the important anticancer phytochemicals in whole grains are likely to be lost during the industrial processes used to make bran flakes. High fibre bran cereals are supplemented with vitamins and minerals lost during manufacturing but many more important micronutrients and phytochemicals are never added back. Bran not only lacks many of the biologically active substances found in whole grains but also the numerous beneficial interactions that result from the complex mix of substances present in whole grains [243].

<u>Low carb and gluten-free diets</u>

Official healthy eating guidelines usually recommend that between a third and a half of energy (calories) comes from carbohydrates. The main type of carbohydrate in plant foods is the polysaccharide starch. Fibre is also a type of carbohydrate, but without most of the calories. To differentiate fibre from starch, fibre is sometimes referred to as "non-starch polysaccharide". In plant foods, starch and fibre usually occur together and so people who adopt a low carbohydrate diet by avoiding carbohydrate-rich plant foods risk reducing their consumption of fibre.

Grains are usually the main dietary source of fibre and in the UK they contribute about 38 - 44% of fibre. This compares with 21 - 32% from vegetables and 6 - 16% from fruit [462]. So it is challenging to eat adequate fibre without also eating grains. Low carb diets usually fail to distinguish between refined carbohydrates - which many people eat too much of and should limit - and whole grains, which most people do not eat enough of. By making a blanket statement to avoid carbs by eliminating grains, low carb diets also risk being fibre-deficient. Diets that eschew carbohydrates from grains, such as low carb diets and the paleo diet, make achieving recommended levels of fibre intake more difficult and so increase the likelihood of diseases associated with not consuming enough fibre. Currently, only 9% of UK adults manage to reach the UK recommended target of 30 g of fibre per day [462].

In the average diet of UK adults, grains also provide about a quarter of dietary zinc and a third of dietary calcium and iron [166]. Bread alone contributes about 11% of the daily intake of protein, 20% of dietary fibre, 16% of thiamine (vitamin B1), 11% of niacin (vitamin B3), 12% of folates (vitamin B9), 16% of iron, 17% of calcium, and substantial proportions of a number of other essential micronutrients [108]. Hence people who avoid grains risk deficiencies in a wide range of nutrients. One group of people who are advised to avoid gluten-containing grains is those with gluten intolerance. This includes most grains and since grains are such an important source of micronutrients, gluten-intolerant people risk micronutrient deficiencies, and these deficiencies are not uncommon in gluten-intolerant people [463].

Diabetics are another group with special carbohydrate needs. The relationship between carbohydrate intake and type 2 diabetes is a good example where dietary advice is not necessarily the same between healthy people and those with a chronic disease. Diabetics are by definition metabolically different to healthy people. Their insulin production is reduced and so they respond differently to carbohydrates in their diet. There is some evidence that low carbohydrate diets may benefit diabetics, for example by reducing the need for medication [95], although the strength of this is benefit is still being debated [464]. Better advice may be to avoid refined carbohydrates but retain whole grains. In healthy people, a blanket recommendation to adopt a low carbohydrate diet that includes restricting whole grains risks significantly reducing intake of fibre and some essential micronutrients. An added risk is that reducing calories from carbohydrates will be compensated for by eating more saturated fat. As with any dietary recommendation, it is always important to answer the question: If I reduce this, what am I going to replace it with? Reducing the amount of carbohydrates in a meal risks leaving people feeling hungry, and of eating too many unhealthy foods.

## Sourdough bread and gluten intolerance

Throughout history, sitting down to eat bread has been associated with friendship and companionship. This is reflected in the word "company" which comes from the Latin word *companio* meaning "one who eats bread with you". Sourdough bread is the traditional bread in the Med diet. It is made from flour that is slowly fermented by natural yeasts and lactic acid bacteria (called lactobacilli) that originated from the air, rather than being made from flour that has been quickly fermented with commercial yeast. Sourdough bread causes far less of a spike in blood sugar levels than white bread (it has a lower glycaemic index). Hence it does not cause insulin levels to rise as much as other breads, so reducing the risk of insulin resistance [465; 466]. This may be because various types of acids produced by the lactic acid bacteria, which create the "sourness" of the bread, alter the starch in the bread and lower its GI compared to normal starch.

The more acidic (lower pH) conditions in sourdough have a second nutritional benefit by reducing "anti-nutrients" in the bread. Anti-nutrients are compounds found in various foods that deplete nutritional value. Flour contains an anti-nutrient called phytate. Phytate reduces the absorption of a range of important minerals like magnesium and iron. As the pH decreases during the fermentation of sourdough, enzymes that break down phytic acid become more active [467]. Reducing phytate in the bread means more iron and other minerals are available to be absorbed compared with bread made by industrial bread-making processes, like the Chorleywood process which has a short fermentation time and where far less of the phytate is broken down [468]. To break down the phytate does require the sourdough bread to be properly fermented for a long time and for this reason not all commercial "sourdough" breads have the same health benefits - some simply mimic the sourness by adding concoctions of acids.

Enzymes that break down gluten also become active during the slow fermentation of sourdough bread. Wheat breeding has created flours with levels of gluten which some people are unable to tolerate and this can lead to conditions such as coeliac disease [469]. [210] A small trial found that sourdough bread where the gluten had been broken down by lactobacilli and fungi, did

---

[210] https://sustainablefoodtrust.org/articles/growing-intolerance-happened-wheat/
https://sustainablefoodtrust.org/articles/sourdough-and-digestibility/

not cause any adverse reactions in people with coeliac disease [470]. However, because sourdough breads vary so widely, and so the amount of gluten broken down is likely to vary, eating sourdough bread is not considered a safe alternative at the moment for people with coeliac disease. Sourdough bread has many benefits and this makes it well worth seeking, but it is important to know that it has been made properly with a long, slow fermentation.

As well as the about one in a hundred people with diagnosed coeliac disease, many others also avoid gluten-containing foods. Some have a genuine intolerance to gluten, a condition referred to as non-coeliac gluten sensitivity. Others simply choose to avoid gluten as they think it will make them feel healthier. Nutritionists usually do not recommend avoiding gluten-containing products unless there is a genuine diagnosis of gluten intolerance. This is because cutting out grains means losing an important source of micronutrients and fibre. [211]

There is increasing evidence that gluten intolerance can present with many different symptoms. This means that people with gluten intolerance may be unaware of it because they have atypical symptoms. Although gluten intolerance is generally considered to affect the lower parts of the gut (the small intestine and the colon) there are some reports that it can also affect much higher up in the oesophagus, causing acid reflux. [212] Sometimes this reflux is just experienced as a sore throat (silent reflux). So for unexplained acid reflux it is sometimes advised to avoid gluten-containing products for a few days to see if this is the reason (although most acid reflux is not linked to gluten intolerance).

Gluten-free ancient grains are now widely available. These include teff, millet, amaranth, quinoa and buckwheat. The latter three are not true grains and are called pseudo-grains. They have very small seeds, which preclude refining and so they are defined as wholegrain. These grains are highly nutritious, climate tolerant and deserve to be consumed much more widely.

---

[211] https://www.scientificamerican.com/article/most-people-shouldnt-eat-gluten-free/
[212] https://glutenintoleranceschool.com/how-gluten-intolerance-causes-acid-reflux/
https://www.glutenfreesociety.org/acid-reflux-linked-to-gluten-intolerance/
https://www.everydayhealth.com/gerd/gerd-gluten-free-diet.aspx

# Whole grains as part of a healthy diet

In the US, only 17% of adults and 6% of children/teenagers consume recommended amounts of wholegrains (48 grams/day) and 18% of adults and 15% of children do not consume any whole grains. Whole grains are sometimes considered to be "heavy", and to cause bloating or sluggishness. But there is no real evidence for this [471].

There are many ways to consume whole grains. For many people, the simplest is to eat more wholemeal bread and wholegrain breakfast cereals. These are the main contributors to whole grain intake in the UK, wholegrain breads providing 44% of all whole grains and breakfast cereals 27% [472]. Most refined cereal products have wholegrain equivalents and so a simple way to increase whole grains is to replace refined versions with wholegrain versions.

Whole grains are a staple in many Mediterranean cuisines. Bulgur is a highly versatile and easy to use whole grain, and is highly recommended. It comes parboiled and dried, making it quick and easy to cook. Bulgur is widely used in Middle Eastern dishes such as *tabbouleh* salad and *kibbeh*. Couscous is made from more refined flour, and does not have the same health benefits. Other whole grains frequently used are oats, pearl barley, wholegrain rice and wild rice (a distinct but related species to normal rice).

If the thought of 100% wholegrain is too much, refined and wholegrain can be mixed, slowly increasing the proportion of the wholegrain version eg by mixing white rice with increasing amounts of wholegrain rice. It will be necessary to precook the wholegrain rice for about 15 minutes before adding the refined rice.

Lack of knowledge about whole grains and their health benefits are major hindrances to increased consumption. Some supermarkets such as Marks and Spencer in the UK are now starting to use logos to help shoppers identify foods that are high in whole grains [471]. A Danish campaign to raise awareness of whole grains with information and a whole grain logo raised consumption by 75% increasing whole grain consumption from an average of 36 g/day to 63 g/day [471]. This shows that the will is there for many people.

More bread is thrown away than any other food. Cheap industrial bread is worthless but good quality wholegrain and sourdough breads go stale with dignity and have many uses. Stale bread can be used for croutons in soups and stews. Breadcrumbs keep in the fridge and are good on top of bakes such as cauliflower cheese. In Spain, breadcrumbs (*migas*) are fried in olive oil and used in many ways. *Panocotto* - literally cooked bread - is a thick Italian soup with many variants and is surprisingly delicious. Left-over whole grains such as bulgur are not limited to savoury dishes and can be sweetened and served with dried fruit and nuts and orange blossom water for a tasty dessert. Transform leftover rice into rice pudding by cooking the rice for a few minutes with milk, sugar, and various combinations of dried fruit, lemon peel, nuts, vanilla essence and orange flower water, and spices such as cinnamon and nutmeg.

# Pulses

## Introduction

For the conscientious eater, finding a source of protein unsullied by its environmental or health credentials seems increasingly challenging. Fish? No longer sustainable and polluted with heavy metals. Dairy? Too full of saturated fat. Meat? Bad for both the environment and for health. The techno food industry has now come up with insects and cultured meat as the next big things. Minimal appeal. Quietly waiting in the wings, and ready to take centre stage to solve the world's protein problems are pulses.

Pulses are legumes that are usually dried. "Legume" is a broader term that, as well as pulses, also includes green beans and green peas that are eaten fresh. Although pulses are now mostly sidelined in wealthier countries, it was not always so. Chickpeas and lentils belong to an exclusive group of "founder crops" which along with a few grains started the whole of agriculture 10,000 years ago in the Levant (Eastern Mediterranean). Later, the Romans cultivated a wide range of pulses, and this was designated in family names such as Fabius, Lentulus, and Piso, which come from the Latin names for beans, lentils, and peas, respectively. Even the Roman emperor Cicero derived his name from his ancestors' cultivation and sale of chickpeas - Cicer in Latin.

Pulses were always prized because they store easily, and grow in harsh conditions, asking little from the soil since they fix their own nitrogen. But the appeal of meat sees societies quickly switch from pulses as incomes rise, as has happened for example in Spain and Greece over the last 50 years. Pulses have been described as "poor man's meat" and while it is true that the protein content is lower than meat (about 8g of protein per 100g in chick peas or lentils, compared to about 30g of protein per 100g in red meat [213]), most people in the west eat more protein than they require. (Some over-seventies are a notable exception and evidence shows that increasing protein intake above levels recommended for the general adult population may reduce older peoples' risk of osteoporosis and sarcopenia - muscle loss.)

To build all the body's proteins we need twenty-one amino acids. The body itself can make twelve of these and the remaining nine - the so-called

---

[213] https://www.nutrition.org.uk/nutritionscience/nutrients-food-and-ingredients/protein.html

"essential" amino acids - must come from what we eat. Vegans and vegetarians often complement beans and grains in a meal in the belief that these foods each lack an essential amino acid: no lysine in grains, and no methionine in beans. In fact, all plant foods contain all the different amino acids, although lysine and methionine are present in relatively low amounts in grains and beans respectively. The current view of some experts is that complementing beans and grains in a single meal is far less important than once thought [473]. As long as beans and grains are both consumed within a twenty four hour period, the body will have enough of all the amino acids it needs to build all its proteins.

Amino acids from plant proteins are generally not absorbed as well as those in animal proteins since some plant foods contain so-called anti-nutrients that reduce absorption. These anti-nutrients include various phytochemicals and some proteins such as lectins. Fortunately many anti-nutrients are destroyed during cooking and it is highly unlikely that a person eating a balanced diet such as the Med diet would become protein deficient because of reduced absorption. [214]

Pulses are composed of a dormant plant embryo and all the food the embryo needs to start growing. Hence pulses are highly nutritious, containing respectable amounts of protein and extremely high amounts of many vitamins, including B vitamins, minerals and a type of phytochemicals called phytosterols. Phytosterols lower cholesterol levels and this may explain why pulses reduce the risk of heart disease.

What really sets pulses apart from other protein sources is their very high fibre content (both soluble and insoluble), which is even higher than in whole grains [474]. Most people in the UK consume insufficient dietary fibre. The high fibre content of pulses, coupled with their low GI, makes them important allies in the fight against insulin resistance. The fibre and minimal effect on raising blood glucose can explain why pulses both lower the risk of developing type 2 diabetes and help manage postprandial glucose and insulin levels in diabetics and non-diabetics [474]. There is also good evidence that foods rich in dietary fibre reduce the risk of colorectal cancer.

---

[214] Https://www.Nutritionadvance.Com/Animal-Protein-Vs-Plant-Protein/

# Practicalities

The main pulses eaten in Mediterranean countries are chickpeas, white beans (such as haricot or butter beans) and lentils (mainly green lentils). In the UK, pulse production is increasing thanks to companies such as Hodmedod's, and locally produced broad beans can replace other pulses in many dishes - they are cheap, and frozen broad beans cook in 10 minutes. Pulses are a very economical source of many nutrients. Restoring the major role for pulses as protein sources would give the world a huge environmental and health dividend. As the world slowly makes the protein transition to more non-animal proteins the slogan "More beans, less beef" is increasingly important.

Canned pulses, pre-cooked and ready to use, are a staple for the Med larder. Canned pulses are cheap, but dried pulses are even cheaper. When buying dry pulses, look for a bright colour and seeds that are not shriveled. Dry pulses keep for several years in tightly covered containers in a cool, dark, dry place. It is best to use them within one year of purchase, though, since the longer a pulse is stored, the drier it becomes and this increases the cooking time and the difficulty of softening them.

## Cooking dried pulses

Here are simple steps for cooking perfect chickpeas and white beans from dry (dried lentils don't need pre-soaking):

1. Soak the dry beans in soft water overnight - this makes the skins softer (use filtered water if your water is hard). Add enough water, as the beans absorb lots.

2. Rinse and add fresh soft water to about 10 cm above the beans

3. Bring to boil and skim off any scum

4. Cook at a simmer (partially covered) until tender (approx. 50 min) (It is quicker in a pressure cooker.)

5. Leave in the saucepan (lid on) to cool (this makes them even more tender)

6. Preparing a large batch (eg 500 g dried weight) justifies the time involved. Unused beans keep for several days in the fridge (very useful as part of a quick cold lunch) and store well in the freezer

Seasonings such as garlic, onion and herbs may be added to the cooking water right from the beginning. But acidic ingredients (such as tomatoes and vinegar) are best added when the pulses are already tender, as acids and salt slow down the cooking process. Some recipes suggest adding baking soda (sodium bicarbonate) to help soften pulses. This is not recommended since it may make the pulses too soft. Also, baking soda is alkaline and some B vitamins are not stable in alkaline solutions (475).

## Digestibility issues

The main culprits that cause digestibility issues with pulses are fibre and a group of carbohydrates called oligosaccharides. These oligosaccharides are something of a double-edged sword. They act as prebiotics (food for beneficial gut bacteria), but some gut bacteria convert oligosaccharides into gases, leading to flatulence. Gas production often decreases with regular consumption as the gut adapts. When pulses do cause gas and bloating, eating small amounts of pulses, drinking lots of water and gradually increasing the amount eaten can help. Pureeing pulses can improve digestibility. There are various products on the market to help eliminate gas, although these are not a part of a traditional Med diet.

A few techniques during the preparation of dry pulses can also reduce flatulence:

1. Change the soaking water once or twice during the pre-soak.
2. Cook pulses thoroughly as undercooked starch is harder to digest.
3. Do not use the soaking liquid to cook the pulses.
4. For tinned pulses, drain and rinse canned beans before use.
5. Look out for skinless beans in ethnic shops – they cook quickly and are more digestible

If flatulence is not a problem, use the cooking liquor as it is full of water-soluble B vitamins. A recent innovation is to whisk up the cooking liquor from chickpeas and other pulses to use as a substitute for egg whites. [215] This is useful for vegans but not necessary when eating a Med diet.

---

[215] https://en.wikipedia.org/wiki/Aquafaba

# Eating

Pulses score poorly for some people in taste tests compared to other sources of protein. But the tastes of pulses are enhanced extremely well by the herbs, spices and other ingredients used in Med pulse recipes. This may require more cooking skills than cooking a steak. But the results are surprisingly good, from lentil burgers that taste as good as meat burgers, to the huge range of soups and stews that have pulses as a key ingredient. For diehard meat eaters, pulses can also be used as "meat-extenders". Roasted chickpeas make a surprisingly tasty snack.

Here are some ideas for digestible Mediterranean pulse dishes:

## 1.Purees

Purees are great as a filling for sandwiches or warmed as a side dish.

### Hummus

This classic chickpea puree with tahini is packed with goodness and keeps well in the fridge if covered. Tahini is an extremely rich source of phytoestrogens that may reduce breast cancer risk. If you have cooked your own chickpeas, ensure they are cool before blending them otherwise they may taste mealy. It is far cheaper to make your own hummus than buying it, and it will be healthier too.

### White bean purees/dips

Can be made with a wide variety of white beans (eg butter beans or cannellini beans). Basically, the cooked beans are whizzed up in a blender with milk-soaked bread and olive oil. Various combinations of garlic and herbs may be added. These purees can be served warm.

## 2. Jars and tins of beans

Spanish pulses in jars are usually very soft and tasty. This is a more expensive way of buying beans and you may have to buy them online if living in the UK. Some jars and tins of beans contain sulphites (sodium metabisulphite, E223) and these are best avoided as sulphites destroy thiamine (an essential vitamin for good brain health and energy [216]).

## 3. Pulse flours

Chickpea (gram) flour slows glucose absorption and is excellent for diabetics [476]. It can be used instead of wheat flour when thickening savoury sauces. (It does taste a bit beany so it is not so good when you don't want this flavour.)

---

[216] https://theconversation.com/are-you-getting-enough-vitamin-b1-to-help-fend-off-alzheimers-71327

# Nuts and seeds

## Nuts

Mediterranean nuts include walnuts, almonds, hazelnuts, pine nuts and pistachios. Nuts, are analogous to pulses in that they are dispersal capsules, in this case for the embryonic tree. These embryos must be provided with all the nourishment needed to start growing, and so nuts, like pulses, are extremely nutrient dense. They are high in protein and their energy source is mostly fat, mainly healthy monounsaturated or polyunsaturated and with very little saturated. The unsaturated fats are protected from oxidation with various antioxidants. Many of these are located in the brown skin, or pellicule as it is known. Just as paint protects an underlying iron structure from rusting by being exposed to oxygen so antioxidant phytochemicals are the protective coating protecting the inner parts from oxidation.

Walnuts contain exceptionally high levels of antioxidant phytochemicals in their pellicule and this may be because walnuts also contain exceptionally high levels of the omega-3 fat ALA, a fat very prone to oxidation. Walnuts are almost always eaten with their skins and so we benefit from these antioxidants. Peanuts on the other hand are mostly eaten without their skin. When options for nuts either with or without skin are available, as in the case of almonds, I would recommend those with their skin. Roasting nuts destroys some antioxidants in the pellicule but new ones also form due to a chemical reaction called the Maillard reaction. This is the same reaction responsible for creating the aroma of roasted coffee. The authors of a detailed study of the effects of roasting nuts concluded that low to medium roasting provides the best balance between health-promoting and potentially harmful nut compounds that can result from too much roasting [477].

Some nuts also contain high levels of antioxidants in their flesh. Almonds are well known for their high levels of the fat-soluble antioxidant vitamin E. This can act synergistically with antioxidant phytochemicals from the skin of almonds to prevent oxidation of LDL-cholesterol [442].

Nuts have well-established benefits against coronary heart disease. This was demonstrated in the Predimed trial. Participants in one arm of this study ate a Med diet supplemented with nuts (15 g per day of walnuts, 7.5 g of almonds and 7.5 g of hazelnuts). Participants assigned to this arm of the study were

37% less likely to have a cardiovascular event such as a heart attack or stroke. Nuts may benefit the cardiovascular system in many different ways. For instance, nuts are a good source of an amino acid called arginine. Arginine gets converted in the body into the gas nitric oxide and this dilates blood vessels, which lowers blood pressure.

Nuts also have cholesterol-lowering effects and this important effect has been confirmed in a meta-analysis of 25 RCTs [478]. This large-scale analysis concluded that eating 67 grams of nuts per day lowered "bad" LDL-cholesterol by 7.4% without affecting "good" HDL-cholesterol. This may be related to the high levels of phytosterols in nuts. Phytosterols are structurally very similar to cholesterol and can bind to the same transporter that would normally take up cholesterol from the gut into the blood stream. When the transporter is binding sterols it is less able to transport cholesterol into the blood stream. These benefits can only occur if the phytosterols are in the gut at the same time as cholesterol [479]. These studies suggest that an aperitif of a few nuts before a meal may have the unexpected benefit of blocking cholesterol subsequently eaten during the meal - another good example of the importance of considering the whole meal pattern.

Phytosterols are widely available as supplements but these will be less effective at blocking cholesterol uptake if they are taken outside of meal times. Phytosterols - whether dietary or from supplements - only have a limited capacity to reduce blood cholesterol, however, because the body eventually compensates when levels get too low by producing more.

Peanuts are not traditional in Med cuisine and are not a tree nut like the others but a legume that fruits underground. Peanuts are also usually eaten without their antioxidant pellicule and are often quite highly salted (in their native state most nuts are very low in sodium). This risks raising blood pressure. Nevertheless peanuts do appear to have beneficial effects against CHD [480]. Peanuts are particularly high in cholesterol-lowering phytosterols, which may be one explanation for this.

Nuts are recommended by many organisations such as the American Heart Association. Despite their high fat content, several studies have found that eating moderate amounts of nuts every day is not fattening [481]. This may be linked to their high protein and fibre content, both of which induce satiety. Almonds have particularly high levels of protein and fibre and when women were given almonds as a midmorning snack they were found to compensate by eating less at lunch [248]. So almonds are a highly nutritious snack food without evidence of leading to weight gain. It is not known if this applies equally with salted peanuts since saltiness can stimulate appetite.

## Practicalities

Nuts are designed by Nature to last well, they are always to hand and they are highly versatile in both sweet and savoury cooking. They are the instant Med diet snack food *par excellence* not only for their own health benefits but also because they can help depose the all-pervasive sugary options. Peanuts are usually the cheapest type of nut but other nuts bring diverse nutrients and help avoid consuming too much salt.

# Seeds

Sunflower and pumpkin seeds are popular aperitif foods in many Mediterranean countries. Sesame seeds are sprinkled on bread in some Med countries especially Greece. Roasted sesame seeds are used as a condiment, for example as an ingredient in *za'atar*. Sesame seeds are also ground to tahini that is widely used in Mediterranean recipes, for example as an ingredient in hummus. Sesame seeds are extremely nutritious. They are a particularly rich source of phytosterols.

Flaxseeds (also called linseeds) are one of the richest sources of plant lignans. Lignans are powerful antioxidants and they may protect against CVD [482]. Lignans may also help reduce detrimental effects of oestrogens including oestrogen-related breast cancer. There is some evidence that consuming flaxseeds reduces the risk of breast cancer and increases the survival of women who have had breast cancer [483]. These seeds are however quite resistant to digestion and so some may pass through the digestive system without liberating any of their useful substances, including their lignans.

Sesame seeds are also an exceptional source of lignans. Indeed, their lignan content is even higher than that of flaxseeds. Unfortunately, there have not yet been any clinical trials to see if sesame seeds help against breast cancer [484]. Apart from linseeds, sesame seeds contain hundreds of times more lignans than any other dietary source and yet sesame seeds have been ignored when examining links between lignan consumption and breast cancer risk [482; 485]. Since the sesame seeds have been ground up in tahini, the bioavailability of lignans is likely to be far higher than in intact seeds. The compelling circumstantial evidence for the potential benefits of tahini warrants clinical trials, especially for breast cancer prevention. A tahini sauce can be made quite simply by thinning tahini with a little water and lemon juice (and maybe with some chopped garlic). It is a great sauce for fish or vegetables.

# Herbs and Spices

Many of the best-known herbs such as rosemary, sage, oregano and thyme originate in the Mediterranean. They help give many Med cuisines their characteristic flavour. For instance, the main herbs in Greek cuisine are oregano, mint, dill and bay leaves, basil, thyme and fennel seeds. Cretan cuisine uses an even wider range of herbs and spices than mainland Greece, by including cumin, coriander and saffron, which are a legacy of invasions from the Byzantines, Arabs, Venetians and Ottoman Turks. Spices are also common in Moroccan and Spanish cuisines, and cinnamon is very popular in the Eastern Med for both sweet and savoury dishes. Herbs and spices can reduce the desire for salt and can even add a savoury note, as is the case with Spanish smoked paprika.

Herbs and spices find their way into many drinks, both alcoholic and non-alcoholic. Alcoholic aniseed-based aperitifs are common in many Med countries, appearing as *anis* in Spain, *pastis* or *anisette* in Mediterranean France, *sambuca* in Italy, *ouzo* in Greece, and *raki* in Turkey. Accompanied by a few olives or pistachios, this drink is part of daily life for (mostly) men in many countries bordering the north shore of the Mediterranean sea.

In Morocco, mint tea replaces alcoholic drinks as the national drink. Many other herbal teas are drunk throughout the Mediterranean region. For example, Mountain tea, a popular herbal tea in Greece and other Eastern Mediterranean countries, is made using the dried leaves and flowers of a plant called ironwort, which is taken against the common cold. It has proven popular during the Covid-19 pandemic in Greece. [217] Herbal teas in Greece are also made from sage, mint and various types of wild oregano. Thyme and rosemary are popular teas in Southern France and are recommended for their beneficial effects on digestion and respiratory problems, respectively. Herbs collected from the wild are particularly prized for tisanes because of their higher levels of phytochemicals. The intense sun, low water and poor soil on rugged Greek mountain-sides stimulate herbs to produce high levels of antioxidant phytochemicals. One herb found growing there is a type of

---

[217] https://greece.greekreporter.com/2020/04/20/is-coronavirus-lockdown-changing-our-culinary-preferences-for-good/

oregano called Dittany of Crete (possibly named after the ancient Cretan goddess Diktynna) and is regarded as a panacea [486].

Despite their widespread folkloric uses, there is still much debate about whether or not dietary herbs and spices contribute to good health. Some argue that the quantities consumed are unlikely to be sufficient to be of benefit. But the amounts consumed vary enormously between people [486], and between different cuisines. Throughout Med cuisine, herbs and spices are an integral part of many vegetable and pulse dishes and so consumption can be high. The small sprinkling of mixed dried herbs added to many western dishes does not reflect the ways herbs are often used in Med cuisine. In *tabbouleh*, parsley and mint are the main ingredients in a salad of bulgur wheat and *za'atar*, a mixture of dried thyme (or oregano), toasted sesame seeds and salt, is used on a daily basis throughout Mediterranean Middle Eastern countries as a seasoning for meats and vegetables.

The benefits of eating pulses and vegetables are supplemented by the herbs and spices used to flavour them. A caper sauce traditionally served with a fava bean dish from the Greek island of Santorini contributed most of the antioxidant phytochemicals in this dish [487]. Likewise, in a simple green bean dish from Greece called *fasolakia* the very high level of antioxidants in the dish was mainly due to the onions and parsley [488].

Drying herbs and spices further concentrates their often already high levels of phytochemicals. One gram of dried paprika powder (a reasonable amount for a person to eat in a Spanish meal) contains the same amount of carotenoids (5 mg) as a serving of half a fresh red pepper weighing about 100 g.

Herbs and spices are excellent at tackling the three Core Risk States. Many of the reported benefits of herbs and spices are likely to be due to their high levels of antioxidants and anti-inflammatory phytochemicals [489; 490]. Cloves, oregano and turmeric are particularly good sources of antioxidants. Some phytochemicals in herbs and spices may also enhance resilience in the body as discussed in chapter 10. Some spices also tackle insulin resistance. This is particularly the case for cinnamon, which has been found in studies to help control blood sugars and increase insulin sensitivity and so this spice may have a role in helping diabetics [491; 492]. Some herbs and spices may benefit health even before they are consumed. Marinating meat with herbs and spices helps reduce the formation of carcinogens when the meat is fried [442].

Although it is easy to demonstrate health benefits, such as anti-cancer effects, for herbs and spices in experimental systems, clinical studies have produced more variable results [493]. In clinical studies, herbs or spices are often given on their own in a capsule, and so are being given to people in a way that mimics taking a drug rather than as a dietary substance where herbs and spices are consumed as part of a dish. Since herbs and spices are usually consumed as one part of a meal, there are many possibilities for synergistic interactions with other dietary substances, something impossible to study in clinical trials with a single herb.

Another limitation of assessing herbs and spices as if they were drugs is that this ignores any effect of food preparation. When herbs and spices are cooked in dishes the heat and liquid - various proportions of water and oil - help solubilise active ingredients. Water-soluble components in herbs and spices will dissolve in watery dishes making them more able to be absorbed by the body and frying herbs and spices with fat will release fat-soluble substances. Rosmarinic acid is one of the most potent water-soluble antioxidant phytochemicals and is present in many herbs, not only rosemary but also sage and thyme as well. Boiling water is added to rosemary to make a herbal tea in some countries and this may enhance the extraction of the rosmarinic acid compared to eating the herb raw. The medical use of these "tisanes" is widely acknowledged in some countries such as Germany. Curcumin, the main antioxidant in the spice turmeric, on the other hand is fat-soluble and absorption benefits from it being with fat. Taking curcumin (or turmeric) in a capsule on its own with a glass of water is probably of limited use since very little will be absorbed.

Dried herbs and spices are essential Med store ingredients. Buying whole spices (such as cumin and coriander) to grind at home using a pestle and mortar is better for shelf life and flavour. A pot of fresh parsley or basil on the kitchen windowsill is extremely useful and much tastier than their dried counterparts. However, a few dried herbs, such as oregano and bay leafs, have even more flavour than when fresh. Sage, rosemary and thyme are great additions to the garden for all year round slug-resistant greenery and for wonderful Spring flowers. When using fresh herbs most are better cut just before use since this limits the loss of volatile essential oils. Adding them towards the end of cooking or just before serving helps preserve their flavour as well. A few, such as parsley and thyme are more robust and can be added at any time. My suggestion for a simple (additive-free) substitute for a commercial chicken stock cube is bay leaves, celery salt and soya sauce.

# Extra virgin olive oil

## The life force of the Med diet

Mediterranean food culture was born with the use of olive oil for cooking. As the 5th century BC Greek historian Thucydides said "The Mediterranean people ceased to be barbarians when they began to cultivate the olive tree and grape vines." Today, olive oil is poured over salads or on bread, forms the base for numerous dips, is used as a marinade for fish and meat, and for frying innumerable dishes. Olive oil enhances taste, and with its oily embrace it unites Mediterranean foods into sublime dishes. It promises good health, and it is the golden life force coursing through the veins of the Med diet. Med cuisine is inconceivable without olive oil. No other oil can match it.

## Olive oil is olive juice

Extra virgin olive oil (EVOO) is produced by simply crushing olives in presses. Olives are the fruit of the olive tree and so EVOO is really a fruit juice. The gentle extraction process retains many of the healthful properties of the olive fruit. It is the beneficial phytochemicals found in EVOO but not in seed oils that endow EVOO with many of its special health properties. Most other cooking oils are made from seeds - like sunflower seeds and rapeseeds - and these seeds yield their oils only reluctantly. Their extractions need chemical solvents and heat and these harsh conditions destroy many of the beneficial substances found in the seeds.

So is EVOO worth the extra cost compared to other cooking oils? Emphatically yes. Thinking of EVOO as a fruit juice makes it seem nowhere nearly as expensive!

## Health benefits

A number of studies from the 1960's suggested that olive oil helped prevent CVD. But these were only observational studies, and it was the randomised control trial called the Predimed study started in Spain in 2003 that really provided the most convincing evidence. Participants chosen for the study were at a higher than average risk of CVD because they either had type 2 diabetes or another risk factor for CVD such as high cholesterol. They were randomised into one of three groups: one group was advised to eat a low fat diet (the recommended diet at that time), the second group were advised to eat a Med diet supplemented with EVOO and the third group advised to eat a Med diet supplemented with tree nuts (almonds, walnuts and hazelnuts). Five years after starting the intervention, the results showed that compared with the low-fat (control) diet, participants eating a Med diet supplemented with either EVOO or nuts had a 30% reduced risk of having a heart attack, stroke or dying from one of these conditions [210]. The Predimed study did not restrict calorie intake or provide any advice of physical activity.

Compared with the low fat control diet, the two test diets supplemented with EVOO or nuts were quite high in fat, especially monounsaturated fatty acid (MUFA) (both EVOO and nuts contain high amounts). (See the Box below for more about fats.) Dietary MUFA reduces the risk of CVD, especially when it is replacing refined carbohydrates in the diet [494]. However not all dietary sources of MUFA are the same, and when the dietary source of MUFA is either pork or even ordinary olive oil this does not give the same cardiovascular benefits as EVOO or nuts [495]. This suggests that the high level of MUFA in EVOO and nuts only partially explains why eating a Med diet supplemented with them helps prevent CVD. This in turn strongly suggests that it is phytochemicals and other substances found in EVOO and nuts, but not in pork fat or plain olive oil, that are important for protecting against CVD. This conclusion has been elegantly confirmed by showing that when EVOO is stripped of its phytochemicals it is less protective against CVD [496]. Just as sea water is not pure $H_2O$ but also contains salt, iodine and other chemicals dissolved in it, so EVOO is a sea of fats (triglycerides) in which many important phytochemicals are dissolved. Many studies have now demonstrated that these phytochemicals are crucial for its protective effects against many different diseases. It is these phytochemicals that distinguish EVOO from all other types of oils, including ordinary olive oil.

---

**Fat facts**

Monounsaturated fat is one of the three main types of fats found in foods, the other two being saturated fats and polyunsaturated fats. A molecule of "fat" is composed of three fatty acids (FAs) attached to a "backbone" molecule called glycerol, a bit like an "E" where the horizontal lines represent the fatty acids and the vertical line is the glycerol backbone. This structure is called a triglyceride (from three + glycerol). The three fatty acids can all be the same or they can be different. Olive oil is "rich" in monounsaturated fatty acids (MUFAs), which means that the majority of the fatty acids that make up the triglycerides in the fat are MUFAs (about 55% -85% depending on the oil). Most of the MUFAs in olive oil are a type called oleic acid (named after *Olea europa* the Latin name for an olive tree).

The other fatty acids that make up the triglycerides in olive oil are various types of saturated fatty acids (SFAs) and polyunsaturated fatty acids (PUFAs). So although we talk about olive oil as a monounsaturated fat, more accurately it is an oil that consists of triglycerides where most of the fatty acids in the triglycerides are MUFA - mostly oleic acid - but that also has some SFAs and PUFAs.

Whereas the majority of MUFA in a traditional Med diet comes from olive oil, this is not the case in the typical UK diet. Here, most MUFAs comes from meat and meat dishes, cereal and cereal products, and potatoes and savoury snacks - these supply 25%, 17% and 12% of MUFAs, respectively, in adults [497].

Inhibiting oxidative stress - one of the three Core Risk States - is probably a very important way that phytochemicals in EVOO protect against CVD.[218] Oxidation of LDL cholesterol is a key event during atherosclerosis and an antioxidant phytochemical found in EVOO called hydroxytyrosol potently inhibits LDL oxidation. This beneficial effect is recognised by the European Food Safety Authority (EFSA). This validation now allows producers of EVOO to make a health claim on their products that EVOO protects against CVD. Very convincing evidence is needed before EFSA awards this kind of approval. Hydroxytyrosol is almost unique to EVOO - wine is the only other significant source. Consuming moderate amounts of these two cornerstones of the Med diet, EVOO and red wine, is an easy and enjoyable way to achieve the recommended daily intake of hydroxytyrosol and so help reduce your risk of CVD [388].

A second key process in atherosclerosis is inflammation - another Core Risk State. Indeed atherosclerosis is often now considered to be as much an inflammatory disease as a disease like arthritis. A phytochemical in EVOO

---

[218] Although many other ways in which EVOO protects against CVD have also been proposed.

called oleocanthal is now attracting a lot of attention for its anti-inflammatory properties. Oleocanthal is responsible for the distinct peppery bite at the back of the throat caused by some EVOOs. The name oleocanthal drives from *oleo* for olive and *canth* for sting. The non-steroidal anti-inflammatory drug (NSAID) ibuprofen also causes this peppery sensation and it was this observation that led to the discovery that oleocanthal acts in a similar way to ibuprofen. Since NSAIDs help lower the risk of CVD, it is possible that oleocanthal may act similarly. A Med diet supplemented with EVOO has also benefitted people with other inflammatory conditions like arthritis and irritable bowel syndrome [498]. However, normal amounts of olive oil may not relieve a headache since 50 ml of EVOO would only contain the equivalent of about 10% of the recommended daily dose of ibuprofen for pain relief.

---

**Unique phytochemicals in the olive**

Members of the same plant family generally produce similar micronutrients and phytochemicals. For example, oranges, lemons and limes - all members of the citrus family - contain high amounts of vitamin C, and all members of the cabbage family, from cauliflowers to kohlrabi, contain beneficial sulphurous compounds. By contrast, the olive tree stands alone as the only member of its family that is eaten - other family members, such as lilac and privet, are far too toxic to eat. This means that olives and EVOO are sources of some unique dietary phytochemicals, and of others found only rarely elsewhere in our diet.

---

The Predimed study has also identified other possible benefits of EVOO. One of the most remarkable results is in relation to breast cancer. Post-menopausal women (aged 60-80 years) from the Predimed study who ate a Med diet supplemented with EVOO had a 62% reduced risk of breast cancer compared to the control group eating a low fat diet [234]. Women who were assigned to the group supplemented with nuts were not protected to the same extent. Some of the world's top nutritionists in a joint statement on the benefits of olive oil in relation to breast cancer recently concluded, "consumption of extra-virgin olive oil seemed to be instrumental for the observed risk reduction" [494]. This statement is reinforced by other studies, which have found that it is only when women consume a Med diet that includes olive oil that their risk of breast cancer decreases. When EVOO is substituted with other sources of MUFA, the health benefits against breast cancer diminish.

The stronger protective effect against breast cancer for the EVOO group in the Predimed study than for the nut group suggests that there is something special in EVOO. The all-important breast cancer-protective substance (or substances) is not known for sure. One possible contributor is a fat-like substance called squalene (which is also found at high levels in shark livers). EVOO is also rich in anti-oestrogenic substances known as lignans. In Spain, EVOO is the main dietary source of lignans [141]. These substances are not unique to EVOO, and it may be that some of the more unusual phytochemicals found in EVOO such as oleocanthal, hydroxytyrosol and oleuropein are important for protecting against breast cancer. As well as their antioxidant and anti-inflammatory properties, some of these phytochemicals also increase insulin sensitivity in the body [130]. This means that the body needs less insulin. Less circulating insulin reduces the risk of breast cancer (see ch. 10). To benefit from a protective effect for EVOO against breast cancer, it is estimated that a woman should obtain 15% of her calories from EVOO (about 30 ml per day) since less than 5% of calories from EVOO conferred far less protection [494]. [219] EVOO may also help reduce the risk of some other types of cancer (such as colorectal cancer), although it is often difficult to know from the studies if the observed effect is mainly due to the benefits of an overall Med diet rather than specifically to EVOO [494].

The possible benefits of EVOO do not end with CVD and cancer. Some of the people recruited onto the Predimed trial were diabetic and the study found that participants who were diabetic and who were assigned to the group advised to eat a Med diet supplemented with EVOO were 22% less likely to need to start glucose-lowering medication. A person becomes type 2 diabetic because they develop insulin resistance, and olive oil may help here too since people consuming olive oil were less likely to be insulin resistant than comparable people who used other types of oils [498].

There are also promising indications for benefits against cognitive disorders. Dementia is often caused by vascular disease and so it is not surprising that a Med diet containing EVOO is linked to decreased cognitive decline and

---

[219] This calculation is based on a daily intake of 2000 cals. 15% of 2000 is 300 cals. Fat contains 9 cals/ml and so 300 cals is equivalent to 33 ml of olive oil/day.

dementia. EVOO may also be an important food in the Med diet for preventing Alzheimer's disease since experimental studies have shown that it reduces a build up of the toxic protein amyloid-beta which is strongly associated with this disease [499].

It is important to emphasise that the most significant benefits of consuming EVOO are achieved when it is consumed *as part of a Med diet*. Treating EVOO like a drug, and as something that can be taken without consideration for the rest of the diet, is likely to be a mistake. This was demonstrated in a study which found that the benefits of EVOO against lowering blood pressure are lost when the olive oil is taken in capsules [500]. One way EVOO may be of benefit as part of an overall Med diet is by helping to solubilise phytochemicals from foods and so make them more bioavailable to the body.

The extraordinary benefits of EVOO demonstrate that it truly is the golden life force coursing through the veins of the Med diet giving more healthy years. And so it will come as no surprise to learn that EVOO has also been found to be associated with extending lifespan [501].

## What about the calories?

Although it may seem counter-intuitive that a high fat diet could help control weight, this is exactly what studies on the Med diet have shown. Even when there is no restriction on calorie intake, participants eating a Med diet supplemented with olive oil lose as much weight as in other dietary approaches and in fact better than a low fat diet. Even more importantly, they retain the weight loss [502; 503]. This effectiveness of the Med diet for weight loss was acknowledged by including it as a recommended dietary approach when the new UK national guidelines for weight management were being drawn up in 2014. [220] However, despite the clear evidence for its benefits in weight control, the Med diet was air-brushed out of the final guidelines. [221] The reasons for this were never made public, but perhaps it was because of concerns that the Med diet constitutes about 40% of total calories from fat compared to UK guidelines which recommends no more than 35% calories. An analysis carried out in 2020 comparing many different dietary patterns has

---

[220] Maintaining a Healthy Weight and Preventing Excess Weight Gain Among Children and Adults Draft Guideline
[221] Maintaining a Healthy Weight and Preventing Excess Weight Gain Among Children and Adults NICE guideline Published: 13 March 2015 nice.org.uk/guidance/ng7

now confirmed that consuming a Med diet may reduce the risk of obesity and, very importantly, retain weight loss over a number of years [504].

An increase in hunger and a slowing of the rate at which the body burns calories are the main reasons why the vast majority of people on diets eventually regain their weight [505]. So key to a successful weight loss programme, and more importantly to one that sustains weight lost, is to control hunger. One of the reasons for the success of the Med diet in weight control is that it is rich in foods such as vegetables and pulses that increase satiety. Studies suggest that oleic acid - the main fatty acid in olive oil - also induces a feeling of satiety. It is thought that this could be being triggered by a substance called oleoylethanolamide which is produced when olive oil is broken down by the body [506]. There is currently a great deal of interest in testing if oleoylethanolamide is an effective anti-obesity agent, and clinical trials are planned. However, a Med diet probably induces satiety in many different ways and eating the whole diet seems more preferable than relying on a single substance.

## Shopping

EVOO is the olive oil of choice because plain olive oil has far lower levels of the all-important phytochemicals. Although EVOO is more expensive than other cooking oils, this is one expense that is really worth it – after all a bottle will still cost less that a half decent bottle of wine, and will last a lot longer. "Light" olive oil means it contains less EVOO, but it does not contain fewer calories!

The levels of phytochemicals in EVOO are strongly influenced by the olive variety and how the trees are grown. Olive oil connoisseurs will describe the colours from pale yellow to green, and flavours with hints of wild grasses, fruits and vegetables... One indicator of the potential health benefits of the EVOO you are buying is from its pepperiness since this is an indicator of its oleocanthal content.

It's probably best to buy EVOO sold in dark glass bottles or tins. This is a recommendation made by the authoritative University of California Davis Olive Center in the US [507]. Clear glass does not block photo- (light-triggered) oxidation of fats and phytochemicals. Plastic containers may be too porous to adequately protect the oil from light, heat, or moisture. Also, small molecules in plastics can leak into the oil further diminishing its quality [(508)].

Some people prefer unfiltered EVOO. There are no known differences in health benefits compared to clear EVOO, but there is some evidence that the olive particulates promote oxidation of the oil so reducing its less shelf life. Although EVOO may go cloudy in cold conditions, this is simply due to fats and waxes in the oil "freezing" and has no detrimental effect on the oil.

As with most plant foods, pesticide residues are sometimes detected in olive oil and so choosing organic is better [(498)]. Loss of biodiversity due to pesticide use on farms is of considerable concern although the impact of olive groves on biodiversity is little studied. Another recently highlighted concern is the large number of birds roosting in olive trees that are killed by vacuum devices used to harvest olives. Not all olives are harvested in this lethal way, and, in the UK at least, most supermarkets and other retailers give "bird-friendly" guarantees for their olive oils. This can be checked out at the Ethical Consumer web site. [222]

## EVOO in meals

Bread with olive oil is two thirds of the Holy Trinity of Mediterranean cuisine. The writer Tomas Graves, son of the poet Robert Graves, devoted an entire book on how *pan amb oli* (bread with oil) is rooted in Majorcan culture. [223] Olive oil greatly increases the palatability of foods. Even stale bread! And as noted by Dr Antonio Trichopoulou a leading authority on the Med diet "It would have been impossible to consume the high quantities of vegetables and legumes, which characterize the Mediterranean diet, were it not for olive oil that is traditionally used in the preparation of these dishes". EVOO is used in dips and poured over foods as a condiment. It is the foundation of Mediterranean vegetable cuisine, aiding digestion and heightening the flavour of vegetables, making eating them a real pleasure rather than a dutiful chore.

Consuming some EVOO raw is the best way to benefit from its phytochemical antioxidants, since some are heat sensitive. Chomping through a plate of raw salad ingredients without first dressing them with EVOO would, anyway, be unthinkable in the Med. While some commercial salad

---

[222] https://www.ethicalconsumer.org/food-drink/olive-harvesting-bird-deaths
[223] Tomas Graves. Bread and Oil: A Celebration of Majorcan Culture

dressings mask the salad's true flavours, olive oil by contrast helps liberate many flavour compounds so that they are better revealed and sensed. Olive oil is the salad *undressing* par excellence!

Dips based on EVOO can enhance the flavour of raw vegetables. Dips can be bought, but many substitute cheaper oils for EVOO. Homemade dips made with EVOO are likely to be far more nutritious. Some examples are *tapenade* which is spread on toast and whose name derives from the Provencal word for capers, the anchovy-based dip *anchoiade* for vegetables, *aiolli* a garlic mayonnaise which is the traditional accompaniment to boiled veg, eggs and fish, basil-based *pesto* and *pistou*, and *romesco* and *taratoor* sauces which include nuts. Not only do these dips have all the benefits of raw EVOO, they are also packed with some of the most nutritious foods you can eat.

Another way to eat EVOO without losing heat-sensitive nutrients is to add it to vegetable stews at or towards the end of the cooking period. This enhances flavour and defines Greek and Turkish *lathera* dishes, which are indeed lathered with olive oil.

Marinating tough cuts of meat with an EVOO-based marinade makes a virtue out of a necessity since, serendipitously, there is now good evidence that marinating with EVOO helps prevent carcinogens called heterocyclic amines from forming when the meat is cooked at high temperatures. More refined olive oils do not have this benefit. Bumping up the level of antioxidants in the marinade by adding herbs and red wine gives even more protection against carcinogens forming [442].

## Frying and cooking

Frying is very much a double-edged sword: on the one side it can generate dangerous substances, and on the other it creates highly desirable flavours and improves digestibility. With the possible exception of meat and meat products, fried food are not considered to be a health risk if consumed in moderation and not fried to a dark colour [509].

The type of oil used and its quality are important when weighing up the health risks of fried foods [510]. Frying subjects the oils to considerable chemical challenges. While gentle simmering of soups or vegetables keeps things pretty much at 100 C, frying raises the temperature considerably: shallow frying is typically at 140-160 C and deep frying at about 180 C. These high temperatures may cause significant chemical changes to the oil. The stability of an oil during frying is influenced by two main factors, namely the types of fat and the presence of antioxidants. Generally speaking, the more unsaturated a fatty acid is the more prone it is to oxidation at high temperatures. SFAs are more stable than MUFAs, which in turn are more stable than PUFAs. When fats break down they can produce toxic substances. Rapeseed oil is particularly rich in the PUFA ALA. This is prone to break down if repeatedly heated to the high temperatures used for deep-frying. One toxic breakdown product is a substance called acrolein, which irritates the skin and eyes, and another called acetaldehyde is classified as a carcinogen [511]. Since saturated fats are more stable than unsaturated fats, this might seem to argue in favour of cooking with saturated fats. However, the danger that saturated fats pose by raising cholesterol levels more than counters this argument.

Cooking oils contain varying levels of antioxidants. These help protect the fatty acids from oxidation. Sunflower oil for instance contains high levels of the antioxidant vitamin E [512]. Although EVOO contains only modest levels of vitamin E, it does contain significant concentrations of other types of antioxidants such as carotenoids and polyphenols [512]. At normal shallow frying temperatures, the antioxidants in EVOO protect the oil against oxidation and so EVOO is better for shallow frying than using ordinary olive oil, which has far fewer antioxidants. Studies have found that despite the presence of vitamin E, the fats in sunflower oil, many of which are PUFAs, are still significantly oxidised when the oil is heated, whereas the fats in EVOO are far more resistant to oxidation [512].

All oils have a so-called "smoke point" which is the temperature at which the oil starts to break down and give a bluish smoke. When used for shallow frying under normal conditions, the smoke point of EVOO is never reached and it is a fallacy that EVOO is not suitable for frying. EVOO is used almost exclusively for shallow frying in Mediterranean cooking and it is not used for deep frying, which is not a common process in Med cooking anyway. The hundreds of studies of the benefits of the Med diet, where food fried in EVOO is an integral part of the meal, are testament to the safety of this oil.

Another group of harmful substances produced in oils when they are re-used too often in deep frying are so-called polar compounds. These compounds are monitored by local government health and safety departments in commercial kitchens that use oils repeatedly for deep frying. Nature has trained our sense of smell to detect dangerous rancid oxidised oils that contain high levels of polar compounds. This is a not unfamiliar smell from fast food shops and pub kitchens, but it is not known if this indicates that recommended levels of these polar compounds are being exceeded. There is currently a good deal of advice from local governments to catering businesses on the correct way of disposing of their cooking oils but perhaps not enough monitoring of how they are being used, and it is of concern that hard-pressed local government workers are not detecting all cases of abuse.

Yet another potentially dangerous compound produced during frying is oxidised cholesterol and it has been hypothesised that oxidised cholesterol derived in the diet from fried foods is an important cause of atherosclerosis and sudden cardiac death [513]. Although this hypothesis awaits further testing, it is generally agreed that minimising oxidation of oils is highly desirable. The biochemist who proposed this hypothesis, Professor Fred Kummerow, recently died at the grand old age of 102 so he certainly worked out how to live more healthy years.

The frying oil used to start Med stews is usually consumed. Even when the frying oil is not consumed, substances from the oil are absorbed into the food and so are eaten. A food fried in an oil high in saturated fat absorbs some of the saturated fat, and so the risk of CVD from eating the fried food goes up. Pan frying is a two-way process, and nutrients can transfer from the food into the oil as well as the other way round. This occurs with frying fish - the most popular way of cooking fish in Med cuisine. In one study, frying sardines in sunflower oil decreased the level of beneficial omega-3 fats in the fish three fold because of loss into the cooking oil whereas levels of less desirable omega-6 fats from the sunflower oil increased nineteen fold in the fish. If the frying oil is EVOO this exchange can have benefits, as significant amounts of antioxidant phytochemicals from EVOO can be absorbed into fish fried in EVOO [3].

## Other olive oil products

Olive oil spreads contain less saturated fat than butter and so they may benefit people who are concerned about their saturated fat consumption. But they are no substitute for EVOO. Only a small proportion of the fat in an olive oil spread is actually olive oil (21 % in one leading brand). Also, the olive oil used is not EVOO and so the spread is likely to contain few of the beneficial phytochemicals that make EVOO so special.

Fish, sundried tomatoes and various other Med products are available preserved in EVOO and these are preferable to these products preserved in other fats or in water. When tuna is canned in EVOO it preserves more of its beneficial omega-3 fats than when the fish is canned in other oils or in brine [514]. This is probably because of the antioxidants in the EVOO preventing the omega-3 fats from oxidising. It is likely that some of the omega-3 fats from the tuna leach into the EVOO and so it would be a shame to simply throw out the EVOO. Although products preserved in EVOO are more expensive, by using the EVOO as well as the product, you get two foods for the price of one.

## Can rapeseed oil replace olive oil?

Rapeseed oil (often called "vegetable oil" in the UK and known as Canola in the US) is sometimes touted as a replacement for olive oil, especially in those parts of the world where olive trees do not grow. [224] Like EVOO, rapeseed oil contains high levels of MUFA. Rapeseed oil does not however contain the all-important phytochemicals such as oleocanthal and hydroxytyrosol found in EVOO [515]. Processing rapeseeds to extract their oil requires a series of harsh conditions including solvent extraction of the oil from the pressed seeds, and refining by degumming, neutralisation, bleaching and finally deodorisation to get rid of the sulphourous smell (oilseed rape is a member of the cabbage family). Not surprisingly these harsh conditions remove most of the naturally occurring phytochemicals. Even more traditional methods of producing rapeseed oil remove most of the polyphenols [516]. Hence rapeseed oil lacks the high levels of the antioxidants found in EVOO.

The benefit of rapeseed oil as part of a Med diet was studied in a landmark RCT conducted in the French city of Lyon. This study, which was started in 1988, used a margarine enriched with rapeseed oil rather than using the oil itself. Also, rapeseed oil-enriched margarine was used rather than EVOO since EVOO is not traditionally eaten in that part of France. The aim was to

---

[224] For a detailed debate on rapeseed oil versus EVOO see Hoffman R and Gerber, M (2014) Can rapeseed oil replace olive oil as part of a Mediterranean-style diet? British Journal of Nutrition 112, 1882–1895

see if the test diet could prevent a second heart attack. Participants who had had a first heart attack were randomised to either a group advised to eat a Med diet and the rapeseed oil-rich margarine, or to a control group [517]. The group receiving the Med diet and margarine achieved spectacular protection against a second coronary event - a 50 -70-% lower recurrence than in the control group. As well as its high level of MUFA, rapeseed oil also contains unusually high levels of the PUFA ALA. There is some evidence that consuming ALA reduces heart arrhythmias and this probably helps explain the benefits seen in the Lyon Heart Study [518].

As well as the Lyon study, there have been a number of other clinical studies examining the benefits of rapeseed oil. However, like in the Lyon study, these have mostly used *raw* rapeseed oil and so do not mimic the normal way rapeseed oil is consumed, which is after frying. Since the ALA in rapeseed oil is very susceptible to oxidation it is not known if heated rapeseed oil will retain the health benefits demonstrated in the Lyon study. A second problem with most of the clinical studies with rapeseed oil is that, apart from the Lyon heart study, they have not measured a clinical outcome such as risk of a heart attack but rather they have measured changes in *biomarkers* such as reduced LDL cholesterol. Although biomarkers are useful, and there have been some beneficial changes in these following consumption of raw rapeseed oil, they are in no way as definitive as measuring a disease outcome.

In relation to other diseases, there is no evidence that rapeseed oil has the cancer-protective benefits that are linked with EVOO. Also, one study suggested that rapeseed oil may impair memory and increase the formation of amyloid plaques in the brain which are implicated in Alzheimer's disease [519]. However, this study was conducted in mice and it is too early to say if this would also apply to humans. [225]

Rapeseed oil is often used for deep frying in fast food shops but there is the danger of oxidation if the oil is repeatedly reused. A number of years ago, the rapeseed oil industry recognised the potential dangers of unhealthy oxidation products from heated rapeseed oil, and developed modified rapeseed oils that are less prone to oxidation. These include a low-ALA version, and although this may be more stable it has also lost a major health component in the oil.

---

[225] https://medicalxpress.com/news/2017-12-canola-oil-linked-worsened-memory.html

Modified rapeseed oils are more expensive that standard rapeseed oil and so are avoided by many small catering establishments, which are operating on very tight margins.

Growing oilseed rape is highly profitable in the EU due to subsidies but this does come with an environmental cost. Oilseed rape fields are heavily treated with pesticides including neonicotinoid insecticides and herbicides such as glyphosate, and these are being phased out in the EU because of the harm they cause bees.

Overall, the jury is still out on the health benefits of rapeseed oil. The high level of MUFA and low levels of SFA in rapeseed oil does make it preferable to some other oils such as peanut oil. Rapeseed oil is also probably preferable to most other seed oils such as sunflower oil and corn oil. These are rich in omega-6 fatty acids, which are consumed at excessive levels by many people in the UK. So although rapeseed oil is probably a healthy option if eaten raw, care needs to be taken when using it for frying especially at the higher temperatures used in deep frying. But why settle for second best anyway when there is so much good evidence for the health benefits of EVOO?

## Other oils

Coconut oil is widely advocated as a healthy oil. It has recently hit the headlines as a possible way of preventing or treating dementia. But there is very little support for coconut oil from nutritionists [232]. Coconut oil is almost all saturated fat. The main saturated fatty acid in coconut oil is called lauric acid. Lauric acid has been touted as having health benefits because it is classed as a medium chain saturated fatty acid (MCFA). Some MCFAs do not raise LDL cholesterol like some other saturated fatty acids. However, although lauric acid is classed as a MCFA it behaves in the body more like harmful longer chain saturated fatty acids such as palmitic acid. In fact there is now convincing evidence that coconut oil not only significantly increases the levels of bad LDL-cholesterol, it does so to a greater extent even than palm oil which is high in palmitic acid [520]. And there is also evidence that it increases the risk of CHD just like palmitic acid [521]. According to one of the world's leading experts of fats, Professor Tom Sanders, emeritus professor of nutrition and dietetics at King's College, London University "the evidence is that coconut oil has the most harmful effect on LDL cholesterol compared to any other fat". [226] This is probably why the UK healthy eating advisory website Change4Life has concluded that coconut oil best fits within the food category "leave these on the shelf! ".

## Summing up

There is a good deal of misinformation on the internet about not using EVOO for frying. At the same time, some potential dangers of using other oils such as rapeseed oil and coconut oil are not sufficiently emphasised. The French poet Georges Duhamel wrote, "Where the olive tree gives up, the Mediterranean ends; with the olive tree stumble all the gods of Athens and Rome" [227]. It is a great shame that some people stumble over incorporating EVOO in their Med diet either because of its price or because of misinformation about its health benefits. I believe the evidence is now very strong that without EVOO the Med diet is deprived of a significant part of its life force. If you do not already use EVOO, adopting EVOO in place of other types of cooking oils is, in my opinion, the simplest and single most important change to make in order to benefit from a Med diet.

---

[226] Quoted in https://www.deliciousmagazine.co.uk/is-coconut-oil-actually-good-for-you/
[227] "Où l'olivier renonce, finit la Méditerranée; avec l'olivier trébuchent tous les dieux d'Athènes et de Rome". Georges Duhamel - Le Temps de la Recherche .

# Meat and Dairy

## Meat, culture and terroir

A few miles from Bordeaux in South West France lies the ancient town of Bazas. Along with its UNESCO-designated world heritage cathedral, Bazas is famous for its beef cattle. The main diet of Bazadais cattle is grass from local pastures, which even in winter provide hay for the barn-kept animals. No antibiotics or growth hormones are used and calves are raised by their mothers and allowed to graze freely. Surplus milk is made into a fine cheese.

Local restaurants under the gaze of the ancient cathedral only cook Bazadais beef and are always packed. Most of the people who go to enjoy the beef are ordinary locals. Of course, raising animals this way costs more. But the locals choose to prioritise their spending on consuming good food such as Bazadais beef over other temptations of our consumer society. These animals embody the local culture and landscape; for the locals at Bazas, this is a price worth paying for.

## Less but better

It is now widely accepted that the levels of meat consumption in the west are too high for environmental reasons (greenhouse gas emissions), for animal welfare reasons (factory farming) and for health (increased risk of many chronic diseases). The argument has now shifted to ask by how much meat consumption should be reduced and indeed if we would be better off not eating any at all. [228] The Med diet is not meat-free, but eating meat in line with the Med diet would reduce the amount of meat eaten to well below the current UK recommended guidelines of no more than 70 grams a day. Some argue that we should go further and completely abolish meat, as this would be best for the environment. But I believe this is rather like saying that we should all abandon our cars - which make a similar contribution to GHG emissions - and use public transport. It is unrealistic and divisive and a diversion from more constructive ways forward. I believe the level of meat consumed in a Med diet is the best target for the vast majority of omnivores in the west as

---

[228]A position for no meat: https://www.theguardian.com/environment/2020/jun/19/why-you-should-go-animal-free-arguments-in-favour-of-meat-eating-debunked-plant-based

there are strong arguments to both reduce meat consumption and yet to retain some.

This is little doubt that the recent trajectory of farming animals has now created a situation that is unacceptable; both because of the harm it causes animals and the harm it causes the planet. We need to reset animal farming within acceptable boundaries. The Bazas farmers demonstrate where these boundaries could be set to maximise animal welfare standards and ensure that meat eating is sustainable. Enjoying high quality, ethically sourced meat rooted in the local environment is not limited to Southern France of course. In the UK, "cow with calf" farming is expanding, [229] and the Pasture-Fed Livestock Association has been created by farmers, butchers and independent retailers to supply and market 100% grass-fed meat. [230] Prioritising quality over quantity is recommended by organisations such as the Campaign to Protect Rural England, and the Eating Better Alliance which has launched its "Less and Better" campaign.

Increasing numbers of people, in the UK and elsewhere in western countries, are switching to eating lower amounts of higher quality meat. [231] One survey found that in March 2017, 28% of Brits claimed to have already reduced or limited their meat consumption in the previous six months and 44% claimed to be willing or already committed to reducing or cutting out meat in the coming year. [232] Even the fast food industry is starting to respond by adapting their menus. [233]

Despite the trends towards eating less meat, the majority of people still choose to eat some, since meat, to borrow a phrase, is considered "Normal, Natural, Necessary and Nice". [234] These beliefs particularly reflect men's views, many of whom see eating meat as healthy, tasty and part of a more masculine attitude [522]. And today, for some men not choosing meat can instill

---

[229] https://www.fwi.co.uk/livestock/dairy/ethical-cow-with-calf-dairy-targets-premium-market
[230] https://www.fwi.co.uk/business/markets-and-trends/meat-prices/pfla
[231] https://www.theguardian.com/environment/2019/mar/16/peak-beef-ethical-food-climate-change
https://www.theguardian.com/business/2018/nov/01/third-of-britons-have-stopped-or-reduced-meat-eating-vegan-vegetarian-report
[232] A Menu for Change report
[233] https://www.bbc.co.uk/news/science-environment-47029485
[234] https://en.wikipedia.org/wiki/Psychology_of_eating_meat

a feeling of shame. [235] By contrast, one UK survey found women were more likely than men to agree that "using animals for food cannot be morally justified" and were less likely to support the idea that a healthy diet should always include meat [(523)]. These opposing views suggest that the wave of vegetarianism and veganism sweeping through western societies is likely to leave many men behind.

A complete ban on meat seems unrealistic and risks a backlash. For instance, a proposal by the Student's Union at the University of East Anglia in the UK to ban beef proved to be unacceptable and led to the reinstating of beef. [236] Similarly, attempting to impose a low meat cuisine through legislation is unlikely to succeed. Few governments are prepared to risk alienating their electorate for the sake of meat through punitive coercion such as taxation. In a BBC report from 2018, the then climate minister Claire Perry told BBC News it is not the government's job to advise people on a climate-friendly diet.[237]

Statistics demonstrate the enormous global impact of meat production on climate change. But proposals for global diets are a rather blunt instrument. One of these, the EAT-Lancet Commission report, was the result of more than two years of collaboration between 37 experts from 16 countries. This report mapped out a healthy and sustainable diet for a planet with a projected population by 2050 of nine billion people [(47)]. The report did give ranges of meat consumption in an attempt to respect different food cultures (between none and 28 grams of red meat a day and between none and 58 grams of chicken or other poultry a day). Nevertheless, this highly influential report was seen by some as a veiled advocacy of veganism since it suggests that for meat "optimal intake might be 0 g/day". [238] Concerns about the report's views on animal products raised the ire of some people. A vociferous outpouring against the report by the Italian ambassador to the FAO/WHO may well have been motivated by concerns for the Italian meat and processed meat

---

[235] https://www.theguardian.com/commentisfree/2018/aug/28/men-vegetarian-meat-eating-social-shame

[236] https://www.fginsight.com/news/student-backlash-prompts-u-turn-on-beef-ban-at-university-of-east-anglia-

[237] https://www.bbc.co.uk/news/science-environment-45838997

[238] The full sentence reads: "Because intake of red meat is not essential and appears to be linearly related to total mortality and risks of other health outcomes in populations that have consumed it for many years, optimal intake might be 0 g/day".

industries in a country where less than 1% are vegetarian [524]. He stated that a diet such as the one proposed by the EAT Lancet commission "would mean the destruction of millenary healthy traditional diets which are a full part of the cultural heritage and social harmony in many nations" [525]. This criticism led the WHO, an organisation that considers that sustainable diets need to be culturally acceptable, to pull its support for a launch event for the report in Geneva [525].[239] The FAO is itself not immune to these concerns and was itself heavily criticised for its 2006 report Livestock's Long Shadow. This report was seen as discriminating against the small farmer with a few cattle rather highlighting the dangers from intensive farming. [240]

These examples illustrate how a global one size-fits-all policy for meat consumption can encounter significant backlashes. So proposals for, say, a vegan world diet may well fit with academic models on GHG reduction but I believe it is very doubtful if this approach would find broad support. A more inclusive way forward is needed. This inclusive approach needs sustainable food production to be tailored to each country or region. Each country is best placed to find its own solution and develop a food and agriculture strategy in harmony with its environment, climate and the cultural food preferences of its people. Trying to make a one-size-fits-all policy in nutrition culturally acceptable across the world makes no more sense than calculating the average shoe size in a population and recommending that everyone wear that size.

## Health

The nutrition case for eating less meat is strong. Although meat is seen as the source of protein *par excellence*, dairy, fish, eggs, beans and nuts are all excellent sources. [241] With all these different protein sources, it is not surprising that most omnivores in the west eat more protein than they need - about 50% more in the case of the UK [526]. The human body cannot store protein, and excess protein is simply converted into energy. Using up precious resources of land and water to feed crops to animals whose protein we simply burn for energy is a very inefficient way to manage scarce resources.

---

[239] https://newfoodeconomy.org/world-health-organization-drops-its-high-profile-endorsement-of-the-eat-lancet-diet/
[240] https://www.telegraph.co.uk/news/earth/environment/climatechange/7509978/UN-admits-flaw-in-report-on-meat-and-climate-change.html
[241] See https://www.nutrition.org.uk/nutritionscience/nutrients-food-and-ingredients/protein.html?start=4 for the actual protein content of a range of foods.

## Animal welfare

There are also strong animal welfare arguments to reduce animal consumption. The industrialisation of raising ever more animals - factory farming - has brought with it huge costs to animal welfare. [242] Animal production has been pushed beyond boundaries of acceptability. Farm animals deserve a life worth living. And yet intensive animal farming systems mean animals are often raised in brutal conditions, conditions that most people prefer not to think about. For many farm animals their lives are in reality not worth living.

Many chickens, pigs and even cattle no longer have access to the outdoors with no opportunity to express their true nature for foraging. Studies suggest that feather pecking in both caged and un-caged hens is redirected ground pecking behaviour. Hens unable to peck as a part of normal foraging instead misdirect this pecking to their flock mates. As a result, many hens have their beaks trimmed, which, according to Compassion in World Farming, can cause significant trauma to the hens. [243] Many farm animals are herd animals but factory farming denies them the ability to socially interact, an important part of what makes their lives worth living.

Studies with farm animals show that concerns about animal welfare are not overly anthropomorphising. One study examined this by seeing how much effort a cow kept in a barn would make to access pasture outside. Despite having fresh food inside the barn, the cows were still prepared to push on a heavily weighted gate to get out. Because feed was readily available inside the barn, the researchers concluded that the cows were strongly motivated to access the outdoors and to engage in social interactions with other cows. Cows prefer being outdoors (527). Studies such as this suggest that one minimal boundary for farming animals is that they have access to conditions that enable them to express their natural behaviours. As long ago as the 1960's "five freedoms" for animal behaviour were defined. These are freedom from:

---

[242] https://theconversation.com/rise-of-the-megafarms-how-uk-agriculture-is-being-sold-off-and-consolidated-104019
https://www.theguardian.com/environment/2020/aug/04/one-thing-ive-learned-about-modern-farming-we-shouldnt-do-it-like-this
[243] Compassion in World Farming ciwf.org Frequently-Asked-Questions-Laying-hens.pdf

(1) hunger and thirst (2) discomfort (3) pain, injury or disease (4) fear and distress and (5) freedom to express normal behaviour. [244]

Just as DALYs (disability-adjusted life years) are calculated for human health, animal welfare can be calculated with ALYS - animal life years suffered - an "animal protection index" that calculates the number of years an animal spends suffering, and by MAL - loss of morally adjusted animal lives. This latter metric considers the living conditions of the animal (such as space), the age at slaughter in relation to overall possible life duration and number of animals required to produce a unit of food. Using this metric, raising poultry for meat and egg production was found to be worst for animal welfare, followed by pork and then beef [(528)].

A concern for animal welfare is the most common reason why people choose to become vegan. Veganism is a coherent position that avoids killing animals. Being vegetarian or "flexitarian" is acknowledging that some animals are killed. For vegetarians, male calves and male chickens present a dilemma, as they are still part of the food chain but not part of the vegetarian diet. Many male calves are simply shot at birth, as this is the cheapest option for a farmer. [245] Raising the calves for veal may be more acceptable but the market for this is very limited in the UK and is not an answer for vegetarians. New technologies that sex animals before birth may resolve the dilemma of what to do with male animals. It is now possible to sex the sperm of cattle so that only females are born, although the technology remains expensive. But maybe vegetarians would be prepared to pay the premium for dairy advertised as "free from all killing", much as buying cosmetics "not tested on animals" is important for many people. Recently, German scientists have perfected a way of sexing chicken eggs so that only female chickens are allowed to hatch and male eggs are used for other purposes. These eggs have now gone on sale in Germany. [246] The meat in fast foods is often from animals raised to poor

244

https://www.canr.msu.edu/news/an_animal_welfare_history_lesson_on_the_five_freedoms
[245] https://www.theguardian.com/environment/2018/mar/26/dairy-dirty-secret-its-still-cheaper-to-kill-male-calves-than-to-rear-them
[246] https://www.theguardian.com/environment/2018/dec/22/worlds-first-no-kill-eggs-go-on-sale-in-berlin

animal welfare standards, although - to their credit - KFC did admit this and is taking action to improve standards. [247]

## Consumers

In 1958, the agricultural economist Willard Cochrane scrutinized the downward spiral that results from farmers adopting ever more efficient farming practices. He showed that although these more efficient farmers become more profitable, other farmers then adopt the same practices. So overall production then goes up, prices - and so profits - go down, and this leads to ever more cost cutting to regain a competitive edge. This race to the bottom is now known as Cochrane's treadmill.

Breaking Cochrane's treadmill is, to some extent, in the hands of the consumer who demands better quality animal products. Although the agricultural trade agreements of some governments risk a race to the bottom, governments will be reluctant to implement policies that do not go along with the popular mood. So consumer attitudes are hugely important. This importance was demonstrated when consumers started demanding a reduction in plastic use following an item on the BBC series the Blue Planet that had highlighted pollution caused by plastics. For meat consumption, replacing quantity with quality hasn't yet reached this level of awareness. To borrow a phrase from the RISE report on EU Livestock: for meat consumption there hasn't yet been a "Blue Planet moment" [529].

Few would disagree that farm animals deserve to be raised as humanely as possible. If consumers demand better quality animal products, then farmers will adapt to support this demand. There are increasing signs that meat eating is embarking on this trajectory. But the question is: how much are we prepared to pay for it? Research indicates that consumers are willing to pay a small premium for animals (especially cattle) raised to high welfare standards [530]. But various options (subsidies/coupons?) need to be debated so that this doesn't discriminate against the poor.

---

[247] https://www.theguardian.com/environment/2020/jul/30/kfc-admits-a-third-of-its-chickens-suffer-painful-inflammation

# Health reasons for retaining some meat consumption

We evolved as omnivores. Throughout evolution the majority of humankind has benefited from meat as a rich source of nutrients. Meat is an excellent source of protein as it provides a good balance of all the essential amino acids. It also provides other important nutrients including vitamin B12 (which is not present in plant foods), zinc and iron. In the west, meat is particularly important for the elderly and others at risk of muscle loss and who may not consume enough protein from other sources. It is of course possible to be healthy by eating vegetarian or vegan diets. But this does require a certain level of nutritional awareness and avoiding meat will, for some, increase their risk of nutrient deficiencies.

# Navigating meat's risks and benefits

The other side of meat's nutritional coin is its links with an increased risk of chronic disease. If vegetables are the green light to healthy eating, then meat signals a rather more cautious red warning sign. Eating large amounts of meat is associated with an increased risk of some types of cancer, type 2 diabetes, CVD and Alzheimer's disease [531]. These studies generally find that processed meats (such as bacon, ham, sausages and salami) pose a higher risk than red meats (beef, pork and lamb) with white meats (chicken, turkey) of least risk. One recent comprehensive analysis estimated that for every extra 50 g of processed meat eaten per day, the risk of oesophageal cancer increases by 81%, stomach cancer by 71%, CHD by 42%, diabetes by 32%, colon cancer by 24% and CVD by 24% [85]. For red meats the increased risks were less: for every extra consumption of 50 g of red meat there was a 36% increased risk of endometrial cancer, 25% for oesophageal cancer and 22% for lung cancer. Moderate intake of poultry meat was generally not significantly associated with these diseases.

In 2015, the IACR classed red meat as probably carcinogenic and processed meat as carcinogenic. Processed meat was grouped in the same category as cigarette smoke. But this does not mean that both are of equal cancer risk to an individual. The classification is based on the strength of the evidence for the association and not on how many cancers the carcinogen causes. Eating bacon sandwiches still carries a far smaller risk of causing cancer than smoking cigarettes. [248]

Cancer risk is used as the basis for many guidelines for maximum meat consumption. The well-respected WCRF/AICR guidelines advise consuming no more than three average portions of red meat per week, which is equivalent to about 350-500 grams raw weight [249] (this is similar to the UK recommendation of no more than 70 grams per day), and very little, if any, processed meat [(532)]. There is generally no separate advice for people already at increased cancer risk although it is possible that this could be important. For example, because eating processed meat significantly increases oesophageal cancer risk, it might be worth thinking twice before biting into that bacon butty if you have been diagnosed with the premalignant state of Barrett's oesophagus (see ch. 11).

## Why does meat eating increase disease risk?

It is particularly important for a person to adhere to dietary advice if they have an increased inherited risk of a disease, or because of a physiological predisposition (such as Barrett's oesophagus). These are non-modifiable risks. But for meat, there are also many ways that its risks can be minimised so that a healthy omnivore can still enjoy meat's taste and nutritional value. So what are these modifiable factors?

### Red meat

Since it is colour that most distinguishes red meat and processed meat from healthier white meats, the red colour is hypothesised to contribute to disease risk. The red colour of meat is due to a protein called myoglobin. White meat such as chicken has about ten times less myoglobin than red meat. In 1958 the English biochemist John Kendrew working at the Cavendish Laboratory in Cambridge, UK reported the structure of myoglobin and demonstrated that tucked inside the myoglobin protein is a chemical entity called haem (Am. heme). At the heart of haem is an atom of iron and it this iron atom that binds oxygen and carries oxygen to muscle tissue. The haem in myoglobin is responsible for its red colour. A year after Kendrew's report on myoglobin,

---

[248] https://www.theguardian.com/science/sifting-the-evidence/2015/oct/26/meat-and-tobacco-the-difference-between-risk-and-strength-of-evidence

[249] https://www.wcrf.org/dietandcancer/recommendations/limit-red-processed-meat

his colleague Max Perutz reported the structure of the related red protein haemoglobin, which is found in red blood cells. Like myoglobin, haemoglobin contains haem. In 1962, Kendrew and Perutz shared the Nobel prize for chemistry for their achievements.

In 2018, the AICR/WCRF concluded that there is "limited but suggestive" evidence that foods containing haem iron are linked to an increased risk of colorectal cancer [533]. A reason for this somewhat cautious conclusion is that not all foods containing haem iron are linked to an increased cancer risk. For instance, haem iron is present at quite high levels in fish. But Japanese men and women who consume a lot of haem iron from fish do not have an increased risk of colorectal cancer [534]. This lack of an unconditional link between haem iron and colorectal cancer risk may be of some reassurance for consumers of the new veg-based burger produced by Impossible Foods that also contains a genetically engineered form of haem iron. [250]

The lack of an absolute correlation between haem iron and colorectal cancer risk highlights the danger of focusing on one factor without considering the bigger picture. Various dietary factors have been shown experimentally to mitigate the carcinogenic effects of haem iron, although conclusive evidence in people is lacking [535]. One of these is the very common dietary factor chlorophyll - the green pigment in vegetables. The chemical structure of chlorophyll is remarkably similar to that of haemoglobin, and (albeit to a lesser extent) to that of myoglobin. This observation led a group of Dutch scientists to discover that in experimental animals chlorophyll reduces the harmful carcinogenic effects of haem iron in the gut [536]. They speculated that when there is a lot of chlorophyll in the gut this out-competes the haem and so prevents the haem from damaging colon cells. The Dutch researchers found that if men who consumed haem also ate green vegetables their risk of colorectal cancer decreased, and the more chlorophyll there was in their diet the more the risk decreased [537]. The effect was quite small and no benefit was found for women. Although this study found an association between high chlorophyll consumption and reduced colorectal cancer from eating meat this does not prove that the two are causally related. There are many other

---

[250] A form called leghaemoglobin, which has been genetically engineered from a vegetable source. http://uk.businessinsider.com/impossible-foods-bleeding-veggie-burger-ingredient-gets-fda-green-light-2018-7

possible explanations why eating a lot of green vegetables might reduce the risk of colorectal cancer and so more studies are need before the protective effects can be attributed to chlorophyll. Calcium is another dietary factor that also binds haem and inactivates it [538], and this could possibly explain why high dietary calcium from dairy products reduces the risk of colorectal cancer. These studies demonstrate that although red meat and haem iron are risk factors for colorectal cancer there are many other dietary factors such as green vegetables and dairy that may potentially mitigate this cancer risk. So the overall risk from eating red meat is probably strongly influenced by the overall diet.

## Processed meats

Although pig meat contains much less haem iron than beef, when pork is cured it poses far more of a cancer risk than beef. This is good evidence that it is not just haem that is a risk factor in cured pork products. One substance strongly incriminated as a cancer risk in cured pork is nitrite. A practice that has been used for hundreds of years is to add potassium nitrate (also known as saltpetre) and salt to cure pork. [251] The potassium nitrate changes into nitrite during this process. Sodium nitrite itself is now usually used in place of saltpetre. [252] Curing preserves the meat, and - it is claimed - protects it from bacteria, particularly *Clostridium bacterium*, the causal agent for botulism. (However this assertion has been challenged. [253]) Nitrites also give preserved meats their desirable pink colour.

The benefits of curing come at a cost. During the curing process and in the stomach, nitrites combine with degraded amino acids to form compounds called N-nitroso compounds (NOCs). Some types of NOCs are carcinogenic and are linked to an increased risk of cancers of the gut and even at other sites in the body such as the lung [533].

There is a slight problem with this argument though. Many vegetables also contain high levels of nitrites (and even more nitrates that are converted in the body into nitrites) but there is no evidence that high-nitrite/nitrate vegetables

---

[251] About 80% of all processed meats are from pig meat.
[252] https://www.theguardian.com/news/2018/mar/01/bacon-cancer-processed-meats-nitrates-nitrites-sausages
[253] https://www.theguardian.com/food/2019/mar/23/nitrites-ham-bacon-cancer-risk-additives-meat-industry-confidential--report

increase cancer risk [425]. [254] So why should high levels of nitrites in processed meats increase cancer risk but not high levels in vegetables? The answer may lie with factors that increase the conversion of nitrite and degraded amino acids into NOCs. Frying is one of these factors and this increases the formation of NOCs in bacon even before it is eaten [539]. Once in the stomach, haem - which is in red meats but not in vegetables - also greatly enhances the harmful effects of nitrites [535]. By contrast, vitamin C and various phytochemicals - which are in vegetables but not in meat - inhibit the formation of NOCs [425].

Meat and processed meat are not only associated with cancer risk. In a study of over half a million participants, researchers from the US found that both red meat and processed meat increased the risk of a wide range of other chronic diseases including CVD, diabetes and respiratory diseases [540]. The US researchers estimated that for processed meats, haem iron and nitrites accounted for much of the harm. For the non-cancer diseases - where the carcinogenic effects of haem iron and NOCs is not directly relevant - the authors suggested that the most likely explanation was that haem iron and NOCs are causing oxidative stress. This implies that dietary factors that either reduce the formation of NOCs (such as vitamin C) or reduce oxidative stress (antioxidants) should reduce the harmful effects of processed meats. In fact, vitamin C (or a derivative of it) is frequently added to processed meats for this reason. So, once again, we see that it is the overall diet that needs to be considered in order to get a more accurate picture of meat's risks. Leaving out the nitrites altogether is possible. Parma ham and UK sausages do not contain nitrites and low or no nitrite bacon is now available. So does this give these meats a clean bill of health? The answer probably depends on another aspect of meat eating. And that is if and how the meat is cooked.

## Cooking meat

The way meat is cooked strongly influences its healthiness. So a good deal of the safety of meat is in the hands of the cook. Cooking at very high temperatures or cooking over an open flame, such as grilling (Am. broiling) and barbequing, carry the greatest risk. In a study of over two thousand women with breast cancer, red meat consumption was associated with an

---

[254] http://www.bbc.com/future/story/20190311-what-are-nitrates-in-food-side-effects

increased risk of breast cancer. When the type of cooking was examined, it was found that the association only held for cooking at high temperature and not for other cooking methods [541]. A greater risk from cooking at higher temperatures was also found in a study of US women where the risk for type 2 diabetes increased when grilled, barbequed or roasted red meat was consumed. There was no risk from eating stewed or boiled red meat [542]. Although this suggests that cooking meat at high temperatures poses the greatest risk, it does not completely exonerate meat cooked at lower temperatures since even this is often associated with an increased risk, albeit usually to a lower extent [533].

So how does cooking affect meat? Complex chemical reactions occur on the surface of meat when it is fried, baked, roasted, grilled or barbequed. The chemical basis for these changes was first demonstrated by the French chemist Louis-Camille Maillard. In 1912, standing before the French Academy, Maillard proudly described some of his new experiments. He had made the very simple observation that a yellow-brown colour develops when amino acids - the building blocks for the proteins in meat - are heated with sugars. This chemical reaction may not seem of great significance. But Maillard realised that it has far-reaching implications since meat and many other foods are teeming with amino acids and sugars. The reaction - now named the Maillard reaction - occurs when meat is cooked at high temperatures and it generates a huge variety of chemicals. Some like new flavour molecules, are desirable. Others are suspected carcinogens.

It was another observation, this time by the Japanese biochemist Takashi Sugimura, which led to the identification of perhaps the most important of the carcinogens that result from cooking meat. In the 1970s whilst on holiday with his wife, Sugimura noticed the smoke coming from fish his wife was grilling in the kitchen. He knew that cigarette smoke contains many carcinogens and so he speculated that the smoke from the fish might do so too. He soon confirmed this in his lab and this led him to discover a group of chemicals called heterocyclic amines (HCAs). Sugimura subsequently identified HCAs on the charred surface of meat as well as fish and he went on to show that they are products of the Maillard reaction [543]. In 1993 the

International Agency for Research on Cancer (IACR) declared that HCAs were probably carcinogenic. [255]

When fat and meat juices drip from barbequed meat and hit the hot coals below they generate another group of carcinogens called polycyclic aromatic hydrocarbons (PAHs). These then rise up from the coals and coat the surface of the meat. These same compounds are found in cigarette smoke. The main PAH, a compound called benzo[a]pyrene, is categorised as a carcinogen by the IARC. PAHs are also produced when meat is grilled or smoked.

Both HCAs and PAHs act as mutagens. This means they damage the DNA of cells. This is the first step -known as initiation - in cancer development. However, further changes need to occur before cancer fully develops. These further changes are caused by tumour promoters. The chemical reactions that occur on the surface of meat cooked at high temperatures are particularly dangerous because they generate not only tumour initiators, like PAHs and HCAs, but also tumour promoters. [256] These tumour promoters are also products of the Maillard reaction and include an important group of substances called AGEs (Advanced Glycation Endproducts). Although AGEs are found in many different foods, meat is the main source of AGEs for most meat-eaters. AGEs stimulate inflammation and this may be how they act as tumour promoters.

The pro-inflammatory properties of AGEs is not their only concern as they can also increase oxidative stress and insulin resistance, the other Core Risk States associated with chronic disease development [544]. All three Core Risk States are important in driving cancer development as was discussed in chapter 10. AGEs also help explain why cooked meat is associated with an increased risk of many other chronic diseases. For example, type 2 diabetes is strongly linked to the levels of AGEs found in cooked meat, and the more the meat is cooked the greater the risk of type 2 diabetes [545]. The risk of Alzheimer's disease is also strongly associated with consuming AGEs [442]. In one study, a high level of AGEs in the blood was shown to correlate with impaired cognition in humans and impaired learning and memory function

---

[255] http://publications.iarc.fr/Book-And-Report-Series/Iarc-Monographs-On-The-Evaluation-Of-Carcinogenic-Risks-To-Humans/Some-Naturally-Occurring-Substances-Food-Items-And-Constituents-Heterocyclic-Aromatic-Amines-And-Mycotoxins-1993
[256] Some studies suggest that HCAs can act as both initiator and promoter.

and enhanced amyloid-beta accumulation in mice [546]. When AGEs were fed to mice, they developed signs of dementia [546]. However, not all scientists are convinced by the role of AGEs in disease pathology. This is because of conflicting results both in preclinical and clinical studies, and because of problems with measuring the AGE content of foods.

In summary, a potpourri of Maillard reaction products develops when meat is cooked. Because these different products interact, there is unlikely to be just one factor that links meat or processed meat consumption to chronic diseases.

---

### How risky is bacon?

Processed meats can mostly be categorised into either "hams and salamis" that are not normally cooked, or into "bacon and sausages" that are cooked, usually at high temperatures by frying or grilling. Current recommendations to minimise eating processed meats because of their cancer risk do not differentiate between these two categories. However, one study found that whereas eating a lot of bacon and sausages increased the risk of colorectal cancer by 14%, there was no risk when all processed meats were lumped together [547]. So is there a greater cancer risk from cooked, compared to uncooked, processed meats? I will examine this by considering oesophageal adenocarcinoma (OAC).

The large European cancer study known as EPIC found that eating relatively high amounts of processed meat more than doubled the risk of OAC [548]. However other studies have not found a link between processed meat and the risk of OAC [549]. These contrary findings suggest that other factors may be involved in modifying the risk. So could the type of processed meat be one of the modifying factors that can explain why some studies have found a link between processed meat consumption and others have not?

If processed meat is a major cause of OAC, countries with high levels of processed meats consumption should have a higher incidence of OAC. But this is not the case. German and Spanish men, for instance, eat far more processed meat than UK men [550], and yet their incidence of OAC is much lower than for UK men - three times lower than for German men and over five times lower compared with Spanish men [301]. UK men, however, eat far more bacon than German or Spanish men, who instead prefer to eat uncooked hams [550]. Dutch men, who also eat a lot of bacon, also have a very high risk of OAC. This supports the hypothesis that the type of processed meat matters.

There are biochemical reasons why bacon could be a greater risk for OAC than hams. Cooking bacon greatly increases the formation of carcinogens such as NOCs and HCAs - well fried bacon has up to ten times higher amounts of HCAs than lightly cooked bacon [551]. AGEs are also produced in particularly high amounts in fried bacon. In a survey of 549 foods, fried bacon was the food with by far the highest levels of AGEs. Levels were nine times higher than a fried steak, which is itself considered to have high levels [544]. Ham contains far lower levels of AGEs than bacon - about a fortieth the levels. This is consistent with the far lower risk of OAC in ham eaters such as the Spanish. Mechanistically, AGEs are considered a risk factor OAC, since AGEs are pro-inflammatory and inflammation in the oesophagus is a driver for OAC.

It is interesting therefore to speculate that the very high levels of NOCs, HACs and AGEs in fried bacon help explain why UK men have the highest rates of OAC in the world. Although there are no epidemiological studies to support or refute this idea, I would suggest that eating bacon is a risky business, especially if you have the precancerous state of Barrett's oesophagus. Bacon is highly prized by many meat-eaters and many would be unwilling to give up eating it. So frying only lightly may at least reduce the risks.

## Why eating meat the Med way reduces the risks from cooked meat

Much is now known about how to control the Maillard reaction and so how to reduce the formation of dangerous Maillard reaction products such as HCAs and AGEs. Probably the most effective way is by reducing the degree of "doneness" of meat by controlling cooking time and temperature. Cooking processes like oven roasting, barbequing and grilling that expose meat to a naked flame, generate far higher temperatures than pan frying or stewing, and are linked to a greater risk of cancer. Appreciable amounts of HCAs only begin to form above 150°C which is the temperature of shallow frying and the most common cooking technique for meat in Med cuisine. Levels increase rapidly at the higher temperatures associated with grilling, barbequing and deep frying. Cooking meat over an open flame truly in-flames it.

Far lower levels of HCAs are produced with stewing, also common in Med cuisine, which is mostly at about 100°C. Stewing meats at these lower temperature also reduces the formation of AGEs. Vegetables added as part of a meat stew add antioxidants that reduce the formation of HCAs and AGEs. Other beneficial phenolic compounds commonly added to Mediterranean stews, such as red pepper, rosemary, black pepper, garlic and wine, have been shown to reduce the formation of HCAs and AGEs. Sulphur compounds in onions and garlic also reduce the formation of harmful HACs when pork is cooked [552]. The potential significance of this finding is enormous since frying an onion is the most common first step in Mediterranean savoury cooking.

Steps to prevent Maillard Reaction Products can start even before cooking by first marinating the meat. Marinating to tenderise tough (and inexpensive) meat is common in traditional Med cuisine, although in our time-pressured society marinating is now far less common. A typical marinade in Med cuisine includes EVOO, an acid like lemon juice, vinegar or wine, and herbs and spices. Cinnamon, garlic and rosemary have all been found to inhibit the formation of AGEs. The acidity of the marinade and the antioxidant properties of herbs, spices and EVOO all reduce harmful products forming by the Maillard reaction. EVOO is far more effective than ordinary olive oil since it contains more antioxidants [442].

The Maillard reaction is responsible for generating flavour compounds as well as for generating harmful compounds. However, this does not have to mean that flavour is compromised since there is evidence that different chemical pathways generate HCAs and flavour molecules and that it is possible to suppress the HCA-generating pathway without compromising the flavour-generating pathway [553]. We also enjoy the flavour produced by the Maillard reaction in many foods other than meat. Fortunately these foods, like roasted coffee and the crust of bread, have lower levels of dangerous Maillard Reaction Products than meat.

Eating less meat is the most direct way of reducing its potential harms. When planning a meal, the first thing many omnivores think about is the meat dish. "What's for dinner?" is more often than not answered by the meat course: "chicken", "beef" etc. It's unlikely to be "Brussels sprouts" or "cabbage". For many omnivores, meat defines the main meal of the day.

Eating meat every day is not part of the Med diet; the weekly allowance only equates to about one to two portions a week (although there is no agreed definition of precisely how much). Eating small quantities of meat is perfectly compatible with a healthy lifestyle. Healthy Greek physically active men eating a traditional Med diet consumed only about 35 grams per day of red meat and chicken combined [554]. The disproportionately high number of meat recipes in most Med diet cookery books gives a distorted impression of meat consumption in the Med diet. But rather than taking centre stage, meat often acts as a flavouring and is mixed in stews with other ingredients such as pulses and vegetables. This means that a small weekly allowance can be spread over several meals. The Med diet is full of recipes that use small quantities of meat to create maximum flavour. As well as many meat stews, there are also zero meat recipes often based on lentils and other pulses that are perfectly good substitutes for hamburgers. [257]

One hugely beneficial legacy of the frugal Med diet is the enormous range of meat-based recipes that maintain the yummy umami flavour of meat even when it is only one of several ingredients in the dish. This is true of meat and bean stews from the South of France (such as *cassoulet*) and Spain (such as *cocido*), Greek *moussaka*, fruit and meat tagines of Morocco and *kibbeh* (mince with bulgur worked into it). Maintaining an umami taste is very important for transitioning to a lower-meat diet, and some sources that can be added to low-meat stews are shown in the Box below.

---

**Ingredients that provide an umami (savoury) taste**

- anchovies; black olives; parmesan, balsamic vinegar, ceps, tomato paste, tomato ketchup
- smoked paprika (a substitute for chorizo)
- various Chinese sauces: soy sauce, mushroom sauce, black beans, miso; umami sauce
- create a savoury stock using soya sauce, celery salt and other umami flavours

---

[257] A good vegetarian cookery site is https://www.forksoverknives.com/#

(Many of these ingredients are also salty, so you may need to reduce the amount of salt in the dish when adding these ingredients.)

In summary, here are some key aspects of eating meat the Mediterranean way:

- fresh meat only (red or white) and avoid meat that has been preserved with chemicals (nitrites)
- if possible, marinate the meat prior to cooking
- if fried, this is with EVOO, for a short period only - and only until a light brown colour develops
- the meat is cooked at relatively low temperatures - which means in stews, boiled or in the oven at less than 140 C
- the meat is cooked together with foods high in antioxidants - eg fruit, vegetables, herbs and spices
- no more than 100 grams is eaten at a serving and no more than two servings a week

These considerations represent a "Mediterranean Meat Eating Pattern". This is analogous to the "Mediterranean Drinking Pattern" that has shown that people who comply with the traditional Mediterranean way of drinking (small amounts of red wine with a meal) do not have the health risks of people who drink in a more typically "western" way (see section on Alcohol). No analogous studies have been carried out with a Mediterranean Meat Eating Pattern, but it would be of great interest to determine if people who follow this way of eating meat do not have the health risks associated with other ways of eating meat.

## Choosing meat

Producing meat to a high standard is a barometer of a society that respects its food. The cattle raised around the French town of Bazas epitomise this concern for quality. Across France, standards for local meat production are maintained with the status of Protected Geographical Indication. More generally in other countries, "organic" status is considered to represent a quality product. Within the EU, meat from ruminants (cattle and sheep) can be designated as "organic" when the animal's diet is least 60% organically grown forage, which means fresh grass, hay or silage. For pigs and poultry, the amount of forage to be consumed is not specified in EU regulations. The feed must be organic but this can be grain or protein crops such as soya beans rather than grass. (This raises the possibility that the soya is from deforested land in Brazil and this is discussed in ch. 14.) In the UK, the "organic" standard as awarded by the Soil Association specifies that the animals must have been allowed time outdoors to eat natural pastures, although the extent of this varies between countries. [258] Having access to pastures increases animal welfare standards and slower growing breeds are often chosen, so giving the animal a longer life. Choosing organic meat also avoids the steroid growth hormones and the presence of antibiotics that can be an undesirable legacy of poor farming practices.

The composition of meat is strongly influenced by what the animal ate. But since the proportion of forage to non-forage varies quite widely even for meat designated "organic", it is not surprisingly that there can be quite wide variation in meat composition. The influence of an animal's diet is most clearly shown by the fat composition. The most detailed study so far conducted found that the meat from livestock raised on organic feed contains a lower proportion of types of saturated fatty acids that raise cholesterol [259] than the meat from animals raised on conventional feed [555]. The proportion of fat in the meat was however similar between organically and conventionally fed animals.

Organically produced beef, lamb or pork was also found to have a higher proportion of desirable omega-3 fatty acids [555]. Meat is not usually thought of as an important dietary source of omega-3 fats. And it's true that fish and especially oily fish are by far the richest dietary sources of the so-called long chain omega-3 fatty acids EPA and DHA. [260] Meat and poultry contain five to fifteen times less of these important fatty acids. However, a typical "western diet" includes far more meat than fish, and so in the overall diet meat can make a significant contribution to the dietary intake of EPA and DHA - up to half in some estimates [556]. So, especially for low or no fish eaters, choosing organic meat can provide a significant part of overall omega-3 fat intake.

---

[258] Soil Association. Feeding the animals that feed us.
[259] These are lauric acid, myristic acid and palmitic acid (which have chains of 12, 14 and 16 carbons respectively)
[260] There is also a third member of this long chain omega-3 fatty acids family called DPA.

The EPA and DHA content of meat is strongly influence by what the animal ate. Pasture fed cattle and sheep do not usually eat EPA and DHA directly but rather they eat the precursor fatty acid ALA found in pasture plants, a small amount of which they can convert into EPA and DHA [557]. Protein concentrates and grains contain only low amounts of ALA and so animals eating concentrates produce less EPA and DHA. In one study, beef from grass-fed livestock contained five times as much EPA and twice as much DHA as meat from animals fed grains [558]. When we eat this meat, this translates into higher amounts of these fatty acids in our bodies. This was shown by the substantially higher EPA and DHA levels in study participants who ate meat from grass-fed animals compared with participants eating meat from concentrate-fed animals [559]. [261]

The omega-3 fatty acid composition of poultry meat and eggs is particularly sensitive to what the animal ate. Even most organic chickens (and pigs) are fed mainly protein concentrates, such as soya products, which are low in ALA. Hence the meat from these animals is low in EPA and DHA even though they are "organic". The idyllic scene of chickens pecking around the farmyard has mostly disappeared. Which is a shame since the weeds and insects the chickens ate were transformed into meat and eggs very high in omega-3 fats. In one study, the eggs from free range Greek chickens were found to contain ten times the EPA and DHA found in the eggs from their less fortunate industrial cousins fed grains [560]. These examples clearly demonstrate that quality meat from animals allowed to forage is nutritionally healthier, substantiating the wise saying that "you are what you eat *eats*".

## Dairy

The benefits of remote lush mountain pastures for grazing dairy animals would have been wasted without cheese, an invention which allowed bulky, perishable milk to be converted into a product that keeps well and transports easily. Making cheeses and yogurt usually includes a fermentation step, which converts the milk sugar lactose into lactic acid that acts as a preservative. This helps increase keeping properties and allowed cheese and yogurt to become dietary staples even in hot Mediterranean countries.

---

[261] https://www.pastureforlife.org is a useful resource for buying grass-fed meat

In the cooler and flatter parts of Northern Europe, transporting milk was more straightforward as pastures were usually closer to habitations. But there was another barrier to consuming milk. And that was the problem of digesting it. During early childhood the gene that enables lactose to be metabolised is normally switched off. So when milk is drunk lactose hangs around unmetabolised in the gut and is fermented by bacteria into gases that cause uncomfortable cramps. Luckily, a few early humans in Northern Europe evolved to retain the gene needed to metabolise lactose. Since the lactose was broken down when they drank milk, there was no lactose left for gut bacteria to convert into gases, and no cramps. These genetically advantaged people thrived on the milk and became the ancestors for most native North Europeans.

Unlike their North European counterparts, Mediterranean people transformed most of their highly perishable milk into yogurt and cheese. These milk products contain much less lactose as it has been used up during fermentation. So there was far less evolutionary selection pressure for Mediterraneans to develop lactose tolerance. To this day, large parts of the populations in Mediterranean Europe, and in other parts of the world, remain lactose intolerant and so consume less milk than people in Northern Europe.

## Healthy dairy

Serendipitously for Mediterraneans, cheese and yogurt - the main types of dairy consumed in the Med diet - are particularly healthy. These fermented dairy foods help support a healthy gut microbiota. This reduces the risk of chronic inflammation in the gut, which, as described earlier, is a risk factor for many chronic diseases. Hence lowering chronic inflammation could be an important reason for the health benefits of cheese and yogurt compared with other types of dairy [561].

All dairy products are highly nutritious. After all, milk is the sole nourishment a mother provides for the early development of her offspring. Dairy products provide fat and protein (mostly proteins called whey and casein) and micronutrients, especially calcium, iodine and some vitamins. Some people who avoid dairy products altogether, such as those on a paleo diet, have been found to be at increased risk of deficiencies in calcium and iodine since finding adequate alternative sources can be problematic [257].

Full fat dairy produce is more calorific than low fat and this is one reason why it is often advised to choose low fat versions. However, it is always important to consider what the replacement is. It is often the case with low fat yogurts for example that the calories are added back as sugar. Some studies in fact show no greater weight increase in people consuming full fat dairy than those on low or no dairy [562]. This could be because people eating full fat dairy compensate by eating less sugar and other calorific foods.

Switching from full fat dairy to low/no fat also reduces dairy as a source of the wide range nutrients found in the milk fat. Some of these such as the fat soluble vitamins A, D and E are readily obtained from other sources, but dairy fat is also a particularly good source of some other nutrients such as vitamin K2 and various unusual fatty fats that are less readily obtained from other sources. [262] A high dietary intake of some of these fatty acids is associated with a reduced risk of chronic diseases [563]. So this is an argument against switching from full fat to low fat dairy.

The major spectre hanging over dairy - and the main argument used for switching to low or no fat dairy - revolves around saturated fat. This is because of links between saturated fat and an increased risk of CVD. In the UK, health guidelines recommend that an average man aged 19-64 years should consume no more than 30 grams of saturated fat a day and an average woman aged 19-64 years should consume no more than 20 grams of saturated fat a day. [263] About 60% of the fats in dairy are saturated fats and dairy contributes about a quarter of daily saturated fat intake in the average UK diet. (Other major sources of saturated fat are meat and cereal products like biscuits and cakes.) Hence many guidelines, such as those issued by Public Health England, recommend low fat dairy in order to help keep overall dietary saturated fat within recommended limits and so reduce the risk of CVD.

But this advice is now being strongly contested. In 2016, a group of European scientists from universities and research institutes (and excluding food industry interests) met in Denmark to develop a consensus position on dairy and health [564]. Their conclusion was that there is no good evidence that eating dairy products increases the risk of CVD (stroke and coronary heart disease) or type 2 diabetes [565]. More recent studies support this conclusion.

---

[262] These fatty acids include conjugated linoleic acid and palmitoleic acid.
[263] https://www.nhs.uk/live-well/eat-well/eat-less-saturated-fat/

For instance in 2018, the results from a nine year study of over 135,000 people in 21 countries showed that people with the highest dairy intake (more than two servings per day) developed less CVD than people consuming no dairy (3.5% of people, versus 4.9% of people not consuming dairy) and the high intake group also had a lower rate of stroke (1.2% versus 2.9%) and death (3.4% versus 5.6%) than the no dairy group [566]. The most likely to explanation for this is that people who avoid dairy simply replace this source of saturated fat with other less healthy sources such as meat or biscuits. The epidemiological studies demonstrate that even full fat dairy is not associated with an increased risk of CVD. The US nutritionist Dr Dariush Mozaffarian, one of the world's leading experts in this field, has concluded, "There is no prospective human evidence that people who eat low-fat dairy do better than people who eat whole-fat dairy." [264]

So how can the saturated fat paradox be resolved? After all, full fat dairy is high in saturated fat, saturated fat increases LDL cholesterol in the blood and high LDL cholesterol is linked to an increased risk of CVD [567]. Moreover, the advice to limit saturated fat because of its links with heart disease is based on 60 years of research starting with the pioneering work of Ancel Keys in late 1950's, and is a recommendation endorsed to this day by leading scientists such as Prof Bruce Griffin from the University of Surrey, UK and Prof Walter Willett from the Harvard School of Public Health, US. [564]

The saturated fat paradox can be resolved by concluding that what matters for health in addition to the *amount* of saturated fat is its *food source*. Current evidence suggests that saturated fat from meat does not necessarily have the same effects in the body as saturated fat from dairy. For example, a 10-year study provided evidence that consuming saturated fatty acids from dairy foods was associated with a decreased risk of CVD, while consuming the same amount of saturated fat from meat was associated with increased CVD risk [568].

Within the general category of "dairy", the evidence for a health benefit is strongest for yogurt and cheese, and some studies have found that not only is there no risk from dairy (within reasonable limits) for CVD but that fermented dairy products may even be protective against CVD [569]. From

---

[264] http://time.com/4279538/low-fat-milk-vs-whole-milk/

studies such as this, the Denmark meeting of scientists concluded that rather than focusing on the level of saturated fat in dairy, the emphasis should be on the *type* of dairy. Their broad consensus was that fermented dairy - yogurt and cheese - are not a risk factor for CVD and diabetes, and indeed may be protective, butter is mostly found to be neutral or not protective [265] and milk occupies the middle ground. This ranking is supported by other experts such as Dr Mozaffarian [570]. In summary, studies have concluded that meat as a source of saturated fat is worse than dairy and within all types of dairy, cheese and yogurt are protective whereas butter may have neutral or detrimental effects.

These differences cannot be fully explained by simply postulating that there are different types of saturated fats found in different types of dairy (and meat). This is because butter and yogurt made from the same milk contain more-or-less the same saturated fat composition. So how can two foods with the same saturated fat content have different effects in the body?

There is increasing evidence that an important cause for these differences is the physical arrangement of the saturated fat in the food. The physical arrangement of nutrients in foods is referred to as the food matrix. In chapter 6 we discussed the food matrix of plant foods and how this influences the rate at which nutrients are absorbed by the body (their bioavailability). The food matrix of dairy may be equally influential.

It is evident from their widely different textures, that milk, butter, cheese and yogurt have quite different food matrices. Many studies have now shown that butter increases LDL cholesterol more than cheese with the same amount of saturated fat, and this has been attributed to differences between the food matrices of butter and cheese [571]. A direct demonstration of the key role for the food matrix was elegantly demonstrated in a study from Ireland. Participants in the study ate either normal cheddar cheese, or they ate a "deconstructed" cheese. In normal cheese, fat is an integral part of the overall food matrix. In the "deconstructed" cheese, most of the fat was separated from the cheese's food matrix by giving a low fat cheese and making up the

---

[265] An example of a meta- analysis finding neutral not harmful effects of butter on CVD is Pimpin et al (2016) Is butter back? A systematic review and meta-analysis of butter consumption and risk of cardiovascular disease, diabetes, and total mortality. PLoS One 11:e0158118.

fat with butter. When the participants' levels of LDL-cholesterol were measured six weeks later it was found that LDL-cholesterol levels had risen far less in the group who ate the normal cheese than in participants who had eaten the same amount of fat in the deconstructed cheese - butter (plus low fat cheese) - where the fat had been freed from its cheesy matrix [571]. This suggests that the cholesterol response to fat in cheese is dependent on the rest of the matrix.

So how can this be? The different effects of butter fat and cheese fat cannot be explained by different types of fatty acids in the cheese and butter since these are essentially the same. Rather, the explanation may come from how much of the saturated fat is absorbed. Studies have found that a lower proportion of fat is absorbed from cheese than from butter. This is shown by a greater amount of fat being excreted in the faeces after eating cheese [565]. Since less fat is absorbed from cheese this translates into less of a rise in LDL cholesterol.

It is not fully established how the different food matrices in butter and cheese influence saturated fat absorption. One attractive idea is that calcium in cheese combines with some of the fatty acids forming insoluble calcium-fatty acids "soaps" that cannot be absorbed and so are excreted [572]. Butter contains far less calcium than cheese, and so these calcium-fatty acids soaps may not be formed to the same extent. Hence, compared to cheese, more of the fatty acids in butter can be absorbed by the body [565].

There is another fundamental difference between butter and cheese. And that is how the fatty acids are present. Fatty acids in "fat" are usually bound in structures called triglycerides - three fatty acids attached to a glycerol backbone. In unfermented dairy - milk and most types of butter - almost all of the fatty acids occur as triglycerides (about 98%). During cheese maturation, bacteria and fungi secrete enzymes that separate some fatty acids from the triglycerides. These fatty acids are said to be "free". The extent to which free fatty acids form varies widely between cheeses, but for some cheeses up to 20% all fatty acids may be liberated from their triglyceride structure. This is especially the case for cheeses such as Parmesan and blue cheeses that are ripened for long periods and have a lot of microbial activity [573]. It is the free fatty acids that form calcium-fatty acid salts. The greater amounts of free fatty acids in cheese could be another reason why there is less fat absorption than for butter. [266] (An additional benefit of the free fatty acids in cheese is that some give flavour, either in their native state or after they have been converted into other compounds.)

So, in summary, even when the overall saturated fatty acid content of cheese and butter are similar, how these fatty acids occur in the dairy matrix can be crucial. So eating the same amount of saturated fat in cheese is not necessarily the same as eating the same amount of saturated fat from meat or elsewhere. In the bigger picture, the "fat content" of a food may only be providing half the story, and it is possible - using the same arguments as for dairy - that the dangers of fat in UPFs may extend beyond the absolute amount of fat and include how the fat is arranged within the overall food matrix.

## Dairy proteins - not all good news

As well as fat, milk is an excellent source of protein. Milk proteins serve not only as the source of amino acids for the baby to build its own protein structures such as muscle. Some milk proteins also act as growth stimulants. Whilst this is of great benefit for stimulating the growth of a growing baby, it may not be so beneficial for fully-grown adults. The signals present in milk stimulate growth in the baby by increasing the amounts of growth hormones such as insulin and IGF1. Whilst these hormones boost growth in babies, IGF1 also has growth-promoting effects on prostate cells and this increases the risk of these cells becoming more cancerous [574]. This may help explain the quite good evidence that dairy products, and milk in particular, increase prostate cancer risk in older men [574; 575]. There is also some limited evidence that cheese increases the risk of prostate cancer but this is thought to be linked more to cheese's high levels of calcium - which is also a risk factor for prostate cancer - rather than because of protein growth signals [576]. For an older man, deciding whether or not to cut back on dairy will be a personal choice based on weighing up these risks in relation to their own personal circumstances.

---

[266] The process of liberating free fatty acids from triglycerides also occurs during the normal digestion of triglycerides in all dairy produce.

# Eating dairy

Cheese consumption varies widely between Mediterranean countries, but can be high. The Greek's consume even more cheese than the French! In Greece, the main cheese is *feta*, a cheese usually made from a mixture of sheep and goat's milk. As well as *feta*, many other Mediterranean cheeses are now widely available such as Spanish *manchego* (made from sheep's milk) and French *chevres* (goat cheeses). Cheese greatly enhances the enjoyment of eating grains and vegetables. Cheese brings together endless vegetable and grain dishes whether it is *parmesan* in risottos or pasta dishes, *feta* in a Greek salad or in many savoury Greek pies such as *spanakopita,* or French vegetable *gratins.* Just as EVOO is the unifier *par excellance* for Mediterranean vegetable dishes, *parmesan* and *feta* have similarly important roles in Italian and Greek cuisines.

The Med tradition for making dairy from the milk of sheep and goats rather than cows may have particular health benefits. Goat and sheep milk are rich in medium chain fatty acid that do not raise cholesterol levels as much as those in cow's milk and so may be better for health. Also, for people who find cow's milk difficult to digest, goat milk is a good option since it is easier to digest than cow's milk. The possible benefit of goat and sheep dairy for helping prevent Alzheimer's disease is discussed in chapter 11. Although milk from ruminants contains low amounts of trans fats, there is no evidence that these naturally produced trans fats have the adverse effects of their industrially produced equivalents [347]. On both health and taste grounds, non-milk alternatives are not equivalent. [267]

---

[267] https://www.theguardian.com/news/2019/jan/29/white-gold-the-unstoppable-rise-of-alternative-milks-oat-soy-rice-coconut-plant

# Seafood

We may owe our intelligence to fish. About 140,000 years ago, early humans living along the African coast started eating more and more seafood and this gave a big spurt to the development of the human brain [577]. Fish, especially oily fish, and shellfish contain high levels of the omega-3 fatty acid DHA (docosahexaenoic acid) - a type of polyunsaturated fatty acid. DHA is the main fatty acid in the human brain and acts like a superconductor speeding up neural impulses and increasing thinking capacity. Having a rich dietary source of DHA allowed the human brain to evolve and as it did so it incorporated more and more DHA into its structure.

At least that's the view of some scientists. Of course, we may never know for sure if this was the main reason why human intelligence leap-frogged over other creatures. But what is clear is that fish is extremely good for health. As well as enhancing brain health and reducing dementia and Alzheimer's disease, eating fish also reduces the risk of heart disease and stroke [578].

DHA is essential for the optimal function of the brain and eye and yet humans have only a very limited capacity to make it themselves. It seems unlikely that evolution would have allowed this precarious state to occur unless early humans had an adequate food source - which strengthens the idea that humans had access to marine sources. Today, though, millions of people don't eat fish, in some cases for cultural or religious reasons, for others because of taste or choosing to be vegetarian or vegan. So what are the health impacts of this?

## Fish and omega 3 fats are not equivalent

Consuming fish is linked to a wide range of benefits. A detailed meta-analysis calculated that eating about one serving of fish per week decreased by about 2% to7% the risk of coronary heart disease mortality, cardiovascular disease mortality, all-cause mortality, stroke, myocardial infarction, acute coronary syndrome, heart failure, gastrointestinal cancer, metabolic syndrome, dementia and Alzheimer's disease [578]. This study included both oily and non-oily fish. Although oily fish are particularly rich in the omega-3 fatty acids EPA (eicosapentaenoic acid) and DHA these contribute only part of the health benefits of fish. Fish contains many other nutrients including easily digested protein, selenium, vitamin D and an amino acid-like substance called taurine, all of which reduce the risk of CHD and stroke [579]. Both fish and shellfish are also excellent sources of vitamin B12. [268] It is likely that it is this collection of important nutrients that together confer the excellent health benefits of seafood.

There is nevertheless widespread agreement that EPA and DHA are an extremely important part of its health benefits. This can be shown by measuring EPA and DHA in people or by calculating how health correlates with intake of these fatty acids from dietary sources - which mainly means fish. When levels of EPA and DHA were measured in people who did not obtain them from supplements, there was an increase in "successful aging" - which meant being without chronic disease or cognitive and physical dysfunction [580]. Studies have also found that dietary DHA is particularly good at preventing heart arrhythmias. EPA may also help prevent arrhythmias. Together EPA and DHA are the oils that oil the heart pump and make the heart more able to respond to increased demand by pumping faster. Studies in experimental systems have also demonstrated that these omega-3 fatty acids have significant anti-inflammatory effects [581]. One way they achieve this is by being converted into anti-inflammatory molecules called "resolvins" which help resolve inflammation. It is highly likely that the anti-inflammatory properties of omega-3 fats are crucial for many of the benefits of consuming oily fish.

Many people do not eat fish, especially oily fish, and compensate by taking omega-3 fat supplements. But these are not equivalent and as discussed in chapter 8 there are concerns about the stability of these supplements. Taking an omega-3 fat supplement can boost the levels of these fats in the body, but this rarely seems to translate into increased protection against disease. Compared to eating fish, the evidence for benefits of omega-3 supplements is weak. For instance, in an RCT from the US, omega-3 fat supplements did not protect against CVD or cancer [582]. These are multifactorial disease processes and omega-3 fats cannot be expected to target all the pathological changes that can cause these diseases. This is why most health authorities recommend eating fish rather than omega-3 fat supplements. One possible exception may be arthritis where supplements may be of benefit in relieving symptoms [581].

---

[268] https://ods.od.nih.gov/factsheets/VitaminB12-HealthProfessional/

A portion of oily fish or a supplement can provide a few grams of omega-3 fats. The daily omega-3 intake of the many people who consume neither oily fish nor supplements is typically about one tenth of this (0.15 - 0.25 g per day). There are a few non-fish sources of EPA and DHA, such as eggs and especially "omega 3-enriched" eggs, but levels of EPA and DHA in these foods are low compared to oily fish. These dietary considerations mean that there tends to be a bimodal distribution of intake of EPA/DHA in western populations - either high from people eating oily fish or taking supplements or low, with far fewer people in the middle.

The third main dietary omega-3 fatty acid called ALA is mainly found in plants. Humans can convert ALA at low rates into EPA and, at even lower rates, into DHA. This amount may be sufficient for a person's needs, and it is possible that when there is not very much DHA in the diet, the body may start producing more from ALA to compensate [577]. This ability to up-regulate DHA production is known to occur in pregnant women so that the mother can provide adequate DHA for her baby's developing brain.

However, there is a cautionary note for vegetarians and vegans who rely on making EPA and DHA from the plant-derived precursor ALA. Along with omega-3 fats there is a second main group of PUFAs, the omega-6 fats. The main dietary omega-6 fatty acid is linoleic acid. Consuming high amounts of linoleic acid slows down the conversion of ALA into EPA and DHA. Linoleic acid is present at high levels in vegetable oils like sunflower oil and intake is often high in vegetarians and vegans. So it would seem advisable for vegetarians and vegans who are relying on making their own EPA and DHA not to consume too much omega-6 containing vegetable oils.

Even though levels of DHA in vegans are only about half those of omnivores [577], some studies have found that vegetarians and vegans have a lower risk of CHD. So it might be argued that they must be getting enough DHA - at least for keeping a heart healthy. Alternatively it could be that other aspects of a vegetarian's or vegan's diet lowers their risk of CHD, such as a low intake of saturated fat or a generally healthy lifestyle, and that this compensates for not eating foods rich in DHA.

One option for vegetarians and vegans is to eat algal sources of EPA and DHA. In the marine environment, it is phytoplankton (marine micro-algae) and not fish that are the actual manufacturers of DHA and EPA. Omega-3 fats in fish and shellfish ultimately come from these phytoplankton. Herbivorous fish eat omega-3 fat-containing phytoplankton and carnivorous fish like salmon get their omega-3 fats from eating herbivorous fish.

Because of their important roles, it seems advisable to have a food supply of DHA and EPA rather than relying on the body to make enough of it. The Med diet recommends fish and so is a reliable source of EPA and DHA. [269]

# Choosing seafood

Even though omega-3 supplements on their own are of limited use, it is still highly likely that the omega-3 fatty acids consumed in fish are extremely important for their health benefits. Oily fish, such as salmon, sardines, mackerel, anchovies, herring and trout, are the best source of omega-3 fatty acids [583]. A serving of salmon or mackerel provides about 1.5 -3.5 g of these fatty acids. Levels do vary according to where and when the fish is caught - DHA has a low freezing point and acts as anti-freeze for fish and so tends to be present in higher amounts in fish caught in colder waters. Canned sardines, mackerel and anchovies also contain high levels of omega-3 fats. Because of the way it is prepared, most canned tuna is a poor source (fresh tuna is better) [583]. Some of the omega-3 fatty acids in canned fish transfer from the fish to the canning oil and so using the oil will prevent wasting the precious omega-3 fats. Buying tinned fish in olive oil is even better as this oil is part of a Med diet. Canned sardines are also an excellent source of vitamin B12 and iron.

Large predatory fish like swordfish, mackerel, salmon and tuna can build up high levels of methyl mercury, and other pollutants, but apart from pregnant women, the benefits of eating fish are considered to outweigh the risks [578]. Even so, there is one way to significantly reduce this concern, and that is to choose small oily fish like anchovies and sardines. Not only are these less likely to be contaminated with heavy metals, they are also more environmentally sustainable. Anchovies are a common ingredient in many Mediterranean dishes, sometimes given prominence in dishes such as *pissaladiere,* and sometimes added more to enhance savoury (umami) flavour, as in sauces where the fishy taste is lost but all the goodness is retained. Unfortunately, the vast majority of anchovies (along with some other small

---

[269] A comprehensive continually updated assessment of omega-3 fats is:
https://ods.od.nih.gov/factsheets/Omega3FattyAcids-HealthProfessional/

fish) are no longer used as a direct food source but end up as fish meal for feeding farmed fish. This is especially the case for anchovies from Peru - the world's largest anchovy fishery. Anchovies are treated as a great delicacy in some countries such as Mediterranean France and here the problem is lack of supply due to overfishing and not lack of acceptance. Attempts to switch some of the anchovy harvest in Peru to food rather than feed has met with only limited success, which is a great loss to sustainable fishing. [270]

Some predict that based on current trends, fishing stocks will be irreversibly damaged within a few decades. Farmed seafood should offer a sustainable way forward but, it has been pointed out, humans are now "making similar mistakes in water that we made on land". [271] Environmental concerns for salmon farming in Scotland are an issue that has been simmering for years. According to a committee of Scottish MPs, expansion of salmon farming in Scotland is damaging the environment "beyond repair". In one report they highlight the high levels of mortality, sea lice and shooting of seals in the vicinity of the farms. [272] Pesticides to control sea lice are an increasing problem and more natural solutions such as wrass (fish that eat the lice) are being attempted. [273] Unfortunately, there is no significant groundswell of public concern to catalyse improvements in conditions - perhaps motivated by a desire to retain the low costs of this once luxury product.

As with other farmed animals, the nutritional quality of farmed fish is strongly influenced by how the animals are raised. Fish get their omega-3 fats and vitamin D from their diet. Farmed salmon were originally mostly fed fish and fish oils (wild anchovies and other wild small fish), but with the expansion of the farmed fishing industry this has become unsustainable and these are now being replaced with vegetable oils [(584)]. [274] However, vegetable oils contain very little EPA and DHA and there is a lower limit of fish oil needed to ensure the fish receives enough dietary omega-3 fats to maintain acceptable

[270] https://www.iffo.net/case-study-peruvian-anchovy-why-feed-not-food
[271] https://www.theguardian.com/sustainable-business/2017/jan/23/aquaculture-bivalves-oysters-factory-farming-environment
https://www.thesolutionsjournal.com/article/seafood-future-bivalves-better/
[272] Dick, S (2018) Fish farm damage "beyond repair". The Herald March 6, 2018
[273] https://www.theguardian.com/environment/2017/apr/01/is-farming-salmon-bad-for-the-environment
[274] https://www.fishfarmingexpert.com/article/how-much-wild-fish-is-there-in-fish-farming-feed/

levels in the flesh of the fish. An alternative approach that is being used is to bump up omega-3 fats by feeding fish oils shortly before harvesting the fish. Because of these various ways of feeding salmon, there is now wide variation in the amount of EPA and DHA in the salmon sold by UK supermarkets. Fish fed mainly vegetable oils can have up to four times less EPA and DHA than the best salmon [585]. Feeding vegetable oils may be better for sustainability but it is less good for our health. An alternative and more sustainable source of omega-3 fats as feed is farmed micro-algae but at the moment this is still in the development stage.

So to eat healthy sustainably produced oily fish can be challenging. One approach is to avoid large carnivorous fish such as salmon because of their requirements for other fish and feed, and instead to eat fish lower down the food chain, which means eating omnivorous and herbivorous fish such as tilapia and carp.[275] At the moment the market in the west for these fish (unlike in many Asian countries) is very limited. Another seafood often of doubtful sustainability is shrimp raised in tropical waters. A quarter of mangrove swamps have been lost since the mid- 1970's to shrimp farming, and high greenhouse gas (GHG) emissions and poor workers rights are additional problems. But there is another alternative, and that is bivalves.

## Benefits of bivalves

When it comes to consuming animals and their products, it is usually more sustainable to eat those lower down the food chain. Demands on environmental resources such as water and land are usually less and there are usually fewer animal welfare issues. Like pigs raised on soya beans, salmon has been raised on feed  - small fish and grains - that could have been directly consumed by humans. When taste, nutritional, environmental and animal welfare grounds are all taken into consideration, there is a strong case that the optimal seafood is mussels and other bivalves such as oysters and clams. [276] During their farming, bivalves eat naturally occurring food and so do not

---

[275] https://tastingthefuture.com/2018/10/01/sustainable-aquaculture-herbivorous-fish-a-solution-for-food-security/

[276] https://www.thesolutionsjournal.com/article/seafood-future-bivalves-better/
https://www.theguardian.com/sustainable-business/2017/jan/23/aquaculture-bivalves-oysters-factory-farming-environment

require fish feed, they are sedentary and so don't need space to move which also avoids animal welfare issues of over-crowding, they suffer little if any pain during their culture and there are far fewer problems of them invading or spreading diseases to natural populations. Mussels produce a fraction of the GHGs of land animals and their GHGs are still only about one twentieth of salmon [586]. Moreover, shellfish sequester carbon in their shells, removing carbon from the atmosphere, and in this regard at least are more like growing plant foods. Mussels are probably the world's most sustainable source of animal protein.

Mussels and other bivalves such as oysters and clams contain good levels of omega-3 fats (although not as high as most oily fish) and are an excellent source of some vitamins and minerals. [277] For example, a portion of 100 grams of mussels contains four times the daily requirement of vitamin B12, three times the daily requirement of manganese and the complete daily requirement of selenium as well as half the day's protein needs [587]. Oysters are a well-known source of zinc and a 100 gram portion provides more than twelve times the daily requirement.

There are a huge number of recipes for mussels including many from Mediterranean cuisine. If the thought of shelling mussels is a disincentive, ready shelled frozen ones are easy to obtain. But it is also worth considering the quality of frozen mussels as discussed in the next section.

## Frozen seafood

Fresh is key to seafood but short storage times can make it difficult to coordinate buying and cooking fish. Frozen or canned seafood are often more practical. It might seem that little harm can be done to seafood by the industry freezing it. But the milky water that seeps out of frozen seafood as it fries is a sign that water has been incorporated into the seafood. This can amount to 10% of the weight of frozen (and canned) seafood. Paying for water isn't the only way the seafood has been devalued. The water is retained by adding the chemical sodium polyphosphate, which acts like a sponge. In 2012 an important publication highlighted the potential health dangers of sodium phosphates [179]. High levels of phosphates in the blood increase the

---

[277] https://health.gov/dietaryguidelines/dga2005/report/HTML/table_g2_adda2.htm

risk of cardiovascular disease because they combine with calcium, hardening blood vessels and other organs in the body. This has raised concerns about consuming foods high in phosphates, and this is especially of concern for people with chronic kidney disease who are less able to excrete phosphates. Not all frozen seafood is equal but sodium phosphate does not need to be indicated on the label and so choosing frozen seafood which does not ooze liquid when cooked is often the only way to know if the seafood contains added phosphates. Most (but not all) fresh seafood is phosphate free and so buying and freezing your own is a good idea.

# Alcohol as part of a Med diet

## Introduction

When drunk as part of a Med diet, alcohol in moderation, particularly as red wine, is considered beneficial for health. It also gives pleasure and relieves stress, which themselves can contribute to good health. In a Greek population, moderate drinking was found to be the aspect of the Med diet that contributed most to decreased mortality [588], and a wider analysis of many different studies has confirmed the important place that moderate alcohol consumption occupies in a healthy Med diet [589].

And yet few subjects in nutrition are as controversial as alcohol. The view that we would all be better off not drinking at all is tacit in UK guidelines, which refer to the current limits as "low risk" guidelines implying that there is still some risk even at these levels of consumption. When the new UK alcohol guidelines were introduced in 2016, the Chief Medical Officer Dame Sally Davies stated that "Drinking any level of alcohol regularly carries a health risk for anyone", although she later toned down her statement. [278] Cancer scientists often take a particularly strong anti-alcohol stance because of links between alcohol consumption and cancer. When the head of Public Health England Dr Duncan Selbie proposed working alongside the alcohol advisory website DrinkAware, the co-chair of PHE's alcohol leadership board Sir Ian Gilmore resigned in protest because of links between DrinkAware and the alcohol industry [590]. Some even insist that to prevent harm from misuse, alcohol should be declared a drug of abuse [591].

But there is also considerable evidence that light to moderate drinking reduces the risk of some chronic diseases, especially CVD [83], and also, possibly, diabetes, cognitive decline and dementia [592; 593]. So is the government message that we would be better off drinking no alcohol at all really in the best public interest? Or is light drinking harmless or even beneficial? Alcohol consumption seems very much a double-edged sword. But are both sides of the sword equally sharp or can we come to some clear recommendations?

---

[278] https://www.theguardian.com/society/2016/dec/30/breast-cancer-warning-wine-dame-sally-davies

No one disputes that many people drink too much alcohol. Heavy drinking and binge drinking increase the risk of liver disease, high blood pressure, various cancers, and brain damage including alcohol-related dementia. The consequences of binge drinking were starkly illustrated in a study that found that heart attacks in Northern Ireland peaked on Mondays and Tuesdays due, it was concluded, to the effects of binge drinking on the previous Fridays and Saturdays [594].

It is light drinking where the disagreement lies, and whether even low levels of consumption are harmful. I will define light drinking as no more than 14 units of alcohol per week for both men and women since this is the upper limit currently recommended by the UK government (in 2020). A daily drink of 2 units equates to about a 125 ml glass of 14% wine (1.8 units) or 175 ml of 11% wine (1.9 units) using UK units. A unit of alcohol in the UK is equivalent to 8 grams of pure alcohol (this is different in some other countries). So drinking within UK guidelines equates to a limit of 16 grams of alcohol per day. This is lower than the amount of alcohol considered beneficial as part of a Med diet which is 5-25 g/day for women and 10-50 g/day for men.

## Cancer

The most contentious area is alcohol's relation to cancer. Some studies conclude that even light drinking increases cancer risk. A recent meta-analysis of studies from around the world found a small, but statistically significant, increase in the risk of cancers of the oral cavity and pharynx, oesophagus and female breast with light drinking (defined as up to one drink per day). However there was considerable variation in the outcomes between studies, especially for breast and oesophagus, suggesting that factors associated with individual studies are influencing cancer risk [595]. (There was no increased cancer risk for cancers of the colorectum, liver and larynx.)

These links with cancer highlight a paradox at the heart of the Med diet. Here is a dietary pattern that includes regular moderate alcohol consumption but which is associated with a decreased, not increased, risk for many of the diseases associated with alcohol consumption, including cancers. To explain this paradox means considering alcohol in the context of the whole Med dietary pattern, and this includes not only other foods but also how the alcohol is consumed.

313

One of the greatest concern around alcohol is its link to breast cancer. Authors of large-scale studies suggest that even low amounts of alcohol increase the risk of breast cancer and that there is no safe lower limit [596]. But there is no evidence that low amounts of alcohol consumed *as part of a Med diet* are linked to an increased risk of breast cancer. For example, conforming to a traditional Med diet - which included an average consumption of about half a unit of alcohol per day - was associated with lower breast cancer risk among postmenopausal Greek women [597]. In an analysis of women taking part in the highly regarded Predimed study, women who ate a Med diet supplemented with EVOO had a 68% *reduced risk* of breast cancer even though almost half were drinking alcohol (mostly up to two units of alcohol a day) [234]. In a large-scale meta-analysis of many studies looking at the link between consuming a Med diet and breast cancer risk, light alcohol consumption had no effect on risk [238].

High alcohol consumption is also linked to cancers of the bowel, liver, mouth and throat, oesophagus (squamous cell carcinoma) and stomach [598]. But again there is no evidence that low levels of alcohol when consumed as part of a Med diet increases the risk of these cancers. In fact, there can be a protective effect [599]. In a study of middle aged Greeks, moderate alcohol consumption (1.5 - 4 UK units) as part of a Med diet was associated with a significantly decreased likelihood of colorectal cancer in men (65% decreased risk) and in women (60% decreased risk) [600]. Higher amounts of alcohol increased risk. Similarly, although high amounts of alcohol are associated with an increased risk of cancers of the upper aero-digestive tract (mouth, pharynx, larynx and oesophagus), Greek men and women with good adherence to a Med diet, had a reduced risk of these cancers even when this included light drinking [601]. Many of the Greeks in this study also smoked and the importance of considering factors, like smoking, that interact with alcohol can be shown by comparing drinking between smokers and non-smokers. In a study called the Million Women Study (which really did involve well over a million women) there was no increased risk of aero-digestive tract cancers in women drinking up to two units a day, so long as they were non-smokers, but if the women also smoked then even low levels of alcohol increased cancer risk [88].

## Dietary factors

The dramatic effect of smoking on increasing the risk of mouth and throat cancers highlights the importance of context when assessing the cancer risk of drinking. So what role do dietary factors play in modifying the cancer risk from alcohol? Many of the large-scale studies suggesting no lower safe link for alcohol consumption did not consider the background diet of the participants. For many, this would have been a western diet. So one possible explanation for differences between studies is that there are cancer-protective dietary factors in the Med diet that are not present to the same extent in the western diet. As discussed earlier in this chapter, one possible protective factor in the Med diet against breast cancer is extra virgin olive oil (EVOO). This protection may be due in part to the high levels of anti-oestrogens in EVOO called lignans [602]. One way alcohol is thought to increase breast cancer risk is by raising oestrogen levels, and so the lignans in EVOO may protect against potentially harmful effects of alcohol by blocking the actions of oestrogens. This suggestion of a protective role for lignans against breast cancer has been demonstrated in some studies. High levels of lignans are present in flax seeds, sesame seeds and rye flour, and eating a diet rich in these was found to reduce the risk of postmenopausal women dying from breast cancer (but no effect was found for premenopausal women) [120; 603].

Another cancer-protective foodstuff is fibre. The average fibre content of the Med diet is double that of the average UK diet (33 g versus 16 g [604]). Fibre in the colon is thought to bind oestrogen and so help carry it out of the body for excretion. This way of sweeping out oestrogen from the body could be one reason why a large EPIC study found that fibre, especially from vegetables, reduced the risk of alcohol-related breast cancer in women [605].

As well as by raising oestrogen levels, alcohol also increases cancer risk because it gets converted into a substance called acetaldehyde. Acetaldehyde damages DNA, a first step in the cancer process. Dietary folates help keep DNA healthy by repairing the damage caused by acetaldehyde. Hence, folates have received a good deal of attention as possible factors in the diet that may help protect against alcohol-related cancer. In a large European study (part of the EPIC study) involving 368,000 women, it was convincingly shown that consuming a diet high in folates protects against breast cancer in premenopausal women [606]. The relative benefits were greatest for women who had at least 12 alcoholic drinks a week. A meta-analysis also found that folate is particularly beneficial against breast cancer for women who drink quite heavily [102]. However, not all studies have found folates to be protective against the adverse effects of alcohol and the latest authoritative verdict from the WCRF/AICR concludes that although there is some limited evidence for a protective effect of folates against breast cancer no firm conclusions can yet be reached [294]. Folates are found in particularly large quantities in the green, leafy vegetables and pulses that characterise the Med diet. Hence it is possible that high dietary folates may be another aspect of the Med diet that helps explain why women who eat a Med diet and drink low amounts of alcohol are not at an increased risk of breast cancer. Finally, another phytochemical very rich in the Med diet and of interest in relation to alcohol-related cancer prevention is the polyphenol quercetin, since quercetin has been shown in experimental systems to block the conversion of alcohol to acetaldehyde in mammary tissue [607; 608].

The benefits of phytochemicals in the Med diet to suppress the harmful effects of alcohol are not limited to breast cancer since folates may also protect against alcohol-related colon cancer. So, summing up, there are many ways that a Med diet could potentially help neutralise harmful carcinogenic effects of alcohol. Disentangling the precise role of each individual nutrient is however difficult, and they are likely to interact. This again demonstrates why it is so important to consider the whole diet when evaluating benefits and risks.

## Other diseases

Many studies have found that overall mortality is lower in people who drink low amounts of alcohol compared to people who have never drunk ("never drinkers"). However, with high amounts of alcohol the risk of dying increases. This trend is represented graphically by a so-called J-shaped curve when weekly alcohol consumption is plotted against the "Hazard ratio" (the relative chance of dying compared to a control group). The data from a study published in the Lancet in 2018, which was a very large analysis that pooled the results from 83 prospective studies, is shown below. The right hand side graph shows all cause mortality. The J-shape is obtained by drawing a continuous line between the point representing the "never drinkers" to the points showing drinking up to 600 grams of alcohol per week. This graph shows that compared to "never drinkers" the risk of dying is lower (lower Hazard ratio) for low amounts of alcohol up to 200 grams per week (equivalent to 25 units in the UK). (Ex-drinkers are also shown on the graph but these should be excluded since they may have had prior health problems and that may explain why they have a higher risk of dying and also why they stopped drinking.)

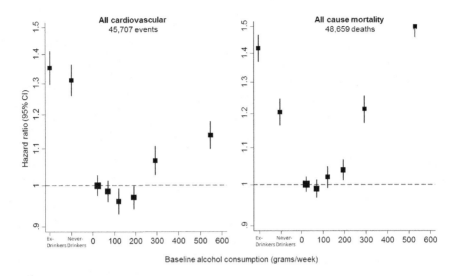

**J-shaped curve showing risk of a cardiovascular event (left graph) or dying from any cause (right graph) compared to people who have never drunk** [279]

The black squares are the values and the vertical lines represent the range of values ("error bars").

The conclusion from this study that for reducing dying from any cause a small amount of alcohol is better than no alcohol at all is at odds with the view that there is no lower limit below which alcohol is safe, and that we would all be better off not drinking. As I mentioned earlier, this is tacit in current UK guidelines of drinking. In fact this was the conclusion drawn from this study published in the Lancet. So how could a conclusion like this have been drawn? The answer is by cutting out the "never drinkers" and "ex-drinkers" from the graph. These means that rather than considering people who have

---

[279] eFigure 10 Supplement to: Wood AM *et al.* (2018) Risk thresholds for alcohol consumption: combined analysis of individual-participant data for 599 912 current drinkers in 83 prospective studies. *Lancet* **391**, 1513-1523.

never drunk as controls, instead the control group - in other words comparison group - is people who drink a small amount. Using this strategy led to many reports in the media that there is no safe lower limit for alcohol [609]. But the data analysis in this Lancet publication has been soundly criticised. For instance, the editor of the highly regarded American Journal of Clinical Nutrition (who for completeness it should be noted has written in support of beer) stated "we believe that the study has little to add to existing scientific literature and cannot contribute to public health advice" [610]. Others have deeper concerns about the way the data in this and similar studies are being manipulated with, it is suspected, the aim of hiding any benefits from light alcohol drinking. An eminent group of epidemiologists concluded that in relation to the Lancet study and similar studies "A growing number of studies seem to be doing their level best to obscure their own data showing that drinking alcohol might have health benefits." [280]

The best evidence that low alcohol consumption has health benefits is in relation to CVD. CVD is the number one killer in the UK and so anything that reduces CVD will also have a major impact on overall UK mortality. The left hand part of the graph shown above compared alcohol consumption to the risk of a cardiovascular event (which mainly relates to having a stroke or heart attack). It demonstrates that compared to never drinkers, risk of a cardiovascular event is lower for alcohol drinkers. In another very large meta-analysis, light alcohol consumption (up to about 1.5 units a day) was associated with a 14 to 25% reduction in the risk of or dying from CVD, coronary heart disease and stroke compared with people who had never drunk, and that with higher amounts of alcohol the reduced risk of stroke was lost [83] It is not entirely clear how alcohol reduces CVD but one likely mechanism is that low levels of alcohol raise HDL cholesterol levels [611].

Some studies have also found that light consumption of wine is associated with a decreased risk of dementia and Alzheimer's disease [593; 611]. One intriguing idea to explain this is that low levels of alcohol help flush away dementia-causing toxins in the brain by activating the brain's unique cleaning system known as the glymphatic system [612].

---

[280] This is the view of many members of the International Scientific Forum on Alcohol Research www.alcoholresearchforum.org/critique-214

318

# The importance of how and what we drink

## Binge drinking

Alcohol occupies a special place in food culture because as well as being consumed with food it is also often consumed on its own in social settings. It is when drinking is decoupled from eating that many of its adverse effects arise. All drinkers know that steady drinking with a meal does not have the same impact as binging on an empty stomach. So it is surprising that many studies choose to ignore this difference. Instead, they simply record weekly alcohol intake and take no account of whether or not the alcohol was all consumed on an empty stomach on a Friday night binge with friends, or if it was spread out over the week and drunk during meals.

There is now convincing evidence that it is crucial to consider the drinking pattern when assessing the effects of alcohol. The 2018 Lancet study mentioned earlier found that drinking about 6 to 25 units of alcohol (48 to 200 grams) spread out over three or more days of the week was associated with a greater protective effect against all-cause mortality ((lower Hazard Ratio) than when the same amount of alcohol was consumed on one or two days of the week [609]. This is shown in the figure on the next page. Many of the adverse effects of binge drinking or knocking back a spirit are thought to be caused by the sudden rise in the blood alcohol concentration (BAC), a spike that is far higher than when a similar amount of alcohol is consumed over a longer period [613]. A sudden spike in BAC raises blood pressure increasing the risk of CVD - as the study on heart attacks in Northern Ireland illustrated well.

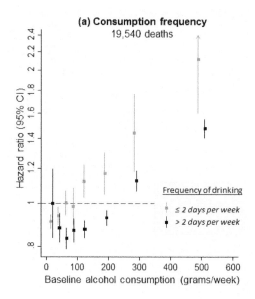

**(a) Consumption frequency**
19,540 deaths

Drinking low amounts of alcohol over more than 2 days (>2 days) per week (black points) reduces the risk of dying from any cause compared to drinking on no more than 2 days ( ≤ 2 days) per week (grey points) 281

Reproduced in accordance with the CC BY 4.0 license.

As well as increasing the risk of a heart attack, binge drinking is also associated with an increased risk of breast cancer. In a study of women who binged (which in this Spanish study was defined as women who drank at least 6 alcoholic drinks in a single day - equivalent to 60 g of alcohol) there was a 76% increased risk of breast cancer compared to women drinking the same amount of alcohol spread over a week [614]. This increased risk could only be confirmed for premenopausal women since there were insufficient postmenopausal women binge drinking to be able to do a separate reliable

---

281 eFigure 17 Supplement to: Wood AM *et al.* (2018) Risk thresholds for alcohol consumption: combined analysis of individual-participant data for 599 912 current drinkers in 83 prospective studies. *Lancet* **391**, 1513-1523. Although the Lancet study also did a separate analysis for "binge drinking" the definition of binge drinking was set at 100 g of alcohol which is well above normal definitions (eg the NHS defines binge drinking as 64 g for men and 48 g for women) and so this will reduce any apparent effects of binge drinking.

statistical analysis for them. So the jury is out here. However, when the statistical analysis was repeated by restricting it to premenopausal women only - rather than pooling data from both groups - this led to the conclusion that the risk of breast cancer in premenopausal women when they binge drank was 100% (two-fold) higher.

There are many possible explanations why binge drinking increases cancer risk. Firstly, it could be related to the way the alcohol is metabolised. It is not alcohol *per se* that is thought to be the main carcinogen but rather its breakdown product called acetaldehyde. Acetaldehyde is classed as a carcinogen by the International Agency for Research on Cancer. Although acetaldehyde is eventually broken down to harmless products for excretion, a sudden rise in alcohol may mean a lot of carcinogenic acetaldehyde is produced before it can be broken down. The dangers of acetaldehyde are clearly demonstrated in people who consume alcoholic drinks that have preformed acetaldehyde. Preformed acetaldehyde is present at particularly high levels in farm-made Calvados and it is thought that the high level of oesophageal cancer found in Northern France was, in the past, linked to this region's custom of drinking calvados [615]. Fortunately, it is mostly commercial calvados that is now consumed and this contains far lower levels of acetaldehyde. It is fortified wines such as sherry that are now more of a worry for their high levels of preformed acetaldehyde [615].

Binge drinking can drive all three Core Risk States. This could be particularly important in explaining the links between binge drinking and cancer. In relation to oxidative stress, a high BAC raises oxidative stress and this raises cancer risk [616]. This is because high levels of alcohol, as well being converted into acetaldehyde, also trigger a second way of disposing of the alcohol that involves the production of free radicals. This free radical mechanism does not get switched on when alcohol levels in the blood remain low. Binge drinking also increases inflammation in the body and insulin sensitivity [611]. These two processes are strongly linked to an increased risk of breast cancer (see ch. 10). Hence all three Core Risk States could be activated following binge drinking and so increase the risk of breast cancer.

## Other aspects of drinking pattern

It is not only no binge drinking that makes drinking as part of a Med diet a far healthier option. In order to encompass the overall benefits of drinking the

Med way, a group of Spanish researchers devised a "Mediterranean alcohol drinking pattern". This scoring system gives points for aspects of drinking that are deemed preferable, such as moderate alcohol intake spread out over the week, a preference for red wine drunk with a meal, little intake of spirits, and no binge drinking. Drinking with a meal lowers the peak BAC compared to drinking on an empty stomach by slowing emptying of the stomach contents into the intestine from where the alcohol is absorbed. Using this scoring system, the researchers found that participants in the study with a high score - achieved because they spread out drinking over a week and were drinking no more than 4 units per day for men or 2 units per day for women - was associated with a significantly reduced mortality compared to those who drank the same amount but did not follow this drinking pattern. [617]. There is also some evidence that better conformity with the Med drinking pattern is specifically associated with lower cardiovascular risk, although the study did not include sufficient numbers of participants to draw firm conclusions about this [618].

Red wine is the quintessential alcoholic Med drink. So is red wine superior to other forms of alcohol? Although one unit of alcohol is the same whether it is from beer, wine or spirits, there is good evidence that drinking wine, and especially red wine, is indeed more beneficial than drinking other forms of alcohol. This applies even when the wine is not drunk as part of a Med diet. For example, the Lancet study found that wine (white or red) was protective against a myocardial infarct (heart attack) and neutral for other forms of CVD such as stroke whereas the same amount of alcohol consumed over a week as spirits increased the risk of all forms of CVD (see graph below) (beer had intermediate effects).

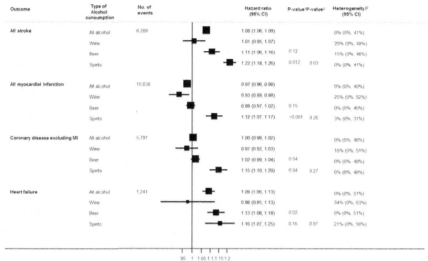

| Outcome | Type of Alcohol consumption | No. of events | | Hazard ratio (95% CI) | P-value¹ | P-value² | Heterogeneity I² (95% CI) |
|---|---|---|---|---|---|---|---|
| All stroke | All alcohol | 8,269 | | 1.08 (1.06, 1.09) | | | 0% (0%, 41%) |
| | Wine | | | 1.01 (0.95, 1.07) | | | 20% (0%, 49%) |
| | Beer | | | 1.11 (1.06, 1.16) | 0.12 | | 15% (0%, 46%) |
| | Spirits | | | 1.22 (1.18, 1.26) | 0.012 | 0.63 | 0% (0%, 41%) |
| All myocardial infarction | All alcohol | 10,038 | | 0.97 (0.96, 0.99) | | | 0% (0%, 40%) |
| | Wine | | | 0.93 (0.88, 0.98) | | | 25% (0%, 52%) |
| | Beer | | | 0.99 (0.97, 1.02) | 0.15 | | 0% (0%, 40%) |
| | Spirits | | | 1.12 (1.07, 1.17) | <0.001 | 0.26 | 3% (0%, 31%) |
| Coronary disease excluding MI | All alcohol | 5,791 | | 1.00 (0.99, 1.02) | | | 0% (0%, 48%) |
| | Wine | | | 0.97 (0.92, 1.03) | | | 16% (0%, 51%) |
| | Beer | | | 1.02 (0.99, 1.04) | 0.54 | | 0% (0%, 48%) |
| | Spirits | | | 1.15 (1.10, 1.20) | 0.04 | 0.27 | 0% (0%, 48%) |
| Heart failure | All alcohol | 1,241 | | 1.09 (1.06, 1.13) | | | 0% (0%, 51%) |
| | Wine | | | 0.98 (0.85, 1.13) | | | 34% (0%, 63%) |
| | Beer | | | 1.13 (1.08, 1.18) | 0.02 | | 0% (0%, 51%) |
| | Spirits | | | 1.16 (1.07, 1.25) | 0.16 | 0.07 | 21% (0%, 56%) |

.95   1   1.05 1.1 1.15 1.2

HR (95% CI) per 100 gram/week higher baseline alcohol consumption

### Risk of a cardiovascular event by type of alcohol [282]

A value of less than 1 on the bottom line (left of the vertical line) indicates a protective effect compared to low levels of alcohol and a value of more than 1 indicates an increased risk. The horizontal lines are ranges of values.

Reproduced in accordance with the CC BY 4.0 license.

A number of other studies have also concluded that drinking moderate amounts of red wine is more protective for health than similar amounts of other alcoholic drinks [619]. One possible reason for the relatively greater benefits of wine could simply be that wine is more likely to be drunk with a meal and so the BAC peak is lowered. The benefits of wine over other alcoholic drinks may also relate to its specific composition. Just as EVOO is much more than just fat, so wine is much more than just alcohol. Both EVOO and wine contain powerful antioxidants, especially polyphenols, which are very important for their health benefits. And just as the fat in EVOO

---

[282] eFigure 18 Supplement to: Wood AM *et al.* (2018) Ibid. The control group for this study was people who consumed low amounts of alcohol rather than never drinkers and this weakens any protective effect of alcohol.

makes the polyphenols more soluble and so easier for the body to absorb (better bioavailability) so too the alcoholic environment of wine may increase the bioavailability of some polyphenols [620]. There is also strong evidence that the far higher amount of antioxidant polyphenols in red wine than in other forms of alcoholic drinks is very important. Red wine contains more polyphenols than white wine, up to ten times more, and this is probably why red wine has additional health benefits over white wine.

It has been possible to demonstrate that the health benefits of wine are due to its polyphenols rather than just its alcohol. This has been shown using red wine that has had its alcohol removed (dealcoholised wine), and also by testing polyphenols after they have been isolated from their normal milieu in red wine. The health benefits of the isolated polyphenols extend to a wide range of diseases including CVD, type 2 diabetes and neurological diseases [621]. One way that antioxidant polyphenols from red wine may work is by reducing the increase in post-prandial oxidative stress that occurs after eating a meal [622]. For instance, drinking red wine reduces the oxidation of LDL cholesterol, a risk factor for CVD. This antioxidant effect can be attributed to the polyphenols in the wine rather than the alcohol since dealcoholised wine works just as well as normal wine [619; 623].

This is not to say that these observations are without controversy. When they are absorbed from the liver, polyphenols (like the vast majority of nutrients) pass through the liver before entering the bloodstream. In the liver, many polyphenols are rapidly metabolised before they even get into the bloodstream and so it is hard to see how the very low amounts that survive intact can exert a direct antioxidant effect in the blood. One possible explanation is that polyphenols work in the gut. By acting in the gut, any effects are occurring before the polyphenols have been absorbed by the body and before they have been metabolised by the liver. Studies have found that red wine consumed with fatty food is able to prevent the generation and absorption in the gut of toxic lipid oxidation products called advanced lipoxidation end-products (ALEs) [624; 625]. ALEs are produced in the gut during the normal digestion of a fatty meal from where they enter the circulation and can promote inflammatory disorders including CVD. Drinking red wine with a meal has been shown to mitigate these dangers and this was ascribed to the polyphenols in the red wine [626].

These examples illustrate the many complex mechanisms how red wine may benefit health. But specific mechanisms for how red wine might work should also be considered in the broader context of the whole diet. This can be illustrated by considering the significance of wine in the French diet. In 1992, two French doctors Serge Renaud and Michel de Lorgeril published a paper highlighting the apparent paradox that despite eating a lot of saturated fat, the French have a relatively low incidence of CHD. They suggested that the amount of wine regularly consumed by the French (2 - 4 units per day) might explain this so-called "French paradox" [627]. This level of alcohol consumption reduces blood stickiness (platelet aggregation), which they offered as a possible explanation for the paradox. Other studies now suggest that the antioxidant effects of the wine polyphenols could also be important. As well as these possible mechanistic explanations, it is important to remember the wider context of the French way of drinking wine. In France this is mainly with a meal and so the BAC will be kept low. Other aspects of the French diet that are independent of wine consumption may also help explain the French paradox. The main dietary source of saturated fat in the French diet is dairy and as discussed previously, cheese and yogurt are not associated with an increased risk of coronary heart disease to the same extent as saturated fat from other sources. So two countries with the same level of saturated fat consumption may have quite different risks of coronary heart disease depending on the dietary source of the fat. Hence understanding the French paradox, and more generally red wine's place in a healthy diet, requires a very broad understanding not only of how the red wine itself works but also its context in the overall diet.

## Practical considerations

Most experts agree that there are no strong reasons for non-drinkers to start drinking as a way to improve health. For people who do drink, personal circumstances can influence risks and benefits. Obvious no-noes are drinking while pregnant and drink driving. When weighing up cancer risk from drinking alcohol, those at more than average risk of cancer may consider not drinking. This includes people with above average risk of cancer such as women with a family history of breast cancer (such as women who have mutations in BRCA1 or BRCA2 genes). [283] This recommendation is currently

---

[283] A good discussion of weighing up personal risk in relation to breast caner and alcohol is at https://www.huffingtonpost.com/julie-chen-md/-alcohol-and-breast-cancer_b_7908604.html

based on the precautionary principle, since there is no consistent evidence that alcohol increases breast cancer risk in women with a genetic susceptibility to the disease [628]. Also possibly at increased risk are women taking hormones such as the birth control pill, other hormonal contraceptives or hormone (oestrogen) replacement therapy. Smoking while drinking greatly increases the risk of aero-digestive cancers. People who flush after drinking are also at increased risk of cancers of the aero-digestive tract [629]. This is particularly prevalent in people of South East Asian origin and is linked to a gene that increases the conversion of alcohol to acetaldehyde. As well as being a carcinogen, acetaldehyde also causes histamine release, which triggers the flushing. This risk is particularly serious in people who only carry only one copy of this gene (heterozygotes) since they are more likely to tolerate the milder flushing effect and so carry on drinking. Students of these ethnic groups are also at higher risk because of peer pressure to drink. An ethanol patch test can be used to test for flushing [629]. Finally, it's worth remembering that alcohol is quite calorific. A small glass (125 ml) of ordinary strength wine (12% alcohol by volume) contains 95 calories. Alcohol may prime the body for fat storage and hinder the burning of fat and sugar. And through a variety of mechanisms, it can increase cravings and appetite. [284]

On the other side of the coin are people who may benefit from red wine consumed in moderation as part of a Med diet. These include middle-aged people who have been assessed as at increased risk of a heart attack, for instance because of being overweight or at high risk of CVD. (In the UK this risk is expressed by a person's QRISK2 score.) Currently, the only (and tentative) support the British Heart Foundation gives for drinking is for very low levels of alcohol (up to 5 units a week), and for women over 55 only. The advice from the BHF is not given in the specific context of consuming the alcohol as red wine drunk and as part of a Med diet. [285]

## How to achieve the optimal drinking pattern

Becoming familiar with the volume of your wine glass can help not exceed recommended amounts. The alcohol awareness organisation DrinkAware sell an alcohol measure cup to help with this. Wine is slightly acidic, like a very

---

[284] *https://betterbydrbrooke.com/alcohol-affects-hormones/*
[285] https://www.bhf.org.uk/heart-matters-magazine/medical/effects-of-alcohol-on-your-heart

refined vinegar, and thinking of wine as a sauce that you drink rather than pour over your food is one perspective to positively link wine with food.

In Mediterranean countries, drinking is closely linked with eating even outside conventional meals. When wine is brought to the table in a restaurant it is usually accompanied with bread. Even alcohol consumed in bars is usually accompanied with some food: a few olives with an ouzo in Greece, a piece of *tortilla* (egg and potato omelette) or some other tempting tapas to accompany a beer in a Spanish bar. What a shame that so few pubs in the UK provide these protective mouthfuls. In the UK, the chances are it will be a packet of crisps or salted peanuts. We must make do with a salty, fatty snack, rather than a nutritious, satisfying one. UK pubs really are missing a trick here - after all what is more appealing to your average UK bloke than egg and potato?

At the beginning of this section on wine, I mentioned that some hold the view that to prevent harm from misuse, alcohol should be declared a drug of abuse [630]. But when taken in moderation, alcohol has many beneficial effects. So it may be more appropriate to view alcohol, not as a drug of abuse, but more as a pharmaceutical drug. It would be rather odd to be prescribed a course of pain killers without it being made clear that only a few tablets should be taken each day - not all of them on a Friday night, which would turn a beneficial drug into an extremely harmful one. Similar precautions also need to be applied to alcohol. This sentiment is encapsulated in that well-known saying attributed to Abraham Lincoln "It has long been recognized that the problems with alcohol relate not to the use of a bad thing, but to the abuse of a good thing."

# 13. Home cooking a Mediterranean diet

## Overview

'Knowing is not enough. We must apply. Being willing is not enough. We must do', said Johann Wolfgang von Goethe. This is clearly true for healthy food: if we want to benefit from it we must eat it. But preventing us eating healthier are many influences on our food choices, especially taste, cost, variety and convenience (most often in that order). Only after these comes health [631]. Home cooking a plant-based diet is key to affordable healthy eating. This chapter shows how to develop the resources needed to be able to home cook healthy Med cuisine. It includes a wide range of practical tips on how to produce tasty, cheap Med dishes quickly and simply.

## The Joy of Cooking

Home cooked, fresh ingredients are at the heart of a healthy, affordable Med diet. Regularly eating home-cooked meals made from good quality ingredients has been shown to greatly increase the chances of eating a healthy diet [632]. Cooking at home demonstrates much more than just having the technical ability to provide a plate of food. It can be a real pleasure, both in using skill to prepare the food and in giving pleasure to someone we care for a tasty, nutritious meal. After all, offering food has been a symbol of hospitality for thousands of years. Cooking with children can help bind a family and return the kitchen to its traditional place as the heart of the home. Cooking is an enjoyable leisure activity for many people. As a way of passing on pleasure to family and friends, cooking is a great way of building self-esteem [633]. All this empowers individuals to eat healthily. Cooking makes cheap ingredients taste good. Cooking improves the nutritional value of foods. Cooking is fun. Cooking shows you care. But cooking is a dying trend. It doesn't make sense, does it? There's something cooking. And it's not only the food.

Increasingly, that something is the multi-billion dollar-pound-euro ready-to-eat meal sector: ready meals, fast foods and takeaways. [286] Every time you cook a meal it's one less meal for them to sell. Advertising tells you to just eat: You don't have the time to cook from scratch! Your time is too valuable! Our meals are for your convenience! This is true for a few people, but it comes with the downside of increasing reliance on ready meals, and it erodes cooking skills placing ever more reliance on ready-prepared food. Cooking from scratch can be much more straight forward than these companies would have you believe, and many meals can be cooked in little more than the time needed to order and wait for a takeaway. And this is no more so than when the food is cooked the Med way.

## Why not ready-to-eat meals?

Cooks have far more control over the quality of the ingredients they buy and prepare than when buying ready-to-eat meals. With ready-to-eat meals we must rely on regulation and labels to ensure that the food we eat is healthy. Food hygiene ranks highly in surveys of consumer concerns and lapses and failings in food hygiene standards regularly make the headlines. [287] In fact the catering sector has long been subject to strict food hygiene and health and safety regulation and inspection, and generally speaking standards in industrialised countries are high. By contrast, animal welfare standards are often overlooked. Unless explicitly stated, it is unlikely that animals will have been raised to high standards. Most eggs and chicken in ready-to-eat meals come from battery chickens and seafood is unlikely to have met MSC standards.

Of more concern in relation to health are the weak nutritional standards and often non-existent labeling around fast food meals bought from takeaways (634). Fast food shops have low start up costs and employ low-skilled cheap labour. This makes these shops relatively simple to open. It also means that the market is extremely competitive, and so keeping costs down becomes a major factor in success or failure. The price paid for the food may be low but the price paid by your health may be high.

---

[286] Sometimes called pre-prepared or convenience foods. Estimated to be worth £10 billion in the UK in 2012. Hucker R. Market report 2013: Fast-Food & Home-Delivery Outlets. 27th ed: Key Note Ltd; 2013. p. 75.
[287] Biannual Public Attitudes Tracker 2015 Food Standards Agency

Quality varies considerably between fast foods served in fast food restaurants, mobile cafes and takeaways. Unlike for packaged foods, these outlets are not required by law to display levels of sugar, salt and fat and calories. And these can be high. A UK study found that pizzas and fish and chips were the worst offenders for calories (worse than Indian and Chinese meals). One meal was found to contain 70% of the entire day's calorie allowance for men and over 90% for women [635]. Pizzas and Chinese meals frequently have very high levels of salt - one serving can provide over twice the recommended daily intake! So it's not surprising that people who regularly eat takeaways typically have a higher than average daily energy intake [636]. In a study based on the UK National Diet and Nutrition Survey, adults eating at least one takeaway meal at home each week consumed 63–87 calories more than the daily average, which is enough to cause substantial weight gain [637].

Some fast foods contain worryingly high levels of saturated fats and trans fats. English meals and pizzas were found to be worst for saturated fats, and kebabs were worst for trans fats. Eating just one meal can quite easily exceed recommended daily amounts [171]. Concerted actions to reduce heart attack-inducing trans fats in shop-bought products have been very successful but the lack of regulation for takeaways is worrying. Although the big players in the fast food market have been taking action, there is very little information on the state of play in the UK with local takeaways and catering vans in laybys. Levels of trans fats in some UK meals of fish and chips or a kebab are higher than the total daily recommended amount of trans fats [638], although there is surprisingly limited information.

UK nutrition surveys paint a rosier picture, and indicate that trans fats only represent 0.7-0.8% of food energy in the UK which is well below the national recommended upper limit of 2% (although it is close to the 1% limit set by the WHO). [288] However this statistic - like so many overall national statistics - hides large variations in society. The UK Office for National Statistics demonstrated that there is a strong correlation between the level of deprivation in an area of the UK and its density of fast food shops. [289] Some deprived areas have five times more fast food outlets than the least deprived

---

[288] National Diet and Nutrition Survey (NDNS) data (combined data from years 1-3 of the rolling programme)
[289] Obesity and the environment Density of fast food outlets (2006) Public Health England

areas. [290] The young are particular fans of fast foods, a BBC survey finding that one in six sixteen to twenty year olds eats fast food twice a day. [291] So nationwide government statistics of fast food and trans fats consumption are likely to mask huge nationwide variations in consumption. [292] There is concern that people from more deprived areas are more likely to eat fast foods on a regular basis and so consume higher than average levels of trans fats than other sectors of the population. This has led authoritative bodies in the UK like NICE and the National Heart Forum to call for government legislation to ban trans fats produced during food manufacture. One estimate is that up to 3500 deaths from coronary heart disease each year could be prevented with policies that improve labeling or simply remove trans fatty acids from foods sold by restaurants and fast food outlets, a policy that would particularly benefit people from poorer socio-economic groups [173].

It may seem unfair to single out small independent takeaways, which are often seen as a valuable part of the community [639]. But operating within very tight budgets means they have limited funding for change and so many are unable or unwilling to switch to healthier foods [640]. Local councils are supplied with "toolkits" to encourage change, but these are of limited value when local council budgets are themselves under such financial pressures. [293]

Deep-fried food cooks quickly and tastes good and so not surprisingly it is the main type of food sold by the fast food sector. Outlets are now being encouraged to replace frying oils high in saturated fat such as palm oil or beef dripping with rapeseed oil. [294] But this policy might not be quite as straightforward as it first seems. Although rapeseed oil contains only low levels of harmful saturated fats, it also contains quite high amounts of the polyunsaturated fat ALA. ALA is particularly susceptible to oxidation. We have evolved to recognise the rancid smell of oxidised fats, and for good reason since they are harmful to health. A rancid smell of cooking fat coming

---

[290] https://www.bbc.com/news/health-44642027

[291] One in six young people 'eat fast food twice a day' http://www.bbc.co.uk/news/health-37511554

[292] Analysis of trans and saturated fatty acids in fats/oils and takeaway products from areas of deprivation in Scotland

[293] Strategies for Encouraging Healthier 'Out of Home' Food Provision. A toolkit for local councils working with small food businesses

[294] Bagwell, S. et al (2014) Encouraging Healthier Takeaways in Low-income Communities
There are some more stable modified RO products but these are even more expensive and less likely to be used by small-scale takeaways.

from the kitchen means it is more than just taste that should be of concern. To keep costs down, there is a risk that rapeseed oil will be re-used beyond the recommended number of times, so increasing levels of oxidised fats. A case maybe of out of the fryer and into the fire.

## Making home cooking easy

Making the decision to eat a ready meal rather than to cook is the outcome of a host of factors such as time availability, cost, and having the ability and confidence to be able to prepare a meal that is acceptable to other members of the household [641]. Confidence is a big factor and removing the apprehension of not knowing how a recipe is going to turn out will remove a major barrier to cooking. Undemanding cooking comes with practice, so it is well worth learning a few basic dishes that everyone likes and will be enjoyed again and again. Following a new recipe can be challenging even for a skilled cook, so building up a repertoire of family favourites is a great way to successful cooking.

There is certainly no shortage of resources demonstrating how to cook - both online and from cookery books. [295] The high number of cookery books on best-seller lists proves that there is a huge appetite for them. Unfortunately there is far less appetite to use them on a regular basis and most cookery books spend far too long languishing on shelves rather than in the kitchen. The 15 minute or 30 minute recipes only take this amount of time if you already have all the ingredients already in the home. Grab your tamarind juice or coconut oil is no good if it's not there to grab. "Simple" recipes based around only three or five ingredients are not simple if they first involve a dedicated shopping trip. And each simple recipe may require quite different ingredients. A ready-to-eat meal can quickly become the more attractive option.

Cooking a Med diet circumvents these issues by using a fairly limited range of ingredients that are always to hand. These come from your "Med store" - a larder/cupboard/shelf stocked in advance with long lasting ingredients. Together with a few fresh ingredients from the fridge-freezer, you will always

---

[295] Jamie Oliver's online cookery courses are available at
http://www.thegoodfoundation.com.au/about-us/

have all the ingredients you need for a variety of nutritious and tasty meals. There is no need to advance plan for a specific recipe. This is a recipe for success.

This certainly does not equate with eating the same old things every day. A Mediterranean peasant may have had access to a relatively limited range of ingredients but this was more than compensated for by their skill and imagination to transform these ingredients into a wide range of tasty meals. Today's cook has far more choice, and can choose from many different Med cuisines: Greek, Italian, Moroccan and so on. These cuisines are built around a similar range of fresh ingredients, and the local authenticity is created with herbs, spices and other flavourings. Because of the multiple ways with a few fresh ingredients, there is far less likely to be waste compared to buying an ingredient that is dedicated to a single recipe.

# The kitchen

### An extra serving of health

A common sight in a traditional Med kitchen is of women - it is still mainly women - cooking for family and friends using the skills handed down to them from their mothers which they in turn have mastered. They do not see cooking as a chore but as an act that brings a sense of purpose and meaning to their lives as they create dishes that bring health and happiness to family and friends. This experience is now being replicated by thousands of women - and men - in the UK and elsewhere who have developed the skills of cooking. Psychologists have a term for the feeling of wellbeing and happiness that comes from a sense of purpose: eudaimonia (from *daimon* meaning true nature). [296] As with developing any skill, such as learning to ride a bike, it takes a bit of practice, but it then brings both mental and physical rewards. There is now a large body of evidence that a high level of eudaimonic wellbeing is associated with healthy aging [642] and in fact the underlying biology of this may be related to reduced inflammation in the body because of reduced stress hormones [643]. So if you are the cook, the health benefits of the Med diet can start even before you eat it!

---

[296] http://positivepsychology.org.uk/the-concept-of-eudaimonic-well-being/

## Practicalities

No matter how small your cookery space (and indeed small spaces can be more efficient), just a few tweaks can make cooking more enjoyable - and so more likely to happen. Some of the following may be self-evident, but I believe they are worth remembering.

1. **The right cooking environment.** Create an attractive space for cooking. This may mean having a space where there is an opportunity for a bit of "me" time: no distractions, maybe some music or the radio, and a glass of wine....

2. **Having the time.** Fear of failure because of unfamiliar or complicated recipes can be a big barrier to ever trying a new recipe - after all it costs money and may disappoint a hungry household. Cooking something new for the first time always takes a lot longer than when you cook the same dish again. So the first time you try a new recipe allow twice the estimated time. The second time round the recipe is likely to be a lot quicker. Also, the result from the first attempt will let you know whether you maybe need a little less or more salt, changing the cooking time and so on. Recipes used again and again become easier and easier.

3. **Building confidence.** Once you build up confidence, you will quickly see how easy it is to incorporate cooking simple meals into your daily life. You will soon be impressing not only any other members of your household that you cook for, but your invited friends as well. And that can make you feel great too.

4. **The right cooking utensils.** Like any good tool, good quality utensils are a pleasure to use. As well as the usual high street shops, there are some excellent on-line suppliers of discount high quality cooking utensils such as Procook in the UK. Some basic essentials are:

- cooker with oven

- microwave - especially for speedy defrosting rather than cooking

- blender

- a good quality non-stick deep-sided frying pan with lid for the many stews that are part of Med cuisine

- other non-stick saucepans - far easier to clean

- sharp, general purpose knife (a Santoku knife is a great multi-purpose knife and its broad blade can be used to carry chopped garlic and herbs to the cooking pan)

- pestle and mortar (for grinding spices, garlic etc)

5. **Cookery books.** There are many excellent Med cookery books. Non-Med cookery books that focus on recipes for vegetables and pulses are also useful. Because the Med diet starts with the ingredient, books arranged by the main ingredient, such as types of vegetables, make it is easier to quickly see the many recipe options for that ingredient. This can be more helpful and inspiring than simply looking up an ingredient in an index. Cookery books based around the seasons can also be helpful. My selection below (by no means comprehensive) includes books that have many uncomplicated recipes using the basics from your Med store cupboard. Many Med cookery books cater to the western palate by including a far higher proportion of desserts and meat-based recipes than is typical of a traditional Med diet. So I have also included a couple of vegetarian Med diet books to help balance things up.

  - The Silver Spoon (Phaidon) - the bible of Italian cuisine, and for me the single most useful cookery book. The cookery book given by Italian mothers to their daughters when they get married. Many of the 2,000 or so recipes are very straightforward and there are multiple recipes for simple, cheap, fresh ingredients that are cleverly combined in different ways. Arranged by ingredient - which makes finding a new way with freshly bought foods from the market even easier.

  - Vefa's Kitchen. The definitive book of authentic Greek cooking. (Phaidon)

  - The Essential Mediterranean cookbook. (Murdoch Books)

  - Food & Cooking of Spain Africa and the Middle East by Pepita Aris and co-authors. (Lorenz Books)

  - Mediterranean Food & Cooking by Jacqueline Clarke & Joanna Farrow. (Lorenz Books)

  - Sud de France The Food and Cooking of Languedoc by Caroline

Conran. (Prospect Books)

- Mediterranean Vegetables by Clifford A Wright. The definitive book for delving into Med vegetable recipes and their history

- Mediterranean Harvest by Paolo Scaravelli and Jon Cohen. A brilliant vegetarian and fish cookbook full of simple, enticing recipes. Mad that it's out of print, but may be available second hand on Amazon

6. **Web sites**

- Dummies Mediterranean diet - useful site for ideas and recipes

- Supercook - a site for searching for recipe ideas using the ingredients you have available - although not just Mediterranean

# Preparing your Med larder

A not uncommon cookery experience is to buy a favourite celebrity chef's latest cookery book, get excited by a dish, write down the long list of ingredients, go to the supermarket, spend a long time searching out those unusual ingredients since they are not on the familiar supermarket shelves, go home and spend twice as long cooking it as the recipe said it would take, and then wait apprehensively to see if the household likes it... It was probably all too much effort and too stressful, and so the cookery book goes back on the shelf. Those unusual (and often expensive) herbs, spices, fruits or veg often don't find another use, and the leftovers end up in the bin. And so it's back to the old standards we are familiar with. That is until the next book comes out...

Mediterranean cooking is not like this since Med cuisine is mainly based around a limited number of ingredients combined in many different ways. After stocking your Med larder there are no complicated one-off shopping lists. The weekly shop is mostly for fresh seasonal foods. Med cooking puts the ingredients first, and the recipe fits around whatever has been bought. A relatively limited range of fresh ingredients is made into a wide variety of imaginative dishes with the aid of flavourings and ingredients from the store cupboard. Shopping just once a week is a big time saver in itself. Covid-19 has been a good teacher of how to limit shopping trips. Using the same fresh ingredients for many different recipes is likely to result in far less waste than from eating around the world's cuisines where different raw ingredients and flavourings are often needed and less often replicated between recipes. This is a big factor in keeping costs down. Waste is not often taken into account when estimating food costs, but typically adds about 30%.

## Basic Med larder staples

Many larder products keep for months or years and just need replacing as and when. Here is a suggestion for a basic Med larder (I have not included many non-Med basics such as salt and pepper):

- extra virgin olive oil (ideally organic)
- anchovies preserved in (ideally olive) oil
- capers
- various jars, tins or dried pulses eg butter beans, chick peas, lentils
- packets/tins of tomatoes/passata/tomato puree
- spices: paprika, cinnamon, turmeric, saffron (turmeric can be substituted to keep down costs)
- orange flower water (used as a flavouring for desserts and salads)
- dried herbs: celery salt, mixed herbs, oregano
- fresh herbs (grow your own if you can): sage, parsley, thyme, rosemary, basil
- fresh garlic
- dairy: butter, cheese (parmesan, feta, goat, others), milk
- eggs (organic and free-range)
- umami flavours such as soya sauce, tomato ketchup, sun-dried tomatoes, anchovies, Parmesan cheese, dried mushrooms (especially wild ones such as ceps).

## Weekly fresh produce

When a group of chefs were asked what would matter most for their next meal if it were to be their last, two main themes emerged. The first was the importance attached to who cooked the meal. And the second was to eat foods that had meaning in the environment. Both these aspects have beneficial sequelae. A meal cooked by a loved one is far less likely to be thrown out than something bought in a hurry from a supermarket. And the relationship to environment is still important in many Mediterranean countries where local fruits, vegetables and cheeses are bought at the market directly from the producers, and local wine is drunk. Awareness that food has been grown by local people makes it less likely the food will be thrown away, just as gardeners, who have laboured preparing the ground, sowing the seed and feeding and watering the growing the plant, are unlikely to want to simply bin all their hard work. Buying fresh local seasonal produce each week also usually equates with cheaper and more nutritious. [297] Knowing a food's provenance is now becoming increasingly important for shoppers who want to appreciate that the food they buy is connected to their environment. Eating natural regional food is an important way that many people connect to their environmental heritage. The French have the word *patrimoine* for this. Factories producing certain branded foods such as Cadbury's chocolate might once have claimed that they retain this link with their locality but there is really little interdependence between a food factory and its surroundings.

## The supermarket

The vast range of produce in the average supermarket is not to everyone's liking and as the number of options increases making the right choice can become increasingly difficult and stressful [644]. A limited range of trustworthy produce is one of the appeals of a familiar local market stall, and, on a larger scale, is one of the reasons for the success of discount supermarkets with limited ranges such as Aldi and Lidl. [298]

Supermarkets are by far the most popular place to shop in the UK. About three quarters of groceries are bought from the "big four" supermarkets. This translates into a significant influence of supermarkets over the food we buy, which in turn means a big influence on our health [645]. This is not always for the better. After adjusting for store size, a study from 2013 found that UK supermarkets had the longest snack food isles amongst eight developed countries (including the US) [646]. Crisps, chocolate and confectionery were the most popular offerings. There is evidence that supermarkets switch what they sell to match the area. A study from Australia found that there was a 70% switch from fresh fruit and vegetables to energy-dense snack foods in more disadvantaged neighbourhoods compared to better off ones [647]. These types of policies are likely to create a vicious circle exacerbating already high social

---

[297] Several websites give lists of in-season fresh foods in the UK such as www.eattheseasons.co.uk

[298] https://www.theguardian.com/business/2019/mar/05/long-read-aldi-discount-supermarket-changed-britain-shopping

differences in food choices. Policy makers need to find ways to encourage supermarkets to help set trends rather than to follow them for commercial reasons.

We mostly navigate supermarket aisles using the same route and buy more-or-less the same ingredients. Taking a different route to make healthier purchases is constantly being challenged by clever marketing and cut-price offers on less healthy alternatives. Supermarkets spend millions designing their layouts to encourage us to buy certain products. [299] Suppliers may be paying more for their products to be displayed at eye level, and the bottom shelf often has an equally good but cheaper version of a product.

Labeling on packaged foods can provide useful information to the consumer, such as the presence of allergens. And there is evidence that labeling foods with calories helps cut calorie intake. [300] But labeling can also mislead. For example, a widely used strategy is to give the amount of an unhealthy nutrient such as saturated fat based on a portion size that is far smaller than the amount the consumer is actually likely to eat (such as basing on one or two squares of a bar of chocolate). [301] How much of this is designed to deceive is a moot point. Highlighting that a packaged junk food is "high in vitamin D" may assuage some reservations about buying the junk food but it is not really doing much for making this a healthy choice. Adding more and more information on labels risks creating information overload during a busy shop. Simplified labeling systems have been invented such as the Nuval system, which simply gives a single number between 1-100 to encapsulate the overall health of a product. Unfortunately, this scoring system was too effective for its own good. It was seen as a threat by food companies who successfully campaigned for it to be discontinued. [302] Fresh foods are not under this threat since they do not carry labels.

## Cost

When he was investigating the eating habits of Mediterranean countries, Ancel Keys (the American scientist who coined the term "Mediterranean diet") was

---

[299] https://www.bbc.co.uk/food/articles/how_supermarkets_tempt

[300] https://theconversation.com/nutritional-labelling-on-menus-helps-cut-the-calories-we-buy-92294

[301] https://www.theguardian.com/money/2019/aug/31/the-fat-shaming-we-should-be-doing

[302] https://www.the-sidebar.com/2017/11/why-did-nuval-nutrition-scoring-system.html

surprised to find that peasant people could be so healthy despite their relative poverty and fairly rudimentary health care. Even today, some of the healthiest people in the world have only low incomes and yet manage to eat extremely healthily. Clearly, wealth isn't a prerequisite to eat well.

And yet headlines seem to contradict this claim. "Four million children in the UK are too poor to have a healthy diet" claims one headline from 2018 [303], which was based on a UK analysis of the costs of conforming to the UK Eatwell Guidelines [648]. A highly influential report called the Marmot Report published in 2010 and updated in 2020 claims the cost of healthy foods is a main reason why less well off people do not eat healthier food. Citing a report from the UK organisation the Food Foundation, the Marmot report claims that "unhealthy foods are three times cheaper than healthy foods" [649]. "Eating healthily is completely unaffordable for many families and individuals" the report stated, and concluded "The exhortations and endeavours to eat healthily that figure in many public health approaches to health inequalities must be seen as rather ineffective". If this is true then it rather undermines efforts to encourage healthier eating amongst the less well off. So what role does poverty play in food selection? And is the corollary correct, that making healthy food less expensive would lead to healthier eating?

Let's start by looking at the claim that healthy food is more expensive than less healthy food. If a pint of skimmed (fat free) milk costs 50 p and a pint of full fat milk costs 50 p, which is more expensive? You're right; it's a trick question. According to most nutritionists the skimmed milk would cost about twice as much. That's because the standard way to calculate the cost of food is based on cost per calorie. Skimmed milk contains half the calories of full fat milk and so to get the same calories in skimmed milk as full fat milk you would have to buy twice as much, hence making it appear to cost twice as much. Of course, this is complete nonsense since both items actually cost the same to buy. Taken to its logical limits this way of calculating costs would mean zero calorie drinks would be infinitely expensive! [304] But - amazingly - it

---

[303] https://www.theguardian.com/society/2018/sep/05/four-million-uk-children-too-poor-to-have-a-healthy-diet-study-finds

[304] Any number divided by zero is infinity. For a demonstration of price parities between many unhealthy foods and their healthy variant see Snowden, C. (2017) Cheap as Chips - Is a Healthy Diet Affordable? IEA Discussion Paper no. 82

is price per calorie that forms the basis for the claim that healthy foods are more expensive than less healthy foods.

There is a historical reason why price per calorie was the method used to calculate food costs, and that is because achieving adequate calories in the diet was once the main challenge. But for most people today the opposite is true (at least in the western world): we eat too many calories. As Christopher Snowden from the Institute of Economic Affairs succinctly put it "For millions of people today, a healthier diet begins with eating fewer calories." (650)

If costing food per calorie does not make sense, then what does? In a food culture such as ours that is awash with calories, a far better way of assessing food costs is to base it on cost per weight or serving. A direct comparison can be made between healthy and less healthy food items when a fat free or reduced sugar alternative exists. One analysis of foods sold in two UK supermarkets found that for most of the foods where like-for-like healthy and less healthy versions are available, such as cereals, dairy produce and soft drinks, prices were similar (650) and this study is backed up by larger scale studies of similar products (651). By contrast, basing cost on a "per calorie" would result in the healthier versions of these foods being declared more expensive. The main exception to this is meat where if healthier is defined as less fatty then healthy meat is more expensive on a weight basis. But this is less relevant to the costs of a Med diet since meat consumption is low.

This comparison cannot be made between versions of other plants foods, namely fruit, veg, pulses, nuts etc since there is no "unhealthy" version to compare them with. When choosing whether to eat these plant foods the alternative is usually junk food. The claim that fruit and veg are more expensive than junk food is the central claim made to explain why less well off people choose the junk food. Again this claim is true if price is calculated per calorie. This is because fruit and veg usually contain far fewer calories per item than junk food - which almost by definition are high in calories - and this makes the fruit and veg appear more expensive since again you have to buy much more to achieve the same calories as a serving of junk food. Junk food is calorie dense and so much cheaper per calorie, whereas most vegetables are low in calories and so are more expensive per calorie. Of course, fruit and veg and junk foods cover a wide price range but I am simply illustrating the fundamental flaw in the way costing are usually presented.

It is important to acknowledge that there is a small sector of the UK population, as there is in other western countries, where achieving adequate calories is the primary consideration when choosing foods. So understandably they will choose the most highly calorific food for the money. But for the majority of people, the opposite is true since most people in the UK consume too many calories, including many less well off people. In the UK, disposable income spent on food is the lowest in Western Europe. At just 8.7% of total spend it is far lower than say in France at 13.6%. [305] This suggests that many people in the UK could afford to spend more on their food if they so chose.

There is little doubt that price has a big influence on the foods people purchase [652]. But I believe cost mainly drives choosing *between similar items* such as which pizza to buy, and it is not the main driver for *deciding between buying junk food or fresh food* - such as whether or not to buy pizza or vegetables. A less well off person may well choose the cheapest variety of pizza, but cost is not the basis for choosing between a pizza and vegetables. So why choose the pizza? I believe this decision is based more on taste and convenience. After all, it would be cheaper to make your own pizza but few do so because of the inconvenience of preparing it and concerns that it would not taste as good as the ready made version.

Preferences around convenience and taste that favour pizza over broccoli can be traced back to broader social influences and cultural attitudes towards food. Influences such as a person's food environment, where popping into a takeaway to buy a pizza from a junk food shop on the high street is more convenient than buying and then cooking vegetables. This is where poverty can have a big impact on choice. Poorer neighbourhoods are often more obesogenic with less healthy food environments such as having more junk food shops and less fresh food shops. These regions are also targeted by the junk food industry creating a vicious circle of more poor quality foods driving more attraction and dependence on them. This dependence can be exerted at

[305] https://ec.europa.eu/eurostat/statistics-explained/index.php?title=File:Table1Price_level_indices_for_food,_beverages_and_tobacco,_2017_(EU-28%3D100).png
https://www.bbc.co.uk/news/business-45559594
https://www.vox.com/2014/7/6/5874499/map-heres-how-much-every-country-spends-on-food

the household level since there may be the added cost to the meal provider of having to convince other members of the household to eat the healthier meal rather than their preferred junk food. And deeply embedded cultural preferences such as taste have been inculcated from an early age and are subsequently strongly reinforced by advertising by the junk food industry.

All this matters profoundly since if it was the case that the main issue is simply not being able to afford healthy food, then making healthy food less expensive and less healthy food more expensive is a logical way to get more less-well-off people to buy them. Often used in evidence to support this argument is the UK sugar tax, which achieved a reduction in the consumption of sugary drinks. However, it only led to a switch to low sugar varieties of soft drinks (which is good as it reduced calorie intake). There is no evidence that it led to a switch to a healthier diet such as eating more fruit and veg. Making food choice a political issue centered around poverty rather than, as I believe, as more of a cultural issue (at least for the majority of people) risks deflecting attention from the true target. Rather than subsidising healthy foods, this money would be better spent on overcoming barriers to healthy eating by promoting tasty healthier alternatives, encouraging home cooking and by reducing the obesogenic environment. As Snowden has said: "The appeal of unhealthy food does not lie in its price but in its taste and convenience" [650].

This is important for the public health debate: if pricing is very important then taxing unhealthy foods and subsidising healthy foods is more likely to be successful to make diets healthier. But if other factors are more important such as taste and convenience then this approach is a regressive tax for the poor who will simply stump up the extra cost and carry on eating less healthy food.

## Cost and the Med diet

The Med diet is sometimes seen as expensive and not a choice for the less well off. Even in Mediterranean countries, studies have shown that low income families are less likely to eat healthily and the main reason given is the *perceived* cost of a Med diet [653]. While it's true than some ingredients such as extra virgin olive oil and fresh fish are more expensive than cheaper alternatives, studies have also found that the cost of the *overall* Med diet is no more than a standard diet [654]. A huge asset of the Med diet is the wealth of recipes that require little time or skill and that turn run-of-the-mill ingredients into healthy meals that can appeal to the entire household. Several cookery books based on the foundations of Med cuisine such as the Italian cookery book the Silver Spoon, and Vefa's Kitchen for Greek cuisine are testimony to this.

Although meat is a relatively expensive food item, very little is consumed in Med dishes and what is consumed is often used in stews, and so cheaper cuts can be bought. Also, because of its wide range of tasty recipes that use inexpensive fruit and veg, there is less need than vegan or vegatarian diets with their more limited food repertoires, to seek variety from expensive "fashionable" plant foods such as quinoa, avocados or mangoes. People eating traditional Med diets rarely feel they are missing out on the latest food trend. Many exotic plant foods also come with a high environmental cost (see ch. 14). As has been commented: "a healthy Mediterranean-style diet can include seafood, salads, and scampi and be expensive, or rice, lentils, and beans and be cheap" [655].

Fruit and veg are at the heart of the Med diet. When it comes to basics such as carrots, potatoes, onions, tinned pulses, apples and bananas, these are not expensive compared to many junk foods [650]. In 2013, Professor Tom Sanders, emeritus professor of Nutrition at Kings College, London, demonstrated that with careful planning an adult could spend as little as £12 per week on a healthy, balanced diet based on starchy foods (bread, potatoes, pasta) and cheap fruit and vegetables including tinned tomatoes and tinned beans and frozen veg, eggs and cheese. [306] These foods align well with a Med diet.

Many households would not find it acceptable to base their diet on these inexpensive yet healthy foods, preferring "tastier" fast foods. Making the healthy foods acceptable means having the skills to turn them into tasty and desirable meals. In an interesting study from Northern Marseille, a small proportion of households with very low incomes and high reliance on social support were identified who for the same cost ate significantly healthier than their neighbours [656]. They didn't so much choose cheaper options of the same foods, since all participants in the study did this, but rather they chose different but healthier things - more fresh foods such as cheap fruit and

---

[306] How little money can a person live on? https://www.bbc.com/news/magazine-22065978

vegetables and fewer products high in fat, salt, and sugar. Having the cooking skills to turn these ingredients into tasty meals was key. Social scientists call these rare people who find solutions despite experiencing similar challenges to their neighbours, "positive deviants". In Northern Marseille, a few positive deviants had found solutions to eating well cheaply that had evaded their neighbours.

Embedded within many large populations are positive deviants who eat healthily for less than their peers. They have overcome the challenge of poor households to access healthy cheap food, and have developed the skills to create healthy inexpensive meals that are acceptable and even preferred by the household. Advice from positive deviants is given as an equal rather than as a superior and so is usually more acceptable to local communities than anything a politician or academic could say. Positive deviants are a greatly underutilised resource in healthy eating campaigns. Many successful celebrity chefs emulate a homely image realising that it is more effective to communicate as an equal rather than coming across as superior.

So it is my belief that the weekly Med diet shopping trolley need cost no more than one for a typical western diet. This would include cheaper cuts of meat and substituting meat with pulses, and less exotic fruit and vegetables, which will balance out the higher costs of extra virgin olive oil and fresh fish. Cheaper types of fresh fish can always be substituted, and tinned and frozen versions are usually less expensive. One saving I would not advise is to replace extra virgin olive oil with a cheaper vegetable oil. Extra virgin olive oil is perhaps the single most important food in the Med diet. After all, it costs less than a bottle of wine and will last much longer. Of course if you can also afford better quality more ethically raised food do so. Cheap food often has "hidden costs" not only costs to health systems but also in terms of labour exploitation and environmental problems. Another cost-cutting factor in a well organised Med diet is the savings brought about by avoiding food waste - which can add up to over a third of the average overall spend. This is discussed later.

---

**Two cheap, simple carrot dishes**

Here are a couple of recipes that illustrate the versatility of an ingredient as humble as a carrot.

## Carrot and orange salad

- one orange
- one carrot
- orange flower water
- sugar

Peel and dice the orange (removing all the white pith) into a bowel
Add sugar and orange flower water to taste
Mix in a grated carrot

## A delicious white bean stew with carrots

- virgin olive oil
- 1 -2 chopped onions
- a tin of white beans eg haricot
- 1 medium potato chopped into dice
- 2-4 carrots cut into thick slices
- a stick or two of celery chopped (or celery powder)
- 3 large cloves of garlic- finely chopped or better still mashed in a mortar and pestle with a little salt
- fresh lemon juice to taste
- a few slices of bread
- 1 teaspoon of sugar
- salt and pepper

Pour a good glug of olive oil into a saucepan and cook the chopped onions slowly for 10 minutes (covered).
Pour in a couple of cups of water, bring to a vigorous boil (this emulsifies the oil) and then add the carrots, celery, garlic, sugar and salt and pepper. Cook for about 10 minutes until the carrots have lost their bite.
Add the potato dice and cook until all veg are tender. Cook uncovered if the stew is too watery - it should be quite thick.
Add the beans and cook for a few minutes more.
Switch off the heat and add lemon juice to taste (about half a lemon). Season to taste with salt and pepper. Add a good glug of olive oil if you like (it does enhance the flavour).

Leave to cool a little.

Toast the bread, or fry in olive oil, put it into bowls and add the bean stew on top.

There are many resources for inexpensive foods (although not all follow the principles of the Med diet) such as the Jack Monroe website https://cookingonabootstrap.com/ and the downloadable US book Good and Cheap Leanne Brown eat Well on $4 a day. French researchers have developed the Good Price Booklet that helps guide people to the best value and most nutritious foods [657]. Pricing food by nutrients per £/euro/$ rather than calories per £/euro/$ should be the way to go.

## Food preparation

Quality kitchen utensils that are effective to use and easy to clean build confidence in food preparation and can mean the difference between home cooking and eating a takeaway. Sharp and well-balanced knives and saucepans that don't stick are invaluable. My own preference is for a Santoku knife with a broad blade that is easy to load with chopped herbs and garlic for transporting to a saucepan. If washing up daunts, a simple grater may be a better option than a complicated food processor. A little time spent learning cutting techniques is time well invested. Jamie Oliver, amongst others, has very helpful videos. Mastery of food preparation elevates it to a craft to be enjoyed and not dreaded. The seemingly effortlessness of TV chefs relies heavily on pre-prepared foods. So if time is short, many veg can be washed, peeled and chopped and stored in the fridge in suitable containers for a day or so, ready for a second meal. Ready prepared veg can also of course be bought but may have been treated (see ch. 12).

The way a food is prepared can transform its taste and nutritional value as much as the way it is cooked. Grating root vegetables releases their sugars changing them from unappealing lumps into sweet pleasures. It's no surprise that the French love their carrot rapé but shun the raw carrot sticks forced on UK schoolchildren. Pureeing aids digestion as well as changing flavour. Chickpeas made into hummus are only one of the many pulses commonly pureed in Med cuisine to add taste and improve digestibility. Marinating is a cooking technique often sacrificed because of time shortages, but it is one well worth resurrecting for its taste and health benefits especially for meat. All these aspects are discussed in more detail in chapter 12.

# Cooking for health and flavour

Cooking makes many raw foods tastier and more digestible and can improve nutritional value. But not all cooking techniques are equal. Boiling can cause water soluble nutrients to leach from veg. Deep frying never became popular in Med cuisine, possibly because the main cooking oil, olive oil, is quite expensive and also because olive oil has a relatively low "smoke point" (the temperature at which it starts to break down). However, the temperature olive oil attains during shallow frying is well below its smoke point. Deep-frying is not intrinsically bad for health and health risks relate more to when the oil is over-heated or re-used too often. These poor practices increase dangerous oxidation products forming in the oil and the food [510]. This is of particular concern with some fast food outlets where margins are tight and temptations to overly re-use oils increase. Boiling and deep frying are not common in Med cuisine and this could be another reason why it is so healthy [442].

The pleasure of flavour comes from an intermingling of taste, smell (aromas), textures, appearances and our emotions. A Med diet satisfies all of these. Fat contributes "mouth feel" and the liberal use of olive oil in the Med diet improves the texture of vegetables, pulses meat and fish to levels that are difficult to achieve with low fat diets. Many classic Mediterranean ingredients have strong, distinctive tastes that add savouriness, saltiness and sharpness. Foods such as garlic, preserved anchovies, capers and preserved lemons are much sought after in Med dishes but can be challenging to palettes used to blander foods. Often though, these foods are used as ingredients in dishes where their taste and flavour significantly mellow. Anchovies melted in warm olive oil create a base for dishes that is quite different to their original pungent fishiness. Many of these ingredients are quite salty and so the amount of salt added to the dish needs to be reduced. These forceful ingredients are among the healthiest in the Med diet, so worth not leaving out.

Receptors on our tongues recognise five basic tastes: sweet, salt, sour, bitter and savoury (umami). Although a bitter flavour is often avoided, it is usually a sign of beneficial phytochemicals (see ch. 6). Too much bitterness can be removed by boiling, or masked with sweetness. Although adding sugar tends to be frowned upon these days, a small pinch of sugar can transform otherwise overly bitter vegetables and is a common addition when cooking vegetables in Med cuisine. (In Arab-influenced Med cuisines dried fruits such as sultanas are often used instead of sugar.)

A craving for the umami taste of meat is often a major barrier for people otherwise willing to reduce their meat intake. Umami has reported to have the duel effects of both stimulating appetite and giving a feeling of fullness (658). [307] Developing the skill to enhance the umami flavour of savoury dishes is a key way to reduce the desire to eat meat. Med cuisine is full of foods packed with umami flavour (see the Meat section for a list). These foods also provide other important nutrients, such as the omega-3 fats in anchovies and antioxidants in sun-dried tomatoes. Many sauces and flavourings from around the world such as soy sauce and tomato ketchup also add potent umami flavour. The skill in using these (some are admittedly not authentic Med ingredients) is to use enough to reveal their umami taste in a Med stew but not so much so that their other flavours come through - a vegetable stew tasting of tomato ketchup isn't very desirable! This balancing act is possible because our taste threshold for the umami flavour is lower than for other flavours. There are also commercial umami concoctions but many contain artificial flavourings and cannot be recommended.

Many popular umami-driven UK dishes have Med equivalents that are far healthier. Bacon and eggs is transformed into *huevas flamencas* where chorizo and eggs are supplemented with healthy red peppers, tomatoes and green beans. Med versions of meat burgers have added healthy herbs and spices such as cinnamon, allspice and mint, and in *kibbeh* the meat is extended with burghul. These healthier counterparts of UK meat dishes make the transition to Med cuisine easier.

When looking for a flavour or aroma, Med chefs naturally turn to their regional aromatic herbs and spices. But if a particular herb or spice is missing from your supplies this does not need to mean the end of the recipe since there is a good chance that another can be substituted. This is because similar aroma compounds are found in the essential oils of many different plants, especially those belonging to the same botanical family. For example, aniseed

---

[307] https://www.nhs.uk/news/food-and-diet/umami-flavouring-may-help-you-feel-fuller-faster/
https://www.theguardian.com/lifeandstyle/wordofmouth/2013/apr/09/umami-fifth-taste

flavour is mainly due to anethole, and this is found in the essential oils of a wide range of umbelliferous herbs and spices including aniseed, star anise, fennel (fresh bulb or seeds) and dill. The lemony flavour of limonene can be derived from lemon juice, lemon rind, preserved lemon, lime, lemon thyme or sumac. Using substitutes may mean that some of the authenticity is lost, but then again you may create a new and even better recipe!

Cooking can be a matter of life and death if it is needed to destroy deadly toxins in foods such as cyanide in cassava. The evidence suggests that not cooking and instead relying on ready-to-eat foods greatly increases the risk of obesity and other chronic diseases [659]. While it may be overstating it to claim that not cooking kills, it is nevertheless a great health asset to have adequate cooking skills.

## Eating together

Meals bring families and friends together. As the Greek philosopher Plutarch famously put it "We do not sit at table only to eat, but to eat together". Meals are a time for hospitality and conviviality, and a time to celebrate a shared cultural food heritage. For many parts of the world these convivial times continue. But, increasingly, fast food culture threatens these times, a culture as much a threat to how we eat as to what we eat. Fast foods are just that: fast. The speed we eat them leaves little time for satiety mechanisms to kick in. And before we know it we have consumed a large number of calories. Eating together around a table with others is usually a far more leisurely affair, often evolving over several courses, each completed at the pace of the slowest eater, punctuated with conversation, and allowing time for a steady rise in satiety mechanisms to help regulate food intake.

Extending the time taken over a meal is now recognised as an important health determinant, not only to allow time for satiety mechanisms to occur and so reduce calorie intake and the risk of obesity [660; 661], but also by lowering triglycerides in the blood, a risk factor for cardiovascular disease [662]. (Unfortunately, one study suggests that these benefits of slow eating do not extend to the overweight and obese, possibly because their satiety signals are not so effective [663].)

Social eating in a relaxed environment also facilitates healthier eating by reducing stress which can induce cravings for "comfort foods" that are high in fats and sugar [664]. The social mores of eating together also helps moderate alcohol consumption and reducing the likelihood of smoking while drinking alcohol. This is a deadly combination that has been shown to boost the risk of oral cancers [665].

## No Waste

The post-war generation were respected for their frugality and not leaving food on the plate: memories of shortages and rationing during and immediately after the war were strong. For subsequent generations, much of this awareness seems to have disappeared. It's not that wasting food is intentional. Much of it just happens without even being consciously registered [666]. The UK anti-waste group WRAP found that 70% of people in the UK believe they have no food waste!

According to WRAP, about a third of food is wasted from cooking, preparing or serving too much, and two thirds from not using it in time. Most drinks are wasted from serving too much. The top foods wasted in UK households are fresh vegetables (especially potatoes) and salads (especially tomatoes and lettuce), drinks (mostly carbonated soft drinks, fruit juice and smoothies), fresh fruit (especially apples and bananas), bread, and meals (homemade and pre-prepared).

Not wasting food is one of the most effective ways of economising on household bills. In 2018, the average cost of food thrown away every month by UK households was £45, increasing to £70 for a household of four. [308] Globally, about one third of food produced is lost or wasted. [667] There are campaigns to raise awareness such as the Love Food Hate Waste campaign organised by WRAP. However, it is unclear if saving money is sufficient to incentivise people not to waste food. Another approach to reduce food waste is to develop a different relationship with the food. In France, school children are taken to meet food producers who use high ethical standards. This helps these children build respect for the food they eat rather than treating it as an industrial commodity. Is it so surprising that an industrially produced chicken is so devalued by consumers, when its life consisted of being de-beaked, detained in a cage and deprived of a natural environment? Dehumanising food is bad for all concerned. Addressing these issues can start from an early age.

---

[308] http://www.wrap.org.uk/food-drink/citizen-food-waste

Wasting food means that growing it, manufacturing it and transporting it were all in vain. Overall food production is responsible for about 30% of total greenhouse gases (GHGs) generated in the UK. By not wasting food, 19 million tonnes of GHGs would be prevented – equivalent to taking one in four cars off UK roads. [309] A lot of food waste is used to generate biogas but this is a very poor return on the energy invested in producing the food in the first place and results in a huge net deficit for the environment. Food not eaten would be far better processed and fed to pigs, but in many countries this is not permitted [668]. The fallacy of the environmental credentials of biogas generation from food waste has been starkly revealed in a damning report from the UK NGO Feedback. [310]

It is quite feasible to achieve no food waste. Choosing less perishable fresh foods is one way to go. In the fridge, grouping items such as dairy, meat, fruit and veg together makes monitoring stocks easier. Having a big fridge and not having too many items stored helps. The Med diet cookery books with a large number of recipes for basic ingredients are a great asset here. Cooking too much is not a problem with most Med dishes since many taste as good if not even better when reheated, and are great eaten the next day. This also eliminates the need to cook.

The same ingredients are used in Med cuisines from different countries and this overlap means less waste because leftovers from different meals can often be combined. Leftovers from one dish can morph into another dish. So two meals can be planned at a time, the meal itself and the subsequent meal that will use up leftovers. One meal begets another meal just as one generation begets the next. And just as generations are depicted in genealogical trees so inter-related meals can be depicted in recipe trees - reciptrees. Experienced chefs have reciptrees in their heads. They already know what they will be doing with the left over boiled potatoes or lentils.

A sustainable food system respects nature's cycles. Recognising and living in harmony with nature's cycles would bring profound benefits to mankind, not least by not accepting waste. There is no waste in Nature. Feeling a strong desire to recycle things is a mindset that can be a more effective way to

---

[309] https://www.theguardian.com/environment/2017/jan/10/uk-throwing-away-13bn-of-food-each-year-latest-figures-show
[310] Feedback (2020) Bad Energy: defining the true role of biogas in a net zero future. London

avoiding waste than financial savings. Our lives revolve around cycles, from the day-night cycle of being awake or asleep to the seasonal production of our food. Cycles are literally programmed in our DNA and building a desire to recycle our food can become another of these. As Joe Moran has said "We find pattern and symmetry pleasing in nature because it gives order and sense to the world." [311] This theme is developed in the concluding chapter.

---

[311] Moran, J (2018) First You Write a Sentence

# 14. The agroecological Mediterranean diet

## Overview

We usually judge food by the health and pleasure it gives to us as individuals. But because food has such a big impact on the environment and on society, it also needs to be judged by how it contributes to the common good for society. A vision of this society was described by the UK organisation for social change the RSA [312] "Imagine a future where healthy, nourishing, delicious food is plentiful and affordable for everyone. Where we can choose from more local and UK produce grown sustainably, and where all the food we buy is grown with care for the planet. Where we have reversed the trend on diet-related illnesses. Where eating food together, at home or in our high streets, is convivial and healthy and strengthens our communities. Where all food is valued, and food waste is eliminated." [(669)]. It is now clear that the diets we eat should not only be *plant* based. They also need to be *planet* based.

This vision is both achievable and realistic. Of course there are many challenges, but as this chapter will demonstrate, there are also well-worked solutions that can turn the vision of a better food and farming system into reality. One of the most widely endorsed sustainable agricultural systems is called agroecology. Agroecology works in harmony with Nature and does not need us to create an alien industrial way of producing our food. An agroecological Med diet is optimum for both person and planet. The only little green men we need are those working in the green and pleasant fields of planet earth.

## Our unsafe trajectory

For many years we have been warned that time is running out. All the signs indicate that we are now at a crux in human civilisation [313], a tipping point in climate change, a point when one change greatly accelerates another, creating positive feedbacks, such as melting Arctic sea ice accelerating the melting of

---

[312] The Food, Farming and Countryside Commission - a team of experts commissioned by the RSA

[313] https://www.theguardian.com/environment/2019/may/06/human-society-under-urgent-threat-loss-earth-natural-life-un-report

permafrost which then releases huge amounts of methane and carbon into the atmosphere which in turn accelerates further global warming [(670)]. [314] Some say we have already passed the point of no return.

To highlight the severity of the scale, pace and implications of environmental destabilisation resulting from human activity, a report published in 2019 described this as the 'age of environmental breakdown' [(671)]. [315] The twenty warmest years since records began in 1850 have been in the past twenty two years; [316] the number of floods has increased by a factor of fifteen, extreme temperature events by a factor of twenty, and wildfires sevenfold. The flames that engulf our planet, from Australia, Brazil and California to Malaysia and the Philippines, are a fitting epitaph for our planet; a planet being cremated by its own forest fires. And going up in flames too are some of our most beloved animal species. Hundreds of koalas were burnt alive in climate change-induced forest fires in Australia during early 2020 that in total affected over a billion animals.[317] And fires are one of the many threats to the survival of orangutans, surely one of the most spiritual of all animal species. The disneyfication of nature on our screens and at "visitors centres" in parks often depicts an image of nature that in reality is long gone, creating illusory reassurances that all is OK with the natural world, when in reality its remnants cling on desperately for survival. [318] Report after report has documented the huge loss of animal and plant species [319].

And the skies are going quiet too, just as Rachel Carson predicted they would in Silent Spring, her famous 1962 polemic on the destruction of nature. We might not like angry wasps buzzing around or biting midges, but they are an essential part of the food web: no insects as food and the birds disappear, no

---

[314] https://www.theguardian.com/environment/2019/nov/27/climate-emergency-world-may-have-crossed-tipping-points

[315] https://www.theguardian.com/environment/2019/feb/12/climate-and-economic-risks-threaten-2008-style-systemic-collapse

[316] https://public.wmo.int/en/media/press-release/wmo-climate-statement-past-4-years-warmest-record

[317] https://www.theguardian.com/environment/2019/nov/26/koala-factcheck-australian-bushfires-survival-species-at-stake

[318]https://www.theguardian.com/culture/tvandradioblog/2006/nov/23/disneyfyingnature
https://georgoconnor.wordpress.com/2017/03/31/the-disneyfication-of-wildlife-documentaries/

[319] https://www.theguardian.com/environment/2019/may/06/human-society-under-urgent-threat-loss-earth-natural-life-un-report

insects to pollinate plants and much of life disappears. [320] A German study found that insect numbers have decreased by 75% over the last 30 years - and this was in nature reserves. [321] This is likely to have a huge impact on the 60% of bird species that eat insects, the 80% of wild plant species that depend on insects for pollination, as well as the many crop plants that need insects for pollination. Although the German researchers could not directly attribute the decline in insects in their study to any one cause, they noted that "agricultural intensification, including the disappearance of field margins and new crop protection methods has been associated with an overall decline of biodiversity in plants, insects, birds and other species in the current landscape." A recent extensive review highlighting "the dreadful state of insect biodiversity on the world" concluded that "almost half of the species are rapidly declining and a third are being threatened with extinction" [672]. Loss of insect eating birds inevitably follows, as shown by the rapid decline in swifts and other birds. [322] Loss of habitat and the use of pesticides are major reasons for this.[323] These are compelling reasons to choose organic foods where possible.

As Ireland's president Michael Higgins eloquently summed up at a biodiversity conference in Dublin in February 2019 "Around the world, the library of life that has evolved over billions of year - our biodiversity - is being destroyed, poisoned, polluted, invaded, fragmented, plundered, drained and burned at a rate not seen in human history... If we were coalminers, we would be up to our waists in dead canaries." [324] Because society has chosen to ignore so many canaries, we are now heading towards massive environmental change, and the social change that will inevitably accompany it. Some changes, such as the loss of the coral reefs and the loss of the 25% of marine life that depend on the reefs, now seem inevitable. [325]

[320] https://www.theguardian.com/environment/2019/nov/13/insect-apocalypse-poses-risk-to-all-life-on-earth-conservationists-warn

[321] https://www.theguardian.com/environment/2017/oct/18/warning-of-ecological-armageddon-after-dramatic-plunge-in-insect-numbers

[322] https://www.theguardian.com/commentisfree/2018/jun/29/natural-world-disappearing-save-it

[323] https://www.theguardian.com/uk-news/2018/may/31/herbicides-insecticides-save-british-countryside-meaows

[324] https://www.theguardian.com/global-development/2019/feb/21/worlds-food-supply-under-severe-threat-from-loss-of-biodiversity

[325] https://www.themonthly.com.au/issue/2019/august/1566136800/jo-lle-gergis/terrible-truth-climate-change

This huge loss of animal and plant species from our bounteous planet has been termed the Sixth Mass Extinction. And because this one is entirely man-made and so profound, geologists have defined a new era for the planet - the Anthropocene. This name refers to the fact that the Earth's current geological time period (*cene*) has been transformed by human activity (*Anthropos* is the Greek for human).

We may have awarded ourselves our own geological time period but we humans are still intimately linked with the world's ecosystems. So as we embark on our current destructive path we are also destroying the ecosystems upon which we, and future generations, rely for survival. Our children and grandchildren will look around their impoverished world and wonder why we did not do better; after all we are aware of the problem and we have the knowledge to find a solution.

We do not need to be victims of this current destructive trajectory. By changing our mindsets we can change from being food consumers who simply choose between the foods we buy to becoming food citizens who actively collaborate in a system that drives change for the better. We have the skills and knowledge in abundance needed to surmount the current challenges. After all, we are not trying to find a cure for cancer or generate energy from nuclear fusion. We are simply talking about producing food in a sustainable way; something that has been achieved by hundreds of previous generations. What we seem to lack is the wisdom to enact what we already know.

As the poet Edna St. Vincent Millay expressed this:

"Upon this gifted age, in its dark hour,
Rains from the sky a meteoric shower
Of facts . . . they lie unquestioned, uncombined
Wisdom enough to leech us of our ill
Is daily spun, but there exists no loom
To weave it into fabric." [326]

At present, there is far too little weaving of the wisdom we already have into the fabric of a society where food and farming are fit for the 21st century. There are solutions but enough people are going to have to want to realise

---

[326] From Huntsman, What Quarry? (1939) by Edna St. Vincent Millay

them, in some cases overcoming short-term self-interest. What is lacking is a sense of urgency. Much like the frog unaware it is being boiled alive by slowly heating water, people are lulled along by their own short term interests as well as the vested interests of the fossil fuel industry, Big Food and others selling products bad for our health and bad for the health of the planet; interests that drown out the warning cries.

## Food production and the environment

Along with transport and the energy sector, producing food is a major contributor to environmental damage. Food production threatens the environment in all directions. In the skies, greenhouse gases (GHGs) are accumulating from crop and livestock production. On land, agriculture is destroying ecosystems. And fresh water is disappearing from our waterways at alarming rates.

The environmental damage is significant. The food chain (which stretches from food production to food transport and to waste) is currently responsible for about a third of all GHG emissions [673]. Forty per cent of the land area of our planet is now committed to agriculture, displacing vertebrate populations whose numbers have fallen by an average of 60% since the 1970s. Tropical rainforests are being cleared to produce ever more palm oil and soya beans. And closer to home, pesticides used for the intensive production of rapeseed and other crops are wrecking havoc on insects. Precious topsoil is being lost ten to forty times faster than natural processes are replenishing it. And in our waterways, much of the 70% of freshwater sucked up for food production is returned polluted with agrochemicals.

This damage is the consequence of poor, unsustainable agricultural practices. The over-production of animal proteins (meat, milk and eggs) is a major cause of environmental damage. Report after report has concluded that current levels of animal production are unsustainable. Animals require large volumes of water, consume huge amounts of feed and generate huge clouds of GHGs. There is a broad consensus that to sustainably feed the projected population of nine billion by 2050, meat consumption in the west must come down. The wellbeing of future generations is being compromised by our current cycle of over-consumption and over-production of animal products.[327]

## Greenhouse Gases

Top of the list of environmental concerns about food production are GHGs. The UK Commission for Climate Change estimates that agriculture produces about 10% of the UK's GHGs [674]. GHGs blanket the earth, warming it up by absorbing energy from the sun, which then drives climate change. Trapping a certain amount of heat created an environment on Earth that enabled life to thrive. But the massive build up of GHGs in the atmosphere and the trapping of heat is now having catastrophic consequences for the planet. The current yearly increases in GHGs show no sign of abating. [328]

Beef and lamb production are major sources of food-related GHGs. This is shown in the graph below (which combines an analysis of GHGs from several hundred studies) [675].

[327] https://www.theguardian.com/environment/2018/sep/15/europe-meat-dairy-production-2050-expert-warns https://www.theguardian.com/environment/2018/may/31/avoiding-meat-and-dairy-is-single-biggest-way-to-reduce-your-impact-on-earth
[328] https://www.theguardian.com/environment/2019/feb/17/methane-levels-sharp-rise-threaten-paris-climate-agreement

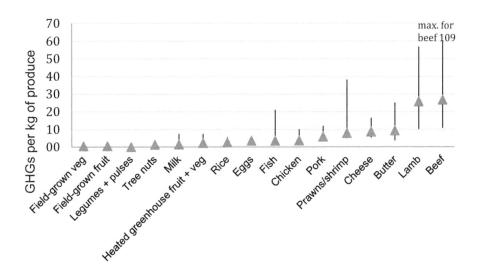

**Greenhouse gases emissions generated from producing fresh foods** [329]

The triangle represents the median (middle) value of all estimates and the line shows the range of values from lowest to highest. (maximum GHGs from beef is off the top of the scale and is 109.) GHGs are expressed as kg of $CO_2$ (carbon dioxide) equivalents.

One of the most striking features of this graph is that for many foods, such as beef and lamb, the amount of GHG emissions per serving varies enormously between production with a low environmental impact and production with a high impact. This is ten-fold in the case of beef. This leads to some surprising conclusions. For instance, farmed prawns and fish if produced badly (such as because of damage to mangrove swamps caused by farming prawns) can generate more GHGs than a serving of beef produced under optimal environmental conditions. So just talking about averages hides huge ranges of possible values. This is another example of the wisdom in the saying "The mean is an abstraction. Reality is variation". [330] This highlights the important

---

[329] Redrawn from data in Clune et al (2017) Systematic review of greenhouse gas emissions for different fresh food categories. *Journal of Cleaner Production* **140**, 766-783.
[330] From Blastland & Dilnot, 2008. The Tiger that Isn't: Seeing through a World of Numbers. Profile Books Ltd: London.

point that *how* a food is produced strongly influences its environmental impact: it is not just the *type* of food that matters.

The amount of GHGs associated with producing a food is calculated using a Life Cycle Analysis. A Life Cycle Analysis considers all the GHGs associated with a food's production, transport and waste. This analysis is complex since there is so much to consider. Undoubtedly, beef production is the biggest overall environmental concern in relation to GHGs. But a Life Cycle Analysis of cattle emissions is complex. To take one small facet: GHG emissions from cattle manure will be far lower if the manure is used for biogas generation than if the manure is left to release its GHGs into the atmosphere. Aspects such as these are not always taken into account. Some researchers do attempt to take into account the whole "ecosystem" in which the livestock is raised. For instance, a whole ecosystem analysis based on the scenario of raising cattle by feeding them pasture and only grazing them in one field for a short period (known as rotational or mob grazing) found that there was a net decrease in overall GHG emissions [676]. This is contrary to estimates of GHG emissions in most studies, which find raising cattle adds to atmospheric GHGs. Similarly, when carbon capture from trees and other farm vegetation was taken into account, sheep and beef farms in New Zealand were estimated as being close to being carbon neutral (no net carbon generation). [331]

There is no doubt, though, that raising livestock using current standard practices is a significant source of GHG emissions. The FAO calculates that livestock are responsible for about 14.5% of anthropogenic GHG emissions [677]. (Other estimates vary between 9% and 15%.) This is about the same as all the emissions from all the vehicles in the world. But this is only a world average and bandying around statistics is often not very helpful; indeed it can confuse. In the US, for instance, it is estimated that livestock contributes only 4.2% of GHGs compared to 27% from transport. [332] It has been argued that because animal production is a relatively small percentage contributor to GHGs in the US, compared to say India, animal production does not need to be a priority area for the US. But this is against the enormous contribution of

---

[331] Case, B (2020) Analysis of carbon stocks and net carbon position for New Zealand sheep and beef farmland

[332] https://theconversation.com/yes-eating-meat-affects-the-environment-but-cows-are-not-killing-the-climate-94968

transport. In absolute terms, the US livestock sector is still a major contributor to GHGs. [333] Global averages are not really very helpful. Because of their poor diets, the cattle from impoverished farmers in sub-Saharan Africa and elsewhere emit relatively high amounts of GHGs. But poor farmers in sub-Saharan Africa don't contribute much to other sources of GHGs such as air transport, whilst at the same time they have a high reliance on their cattle to survive. So the issues surrounding how to reduce the environmental impact of GHG emissions from these farmers are quite different to those in more affluent countries. My discussions are only relevant to Northern Europe and US.

---

**Simplifying the statistics on GHG emissions**

It is easy to be confused by the various stats around GHG emissions and food production. It is important to be aware of which part of food production is being discussed: Is it:

All aspects of food production?
A quarter of all GHGs come from food

⬇

Animal products only?
More than half (58%) of food GHGs come from these

⬇

Beef and lamb only?
These represent half of farmed animal GHGs

---

[333] https://caes.ucdavis.edu/news/articles/2016/04/livestock-and-climate-change-facts-and-fiction

## The big three GHGs

The three main GHGs emitted during farming are methane, nitrous oxide and carbon dioxide ($CO_2$). In the UK, methane accounts for about 57% of agricultural GHGs, nitrous oxide 32% and $CO_2$ 12% [674]. Trends in GHG emissions from agriculture have remained more or less flat over the last decade. This contrasts with some other sectors such as electricity generation where there has been much more progress in reducing GHG emissions. This demonstrates that current policies to reduce GHGs from agriculture are not working [678].

GHGs warm the planet to different degrees depending on (a) the amount of heat they trap and (b) how long they persist in the atmosphere. To allow comparisons between GHGs, each gas's "global warming potential" is expressed relative to that of $CO_2$. Methane acts as a far thicker warming blanket than $CO_2$, but it is broken down in the atmosphere more quickly, persisting for only twelve years compared to the hundreds of years for $CO_2$. [334] The overall global warming potential of methane is estimated to be 28 times greater than that of $CO_2$. By comparison, nitrous oxide's global warming potential is a whopping 300 times more than $CO_2$.

Nitrous oxide

Maintaining nitrogen levels is essential for soil fertility. Unfortunately, attempting to do this is responsible for about a third of the current GHG emissions from UK agriculture. Nitrous oxide is released during the manufacture and use of synthetic nitrogen fertilisers, and nitrous oxide is also one of the main GHGs (along with ammonia) released from unwanted slurry from the industrial farming of animals.

Methane

Methane is the main GHG produced by farming. Much of it is produced by ruminants during their digestion of grass and grains by a process called enteric fermentation. Pigs and chickens are not capable of enteric fermentation and so this is not a source of methane. What methane they do produce mainly comes from their manure and during the production of their feed. Hence,

---

[334] https://www.epa.gov/ghgemissions/overview-greenhouse-gases

methane production per kilogram of protein from pigs and chickens is far lower than for ruminants. (Producing pork and chicken generates about six and eight times less GHG emissions respectively than beef [679]).

As mentioned earlier, there are many steps in animal agriculture and so estimates of GHG emissions for a particular food product will vary widely depending on how many stages of the production cycle have been considered. Depending on the type of farm animal, these stages might include methane from enteric fermentation; nitrous oxide and methane emissions due to manure management; various GHGs from the production of animal feed and forage; emissions of nitrous oxide associated with fertilizer application; $CO_2$ emissions from land use changes - such as destroying mangrove swamps and rainforests; $CO_2$ emissions from transporting animal feed, livestock, and food animal products; and emissions associated with imported food animal products. [335]

The example of beef production, given earlier, whose GHGs emitted to produce a kilogram of protein can vary ten-fold or more depending on the farming system [680], re-emphasises the point made earlier that presenting GHG emissions as fixed values can be misleading. Cattle raised on the rain-watered pastures of English meadows, which then return a significant part of the carbon to the soil as manure, are far less environmentally damaging than cattle raised on lands that were once rainforests.

There is also a lively debate about the relative merits of grass-fed cattle versus animals given feed in terms of their contributions to GHG emissions. [336] Some estimates suggest that grass-fed beef cattle produce about 20% more methane than cattle given feed (mainly grain) concentrates. Reasons given for this are that grain feeds are easier to digest (and so less methane is produced by enteric fermentation) and also that the average time to market of grain-fed cattle is shorter and so they are not around so long to produce GHGs. However, there is such huge variation between different farming systems that some estimates give lower overall GHG emissions from grass-fed cattle when all factors are considered [681]. For instance, GHG emissions from growing the

---

[335] https://www.jhsph.edu/research/centers-and-institutes/johns-hopkins-center-for-a-livable-future/_pdf/about_us/FSPP/letter policymakers/20160512_Mitloehner_Response12.pdf
[336] http://newzealmeats.com/blog/grain-fed-vs-grass-fed-beef-greenhouse-gas-emissions/
https://sustainablefoodtrust.org/articles/grazed-and-confused-an-initial-response-from-the-sustainable-food-trust/

feed for corn-fed cattle are not always taken into consideration (these emissions come from the fossil-fuels needed for the fertilisers, pesticides and transport). Local pasture does not have these emissions. Another important difference between pasture-fed and barn-raised animals is what happens to the manure. Pasture-fed animals return much of the carbon and nitrogen in the manure to the soil. By contrast, the management of manure from animals in barns can generate huge amounts of potent GHGs (especially the very potent GHG nitrous oxide). Another interesting, but not clearly quantified, part of reducing methane produced by ruminants is by so-called methanotrophs. Methanotrophs are soil bacteria that absorb and break down atmospheric methane. When cattle sit amongst pasture chewing the cud, some of the methane is absorbed into the soil and is broken down by methanotrophs in the soil. This is not possible for cattle kept in barns.

One of the main contributions to the debate on GHG emissions from cattle, and the relative merits of corn-fed versus grass-fed cattle, was a report called Grazed and Confused [682]. And yet, despite the authors' best efforts, there is still much confusion surrounding this topic, some suggesting that corn-fed emit fewer GHGs whereas others suggesting it could be the other way round [683; 684]. There is however no confusion that pasture-fed cattle are more likely to be raised to high welfare standards and as discussed in chapter 12 there is good evidence that grass-fed meat and dairy is better nutritionally.

## Sustainable land use

The British countryside alone cannot feed the huge numbers of factory-farmed animals in the UK. So to satisfy the demand for cheap meat, vast tracts of rainforests in Argentina and Brazil are being ripped up or burnt, an ecosystem that will soon disappear forever, one that for our grandchildren will simply be a part of ancient myths. All this just to grow ever more soya beans to feed the chickens, pigs and (to a far lesser extent) cattle which our own farming system cannot support. And all too often these animal products are treated with little respect: the tastiest morsels consumed, the rest thrown away. [337]

---

[337] https://www.theguardian.com/environment/commentisfree/2019/jul/02/barter-amazon-rainforest-burgers-steaks-brazil
https://www.theguardian.com/environment/2019/jul/02/revealed-amazon-deforestation-driven-global-greed-meat-brazil

Even when chicken and pig feed is grown in the UK, this is still using land that could have been producing food for direct human consumption. So there is a trade-off between using the land for feed (for farm animals) and food (for humans). Feeding pigs food waste would be one solution although this is currently illegal in some countries such as the UK.

Beef is often cited as having a high demand for water. But if this is rain falling from the sky ("green water"), then water use is having a negligible impact on the environment. Water extracted from rivers and aquifers ("blue water") can have a far greater impact. Irrigating almond orchards in California has a far greater impact on water reserves than farmers raising beef cattle in the rainy west of Ireland.

Land use needs to be considered in relation to its other possible uses. Compared to the amount of land needed to produce 1 kg of protein from plants, three times more land is needed to produce 1 kg of protein from pigs and five times more for beef [529]. But this is not *ipso facto* an argument to allocate all land to growing arable crops. Ruminants can be raised on marginal land not suitable for arable farming. Sustainably produced cattle can live mainly off grassland and are consuming a plant humans cannot eat that has been grown on land unsuited for food crops, using freely available water.

Pasture-fed ruminants also directly return carbon as fertilising manure to the land, whereas intensively farmed animals create huge amounts of excrement for which there may be no immediate use. In the US, it has been estimated that intensively raised livestock produce 500 million tons of manure per year, which is three times the annual amount of human sanitary waste [685]. The waste emits huge amounts of GHGs and can easily end up polluting waterways. Sustainable farming minimises its impact not only from the gases it emits into the skies but also how it influences the land and the rivers. This is achieved by farming in a way that is most compatible and sustainable with the local environment. How animals are raised is an important determinant of sustainability.

## Towards more sustainable farming

The massive negative impacts of industrial farming on animal welfare and the environment, and the epidemic of obesity and chronic diseases caused by UPFs demonstrate that our current food system is broken. We have now become desensitised to the factory farming of pigs and chickens, a way of farming that continues to expand and now includes an estimated "20% of cattle that never see the sky". [338] From the inhuman ways of rearing and transporting animals to the vast amounts of polluting animal excrement, animal production has been pushed beyond acceptable boundaries. And the pesticides used on crops endanger farmers and pollute the countryside. A better way of farming is long overdue.

A growing number of people care for the environmental, health, social and ethical issues associated with food production. Even though most people live in urbanised areas, they still want to feel close to their food. They want food that is fresh, less processed and sustainably produced. The ground swell of dissatisfaction with much of today's way of eating can help sweep us to a more compelling future, one where the food we eat is produced with care for the planet, where food is valued and food waste eliminated. A diet that is both plant-based and planet-based. Consumers should be empowered to make sustainable food their food of choice and enabling this should be both the responsibility and an opportunity for food providers. Sustainable food should be the cheapest option not only for the customer to consume but also for the farmer to produce.

There are, of course, many barriers to achieving this. For a start, not everyone is dissatisfied with the current situation and, in fact, some benefit from the *status quo* by plundering natural resources. These entrenched positions are being challenged by radical action by movements such as Extinction Rebellion. [339] But each individual also makes the choice to be part of the problem or part of the solution. Being part of the solution for a sustainable food system starts with eating more sustainably produced foods. This in turn puts pressure on retailers to choose more ethical suppliers, creating a virtuous circle that benefits the entire food chain. The writer and environmental activist Wendell Berry linked together the two ends of this chain in his famous phrase "Eating is an agricultural act"- in other words the foods we choose will ultimately impact of the type of agriculture used to produce it. [340] Michael Pollan in his book In Defense of Food extended the food chain even further

[338] https://www.theguardian.com/uk-news/2017/mar/12/free-range-milk-farming-revolution-dairy-industry-decline

[339] https://www.theguardian.com/commentisfree/2019/apr/15/rebellion-prevent-ecological-apocalypse-civil-disobedience

[340] https://www.ecoliteracy.org/article/wendell-berry-pleasures-eating#

by declaring "eating is a political act". In other words, that the heart of governance can ultimately be influenced by how little meat we choose to eat, whether we eat only ethically produced meat and whether we choose organic fruit and veg. As food citizens we have the power to lead, not follow.

The food industry has been known to piggyback on people's desire for locally produced natural foods by branding their products with the names of fake farms. Tesco's fake "Woodside Farms" gave the image of the produce being from local farms whereas some of the products carrying this label actually contained imported foods. [341] It does not seem very likely that a supermarket would happily show the true provenance of their cheap eggs or meat with images of battery chickens or cattle cooped up inside. Well-cared for animals do matter to shoppers.

More and more national governments now recognise the need for more sustainable approaches to food production and consumption. The Dutch national guidelines for example now factor in ecological considerations when making dietary recommendations for red meat [(686)]. This is not yet the case in the UK, where the current guideline for red meat consumption of no more than 70 grams per day is based only on nutritional considerations. However, in August 2019, the UK government launched a National Food Strategy, which amongst its objectives is to "restore and enhance the natural environment for the next generation in this country" based on a strategy that is "built upon a resilient, sustainable and humane agriculture sector". [342] A resilient food system is one that can absorb changes in circumstances - such as the Covid-19 pandemic - and then adapt and transform into a new system able to cope with the new conditions [(687)]. How much of the UK's National Food Strategy will simply be lip service time will tell.

Governments' role in food extends well beyond setting national dietary guidelines (which few people are aware of anyway) to also include legislating bottom lines of acceptability in areas such as pesticide use, animal welfare and imports of produce grown on ex-rainforest land. By our actions, we as

---

[341] https://www.theguardian.com/environment/2017/dec/13/tesco-faces-legal-threat-over-marketing-its-food-with-fake-farm-names. (an action subsequently legally challenged)
[342] https://www.gov.uk/government/publications/developing-a-national-food-strategy-independent-review-2019

consumers can help influence these laws. Our eating is then both an agricultural and a political act.

Unfortunately, there is evidence of the food industry acting in the political arena to actively undermine sustainable food production. A commission of experts identified that the food industry has, through political pressure, succeeded in keeping sustainability out of national dietary guidelines in the US and Australia [688]. The fears of the commission that the food industry is undertaking actions that endanger planetary health were endorsed by Fiona Sing of the World Cancer Research Fund who said: "We support the implementation of a global treaty to limit the political influence of big food. How we produce and consume food is possibly the most important determinant of both human and environmental health worldwide." [343]

Diets need to align within the capacity of a sustainable farming system to provide the foods for these diets. As most current national dietary guidelines show, too much current dietary advice starts from the opposite end. That is, the advice starts with dietary recommendations regardless of whether or not these recommendations are feasible within a sustainable farming system. The dietary advice is detached from farming reality. Operating within environmentally sustainable boundaries is one of the defining features of the United Nation's Seventeen Sustainable Development Goals that offer a "shared blueprint for peace and prosperity for people and the planet" [344]

To achieve this vision for food production we need, as the medical journal the Lancet suggests, to reconnect with Nature. "Our connection with Nature holds the answer and if we can eat in a way that works for our planet as well as our bodies, the natural balance of the planet's resources will be restored [689]". For centuries, the quintessential image in many North European countries of animals grazing in fields has forged important links between the countryside and our food heritage. Linking people with the farming countryside is a key way to preserve it.

---

[343] Quoted in https://www.theguardian.com/society/2019/jan/27/food-industry-obesity-malnutrition-climate-change-report
[344] https://sustainabledevelopment.un.org/?menu=1300

# Agroecology: sustainable, nature-based farming

There is an agriculture and food system that does reconnect people with Nature, that is in harmony with the natural environment, a farming system that respects the huge diversity of diets around the world, one respecting ecological boundaries by staying within the productive capacity of sustainably managed farmland and that farms animals to acceptable welfare standards. This system is called agroecology. [345] Agroecology can produce all the food Europe needs and still achieve net zero carbon by 2050 [690]. It is a system based on recycling. By recycling nutrients and recycling waste it minimises the need for external inputs.

Agroecology is not a niche undertaking for a few high-end products but a system for all foods and one that fundamentally reconfigures how farming is undertaken so that it benefits the environment, health and jobs. Agroecology is recognised by the UN in its Sustainability Development Goals as a sustainable system [691]. And many expert committees and think tanks in the UK and internationally have concluded that agroecology is the food system that best serves the interests of the environment and society, from farmer to customer. [346] The EU Commission in its 2020 report "A Farm to Fork Strategy for a fair, healthy and environmentally-friendly food system" identifies agroecology as a future area for major funding [692] and their recommendations will be the subject of a legislative proposal on sustainable food systems (by 2023) for the European parliament. [347] Closer to home, the Food, Farming and Countryside Commission convened by the RSA in their report Our Future in the Land strongly endorsed agroecology stating that "the principles of agroecology best sum up how farming will need to change globally to address the challenges and opportunities" for the future of farming. [348]

---

[345] https://sustainablefoodtrust.org/articles/linking-our-diets-with-the-outputs-of-sustainable-farming-in-the-uk/

[346] Committees supporting agroecology include the International Panel of Experts on Sustainable Food systems in their policy report Towards a Common Food Policy for the European Union and the Institut du Développement Durable et des Relations Internationales (IDDRI) in An Agroecological Europe in 2050: Multifunctional Agriculture for Healthy Eating.

[347] https://www.iddri.org/en/publications-and-events/blog-post/towards-sustainable-european-food-system-successful

[348] RSA Food, Farming and Countryside Commission (2019) Our Future in the Land

Agroecology can provide all the foods needed for a broad range of healthy diets; by aligning with nature it is good for the planet and boosts biodiversity; and it offers a feasible route for farmers to transition towards more sustainable farming practices. [349] It is a way of farming that adapts to the environmental conditions, ecologies and cultural values of different countries. It is now increasingly recognised that hunger in developing countries is fundamentally tied to factors such as poverty and social exclusion and that, rather than relying on imports, increases in productivity have to occur predominantly within these countries if they are to have an impact on food and nutrition security, particularly among the poorest [693]. One example of a country applying agroecology to benefit domestic food production is Cuba, where it is estimated that family farms practicing agroecological farming may account for as much as 65% of the domestic food supply [694].

## Animal protein and agroecology

Agroecology is a middle way that respects the desire of the majority of people for moderate amounts of animal protein. Grassland occupies about a third of agricultural land in Europe and much of this is marginal land not suited to growing food crops. Within the UK, the devolved countries of Northern Ireland, Scotland and Wales are especially rich in pastureland. Ruminants are efficient at converting this pasture into nutritious food for human consumption and there is little competition for this land between ruminants and humans.

Pigs and chickens, by contrast, are usually fed grain and protein-rich feed. Whether grown locally or imported, this could usually have fed humans. It is estimated that over a third of the world's grain is fed to poultry [695]. Agroecology avoids importing feed. This means growing the feed locally and the extent to which land should be devoted to growing this feed is a matter for debate. Pigs are omnivores and will eat waste from human consumption and surplus food production [668]. Pigswill was widely used in the past and its revival is long overdue when disease transmission concerns diseases have been addressed. This would be a far more efficient use of waste food than simply turning it into biogas, as is now often the case.

---

[349] https://www.theguardian.com/environment/2019/feb/20/european-farms-could-grow-green-and-still-be-able-to-feed-population

GHG emission considerations and land available for grazing and to produce animal feed (mostly for pigs and chickens) will impose limits on how much livestock can be raised without environmental harm and so how much animal protein can be eaten as part of a sustainable diet. It is clear that meat consumption will need to come down since sustainable agriculture cannot support the current huge numbers of industrially raised chickens, pigs and cattle. An optimistic and constructive report from the Rural Investment Support for Europe (RISE) foundation has set out these limits, defining them as the "Safe Operating Space" (SOS) [529]. The SOS operates between a minimum livestock population that provides adequate nutrients and an upper limit beyond which there will be damages to the environment. The report concluded that even with all available technologies to mitigate the effects of GHG emissions, a reduction in the numbers of livestock is also needed if target reductions are to be achieved. [350] The report estimated that ruminant numbers are between one-third and two-thirds above the levels necessary to occupy and sustainably graze the permanent pastures of the EU. [351] This level of livestock reduction is entirely compatible with a Med diet. Reducing livestock by half would free up 23% of cropland in the EU, and globally it would also free up a further 23% of cropland globally. This creates big opportunities for the land to be used to regrow forests, produce crops or biofuels, re-wild it, or use it for human habitation. [352]

## How farm animals enhance farming

Increasing numbers of people are choosing vegetarianism or veganism. Which is a great help to counter-balance the excessive meat consumption by some people. Increasing numbers of voices (often the self-same vegetarians and vegans) advocate that no one should eat meat. [353] I do not believe this is acceptable culturally and is highly unlikely to become a reality. In a survey of Europeans, 82% declared that they were willing to eat less but better quality meat whereas only about half would be willing to go a step further and replace

---

[350] What is the safe operating space for EU livestock? p. 10
[351] What is the safe operating space for EU livestock? p. 76
https://www.theguardian.com/environment/2018/sep/15/europe-meat-dairy-production-2050-expert-warns
[352] What is the safe operating space for EU livestock? p. 72
[353] https://www.theguardian.com/environment/2020/jun/19/why-you-should-go-animal-free-arguments-in-favour-of-meat-eating-debunked-plant-based

most of the meat with vegetables [696]. Banning meat risks becoming counter-productive by creating antagonism from meat-eaters and jeopardising the more widely acceptable route towards reducing meat consumption but not completely banning it.

A farming system that only grows crops would require large amounts of external inputs such as artificial fertilisers. These often end up contaminating waterways, they do nothing to improve soil structure, and their production and use generates large amounts of GHGs (especially nitrous oxide). It is true that because of their soil and climate some agricultural areas, such as the East of England, are best suited to crops. But even these areas benefit from using animal manure as fertiliser and to improve soil structure. For many other parts of the UK, mixed crop-livestock farming offers an attractive way forward. And it is mixed farming that best aligns with agroecology.

Mixed farming is an economic and environmentally friendly way of farming. Leftover parts of crops are fed to farm animals and animal waste fertilises crops. This way of cycling farm products is the way farming has successfully operated for centuries. And studies suggest that even today in our era of specialised intensive monoculture farming, mixed farming is economically viable. A study of farms in the South West of France compared dairy farms, beef farms, crop farms and mixed crop livestock farms [697]. The study identified that the mixed system was particularly favourable in helping to ensure financial security since the farmer needed to buy far less fertiliser and feed and so was less influenced by price fluctuations in these commodities. By mixing the use of the land, mixed farming also reduces the likelihood of nutrients either becoming overly depleted or saturated. Also, as the authors of the study noted, mixed farms are particularly favourable for birds and insects. Overall, the mixed farming system compares very favourably with more specialised monoculture farms.

Unfortunately, it is specialised monoculture farms that dominate farming at the moment with their intensive monocultures of crops requiring huge inputs of fertilisers and pesticides, or factory farms for animals. The natural cycles between plants and animals have been lost in these systems and so they are not compatible with agroecology.

The switch from the diversity of mixed farms to the uniformity of monoculture farming also comes with risks when a single cultivar is grown.

One of the best-known examples was the monoculture of potatoes that exacerbated the Great Irish Potato Famine, which started in 1845. More recent problems include a fungal disease in banana plantations which all grow the same Cavendish cultivar. Similarly, recent major outbreaks of swine fever in Nigeria and China illustrate the dangers of huge numbers of genetically identical animals. [354]

The switch to monoculture is driven by economies of scale. The junk food industry is also a driver of monoculture farming by demanding large volumes of uniform commodities such as vegetable oils and corn-based sweeteners. These mega-farms are often bad for the environment, just as their products are bad for our health. Large-scale factory farms are also swallowing up smaller more mixed farms. [355] The small farms that shaped our landscapes are dying out, replaced by a countryside of mega farms, many of which are tantamount to open-air factories. In the EU this has been made worse by subsidies incentivising farmers to enlarge their farms leaving mixed crop-livestock systems marginalised on less productive land. New payment structures for environmental protection such as those introduced in the EU's Common Agricultural Policy (CAP) in 2018 and further proposals made for the post-2020 CAP may help change this and hopefully also lead to an increase in mixed farming [698]. A step back to the future.

## The importance of cycles in agroecology

Agroecology-based mixed farming is a way to rekindle old traditions. In agroecology, crops and livestock are brought back together, and so natural cycles can operate again in sustainable and ecologically balanced ways. [356] Animals fertilise plants with their manure, and plants feed the animals. Animals feed on land best suited for pastures and food plants are grown on land able to support their growth and productivity. These cycles are illustrated in the figure.

---

[354] https://www.theguardian.com/environment/2020/jun/18/worst-outbreak-ever-nearly-a-million-pigs-culled-in-nigeria-due-to-swine-fever

[355] https://www.theguardian.com/environment/2019/mar/09/american-food-giants-swallow-the-family-farms-iowa

[356] In the UK, Knepp farm is much discussed as a model mixed farming system
https://www.theguardian.com/commentisfree/2018/aug/25/veganism-intensively-farmed-meat-dairy-soya-maize

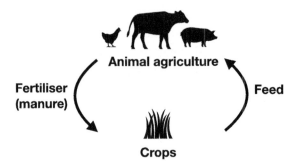

Fertiliser (manure)

Animal agriculture

Feed

Crops

**Basic cycle between farm animals and crops**

The concept of cycles is fundamental to understanding agroecology. Agroecology works within the constraints of closed systems, recognising that planet Earth is finite and not a bottomless pit. Rather than irreversibly plundering the Earth of its finite resources, it is a system that puts back what it takes out, one that regenerates the planet for future generations. Hence agroecology is sometimes called "regenerative farming". By being regenerative and self-sustaining, agroecology is recognising that the planet does not have infinite resources to be plundered. Sir David Attenborough summed this up in his President's Lecture in 2011 at the RSA: "Anyone who believes in indefinite growth in anything physical, on a physically finite planet is either mad – or an economist ... We need to ... shift to an economic model that accounts for the fact that we operate within a closed system – planet Earth – and that our economic growth is limited by the ecological limits of the planet". [357]

Much of farming today in Europe and North America is not regenerative since it relies heavily on external inputs of synthetic fertilisers for crops or imported feed for animals. The EU is a massive net importer of soya to feed cattle in Germany, chickens in Spain and many others. [358] European agriculture imports the equivalent of almost 35 million hectares of soybean. This equates to the EU using 20% more agricultural land than is contained

---

[357] David Attenborough in his speech to the RSA: People and Planet was quoting Kenneth Boulding, President Kennedy's environmental advisor
[358] https://theconversation.com/message-to-the-eu-you-have-the-chance-to-stop-fuelling-devastation-in-the-amazon-115465

within its own borders. In the UK, at least 90% of soy imports from South America are fed to animals, particularly pigs and chickens. Only 20-30% of this is certified as not grown on recently cleared land and the UK's soy imports are associated with considerable amounts of land clearing in Brazil. [359] It is now well-documented that cultivating soy is a major driver of damage to many natural ecosystems including the Amazon, Cerrado and Chaco regions of Brazil – home to spectacular wildlife like jaguars and to staggering biodiversity. The deforestation not only causes immense loss of biodiversity, it also increases GHG emissions through burning and loss of the forest as a carbon sink. It is estimated that a third of imported soya comes from deforested land or land that was originally savannas. When president Bolsonaro assumed power in Brazil on 1st January 2019 he started reversing environmental protection of the rainforests allowing further destruction for growing yet more soya. [360]

Agroecology does not require inputs from far off external sources that destroy the environment: there is no place in agroecology for chickens fed soya that has been grown on deforested lands in the Amazon. By abolishing imported soybean feed, in agroecology the associated GHG emissions are zero.[361] Since imported soya is associated with an enormous loss of biodiversity when this land is converted to agricultural use, not contributing to this would make a huge environmental statement.[362]

Halting plant protein imports would drastically reduce the level of imported tropical deforestation in the EU. By feeding animals locally grown cereals and pulses rather than imported animal feed, agriculture once again becomes harmonious with its environment. According to an article in the trade journal Pig World, pork is already available from pigs fed sustainably produced soya

---

[359] https://fcrn.org.uk/fcrn-blogs/soy-uk-what-are-its-uses
[360] https://sustainablefoodtrust.org/articles/the-forest-is-burning/?utm_source=SFT+Newsletter&utm_campaign=418d6e75ae-Newsletter+214_COPY_01&utm_medium=email&utm_term=0_bf20bccf24-418d6e75ae-105160197
[361] Auber et al (2019) Agroecology and carbon neutrality in Europe by 2050: what are the issues? p. 20
[362] The 10% figure from the UK Committee on Climate Change for GHGs emitted by agriculture as a proportion of all the UK's GHGs is based on domestic production only and does not take into account the significant GHG footprint of imported feed and transport costs. https://anewnatureblog.com/2019/09/23/climate-action-food-and-farming-a-seismic-shift-for-the-nfu/

from the EU and from pigs fed other pulses. It is more a lack of demand, they say, that is the issue. [363] Unfortunately at present there is no adequate labeling system to raise the awareness of consumers to allow them to make this choice. The success of recent campaigns to raise awareness of products that are palm oil free suggests that there would also be a market for animal products not implicated in rainforest destruction.

As well as the more visible cycles between animals and plants in agroecology, there are less visible self-sustaining cycles for critical chemical elements such as carbon, nitrogen and phosphorus. These closed cycles have become distorted by human activity over the last hundred years or so. No longer circular, many now point in a direction that ends in an accumulation of unwanted and harmful products. We need to re-close these cycles. The most significantly distorted cycle is for carbon and its accumulation in the atmosphere as GHGs.

## The carbon cycle

In the carbon cycle, atmospheric $CO_2$ is captured by photosynthesising plants and transformed into carbohydrates. Animals consume these carbohydrates and use them to generate energy, breathing the carbon back out into the atmosphere as $CO_2$. Decaying plants and animals also return carbon as $CO_2$. Plants recapturing the atmospheric $CO_2$ close the cycle. This closed, balanced cycle has operated successfully since time immemorial.

Over millennia, the carbon cycle has kept atmospheric $CO_2$ within safe limits. However, over the last few decades the carbon cycle has been distorted because of human activity and is leading to ever increasing levels of atmospheric $CO_2$. The burning of fossil fuels is the major culprit since it adds to atmospheric carbon by putting into the atmosphere carbon that was previously in permanent storage. So this is a one-way process, generating $CO_2$ but not recycling it.

Excessive numbers of cattle is another reason for the current build up in $CO_2$ and this is at the heart of the debate around whether or not we should be eating meat. But ruminants - unlike fossil fuels - have the potential to be part of a carbon cycle. Pasture-fed cattle consume all their carbon from that captured by photosynthesis by the plants on which they graze. So in principle

---

[363] http://www.pig-world.co.uk/news/why-the-pressure-is-on-to-change-our-soya-habits.html

they can be part of a carbon cycle that keeps atmospheric $CO_2$ within safe limits. This was the case before the rapid rise in ruminant numbers.

A cow's main carbon source is cellulose, a major constituent of the grass it eats. [364] Bacteria in the cow's rumen (the rumen is the first of the four chambers of its stomach) break down the cellulose to glucose. The bacteria along with other microorganisms then ferment the glucose by enteric fermentation. Methane is a by-product of enteric fermentation.

The cow's bacteria provide it with most of its nutrient needs. Glucose molecules fermented by bacteria are converted into precursor molecules that cows use to produce fats. Bacteria are also a major source of protein for the cow since cows break down the protein-rich bacteria. (This occurs after the bacteria have passed from the rumen into the cow's fourth stomach chamber called the abomasum.) So most of the grass a cow eats is used to feed bacteria in its rumen, and it is products of these bacteria that are the main source of nourishment for the cow. Much is made these days of human's reliance on bacteria for good health, but this reliance is small compared to a cow's reliance on the bacteria in its rumen. The ability of ruminants, with the aid of enteric fermentation, to convert the cellulose in grass into sugars, fat and protein has allowed humans to derive food from the vast amounts of cellulose stored in the pasturelands of the world. We consume some of the fats and proteins manufactured by cows as dairy products and meat. Since both the protein and fat in dairy and meat contain carbon (fat is mainly carbon and hydrogen), we are also part of this carbon cycle.

In agroecology, as much as possible of the carbon that a cow consumes comes from pasture, either pasture eaten directly from grazing land or pasture that has been made into hay or silage. Cows fed only pasture from the farm are part of a carbon cycle and cannot produce more carbon than is captured through photosynthesis by the pasture plants. [365] Well managed pasture grazed by livestock also traps carbon in long-term storage, removing carbon from the carbon cycle. This process is called carbon sequestration and is an important way that cattle can contribute to carbon neutral farming.

---

[364] Cellulose is a polymer of glucose molecules and each glucose molecule contains six carbon atoms. It has the chemical formula $C_6H_{12}O_6$.

[365] Small amounts of carbon are also released into the atmosphere by respiration by pasture plants and by $CO_2$ emissions from the burning of fuel to transport the milk and cut pasture.

## Carbon sequestration

Estimates suggest the that the amount of carbon in the soil - the soil carbon pool - is over three times greater than the amount of carbon in the atmosphere [699]. Since soil carbon sequestration takes out atmospheric carbon (mostly $CO_2$) from the carbon cycle into long-term storage, depositing carbon in soil can, at least in theory, reduce the amount of carbon in the atmosphere. Achieving net zero carbon in farming - which means that farming adds no more carbon to the atmosphere than it removes - is a major goal for climate control. And carbon sequestration is receiving a lot of attention as an important way of helping achieve this. Soil carbon sequestration is a natural process and has none of the uncertainties of more technical geo-engineering ideas. Soil carbon sequestration simply returns carbon to a place where it belongs: in the soil.

Much of the carbon sequestered in soil derives from plant roots that have died. Some also comes from soil microorganisms, leaf litter and, in grazed pastureland, from animal manure. The carbon from these plants, microorganisms and manure is converted into a substance called humus, one of the building blocks of soil. The carbon in humus is very stable since it can remain bound up in humus for hundreds of years. So carbon that becomes part of humus is in effect taken out of the carbon cycle.

Farming practices that create healthy soils promote the formation of humus. In agroecology, these practices include mulching, reduced tillage, agroforestry (combined growing of trees and crops) and growing cover crops. Converting land to organic agriculture as part of a transition to agroecology has also been shown to significantly boost soil carbon. Agroecology encourages the use of deep-rooted plants in pastureland and this has the benefit that after the roots die they add carbon to the soil at greater depths than is normally achieved in conventional farming. This is an important way of increasing the overall capacity of a soil to store carbon. When deep-rooted grasses were planted in the savannas of South America to improve the local agriculture, these plants also greatly increased soil carbon sequestration: a win-win for both farmers and the climate [700].

Estimates suggest that soils eventually (after about 20 to 50 years) become saturated with carbon. This period varies enormously depending on the initial amount of carbon in the soil and how the soil is managed. It is sometimes stated that because soil will eventually becomes saturated with carbon, soil sequestration should not be considered as an effective way of helping tackle $CO_2$ levels. But this is somewhat disingenuous since it is our next few decades that are critical for managing $CO_2$ levels.

Even though soil carbon sequestration sounds very promising, the amount of carbon that can be sequestered in soil and the stability of the carbon in humus are matters of intense debate. This is because there are so many factors involved. So it is not surprising that claims for estimates of the capacity of soil to sequester carbon vary widely. The former Quality Meat Scotland chairman Jim McLaren has stated his view that with proper accounting for pasture-based livestock farming's considerable ability to soak up $CO_2$ this could legitimately present the industry and its products as net-zero. [366] Scientists in New Zealand have taken a more nuanced view of their soils and estimate that the topsoil in many of their pastures (which means the top 15 cm) is already reaching saturation, but that this is not the case at lower depths. So to improve soil carbon in these New Zealand soils, the best strategy may be to sow deep-rooted plants that deposit their carbon at these depths when they die. [367] Another strategy shown to increase soil carbon sequestration is by grazing animals in one field for a short period and then moving them on (rotational grazing). This stimulates plant growth and deposits more carbon in the soil than conventional grazing.

One detailed report estimated that with current farming methods between 20-60% of GHGs produced by cattle could be offset by soil carbon sequestration [701]. This would suggest that cattle are still overall net contributors to GHGs. But this estimate excludes a consideration of the entire farming system. For instance, grassland can also be used to generate biofuel. An agroecological farming system that includes ruminants has been modeled to achieve a net zero carbon system when the entire system is considered. This is discussed in more detail later.

---

[366] https://www.thescottishfarmer.co.uk/news/17794768.scotland-39-s-grass-fed-livestock-carbon-neutral/
[367] https://www.nzagrc.org.nz/soil-carbon,listing,595,grassland-soils-have-potential-to-offset-ghg-emissions.html

## Agroecology and GHG emissions

Whilst there is broad agreement that current levels of meat production and consumption need to come down (by about half), there is disagreement about whether the main consumption should be from ruminants or pigs and chickens. Agroecology favours maintaining meat from ruminants. This may seem to be incompatible with reducing GHGs because of ruminant's high methane emissions. However, these emissions are just one part of the farming process, and when this process is considered in its entirety (by conducting a Life Cycle Analysis), agroecological production of ruminants can be seen as part of a path to carbon neutrality [690]. The grazing land for cattle and sheep are a crucial part of this Life Cycle Analysis. Large amounts of carbon from animal manure become sequestered in the soil of these grasslands in plant roots and soil microbes (although as I have mentioned the extent of carbon sequestration by grassland is much debated. [368]) Grass and animal manure can also both be converted into biogas by a process called anaerobic digestion and used to generate energy. So grasslands play an important role in regenerative farming. And let's not forget that they can also create beautiful landscapes and rich biodiversity.

Manure is the main source of soil fertility in agroecology and retaining soil fertility is a major concern for many farmers. We call the very planet we inhabit "planet earth", and without soil, life on earth could not exist. And yet we treat soil with wanton disrespect. Soil is a natural system being pushed beyond its limits and loss of productive soil is already a serious threat to the world's agriculture. [369]

## Agroecology is organic

As an organic system - one not using synthetic fertilisers and pesticides - there is little doubt that agroecology is better for the environment. There are now widespread concerns about synthetic fertilisers and pesticides, and the EU has set the objective of having at least 25% of its agricultural land under organic farming by 2030 [692]. Run-offs of nitrogen and phosphorous fertilisers from

---

[368] Grazed and Confused (which says grazing is not sustainable) and the response from the Sustainable Food Trust to this at https://sustainablefoodtrust.org/articles/grazed-and-confused-an-initial-response-from-the-sustainable-food-trust/
[369] https://theconversation.com/soil-is-our-best-ally-in-the-fight-against-climate-change-but-were-fast-running-out-of-it-

fields cause eutrophication (excess algal growth) of waterways which damages freshwater and marine ecosystems around the world [702]. In Europe, in 2016, GHG emissions from agricultural soils, especially of nitrous oxide from artificial nitrogen fertilisers, accounted for almost 37% of direct agricultural emissions. These emissions would be eliminated with agroecology since it does not use artificial fertilisers.

Pesticides are also of great concern. [370] There is now little doubt that pesticides and herbicides harm biodiversity, as Rachel Carson in Silent Spring so eloquently forewarned, and that has now been confirmed in various recent studies such as the one conducted over 27 years in Germany which found that insects had declined by three-quarters over the period of the study [703]. The need for so many pesticides has been challenged at the highest level. A UN report denounced as a "myth" that pesticides are necessary to feed the world and criticised global manufacturers for their aggressive practices that obstruct reforms in pesticide use. [371] One of the recent high profile links between pesticide use and the decline in insects is between neonicotinoid pesticides and the decline in the bee population. This has led to an EU ban on some types of neonicotinoids. [372]

Phasing out the synthetic pesticides and fertilisers used in industrial farming is seen as essential to prevent the decimation of insect populations. [373] At the moment, each attempt to ban a suspect pesticide is met with fierce resistance from the agrochemical industry. Agroecology circumvents these continual challenges and delaying tactics by the agrochemical industry by simply proposing a complete ban on all chemical warfare.

Lower yields from organic farms have long been of concern. In 1971, Earl Butz then US Secretary of Agriculture declared, "Before we go back to organic agriculture in this country, somebody must decide which 50 million

---

[370] https://www.theguardian.com/environment/2018/jun/17/where-have-insects-gone-climate-change-population-decline

[371] https://www.theguardian.com/environment/2017/mar/07/un-experts-denounce-myth-pesticides-are-necessary-to-feed-the-world

[372] https://www.theguardian.com/environment/2018/apr/27/eu-agrees-total-ban-on-bee-harming-pesticides
https://ec.europa.eu/food/plant/pesticides/approval_active_substances/approval_renewal/neonicotinoids_en

[373] https://www.theguardian.com/environment/2020/jan/06/urgent-new-roadmap-to-recovery-could-reverse-insect-apocalypse-aoe

Americans we are going to let starve or go hungry." While it's true that yields from organic farming are often reduced - by up to 25% in some cases, this needs to be seen in context of the overall farming system. By reducing the amount of land devoted to growing crops to feed animals, more land can be devoted to growing crops for direct human consumption. [374] Also, diversified organic agroecological systems usually out-perform conventional farming during climate stress such as drought years, and these are becoming increasingly frequent in many parts of the world [685].

Even though a policy of banning chemicals from farming may seem radical, increasing numbers of farmers see organic farming as the future and it is rapidly expanding in Europe. [375] The UK lags behind many other European countries with only 2.8% of crop area organic compared to 5.3% in France, 14% in Italy and 57% in Denmark. [376] Yields from organic farms may be lower, but profits are on average about a third higher than in conventional farming [702]. In 2014, France put agroecology at the heart of its agricultural policy. [377] In a country which has traditionally used high levels of pesticides, the French government is making €1.1 billion available for agriculturalists who wants to switch to organic production. The French *Ambition Bio 2022* (Organic Ambition 2022) programme developed by the French Minister for Agriculture and Food has given itself two goals: reach 15% of agricultural surface producing organic products by 2022 and have 20% organic products in institutional catering (which includes cafeterias in administrations, schools, hospitals, nursing homes, etc). [378]

## Integrating agroecology in farming

Agroecology considers that too much food production is being forced into inappropriate ecological niches. It is wrong to raise animals in factory farms and it is wrong to grow their food on land that was once a tropical rainforest. Animal rearing is becoming more and more disconnected from the landscapes

---

[374] https://www.theguardian.com/sustainable-business/2016/aug/14/organic-farming-agriculture-world-hunger

[375] https://ec.europa.eu/info/food-farming-fisheries/farming/organic-farming
https://ec.europa.eu/agriculture/organic/eu-policy/data-statistics_en
http://www.fao.org/organicag/oa-faq/oa-faq5/en/

[376] http://www.europarl.europa.eu/news/en/headlines/society/20180404STO00909/the-eu-s-organic-food-market-facts-and-rules-infographic

[377] cited in RSA Food, Farming and Countryside Commission (2019) Our Future in the Land

[378] https://frenchfoodintheus.org/3825

and from local sources of food. Growing fruit and veg out of season in heated greenhouses is also something to minimise. The UK certainly needs to increase its fruit and veg production since at present only 54% of veg and 17% of fruit is home-grown. [379] Some fruit and veg such as oranges and bananas will always need to be imported. But much more could be done to grow and promote the consumption of home-grown fruit and veg. There is a strong argument to rebalance the relative amounts of international to local foods in a more sustainable way. This becomes financially feasible for farmers when consumers develop a preference for local, seasonally grown produce rather than out of season imports. This requires campaigns providing advice on what is locally in season and advice on how to prepare this food. Based on the experiences of the Covid 19 pandemic, governments are now recognising that food security and minimising reliance on food imports is not just of theoretical interest.

Food security is often seen as a somewhat abstract concern, relevant to less developed countries and not something that need concern wealthy industrialised countries, such as the UK, which are able to buy their food from abroad if needs be. The Covid-19 pandemic has changed all that, exposing weaknesses and vulnerabilities in countries that rely on others for their food. Self-sufficiency and resilience are now the names of the game and agroecology is a system that can help achieve this. It will never be about growing coffee beans or bananas in Northern climes but it will enable a country to know that it can produce its basic produce in times of crisis. [380]

Dietary recommendations conducive to good health are not necessarily compatible with a sustainable way of farming. A farming system that supports veganism is likely to require large amounts of synthetic fertilisers, since no nitrogen is available from animal manure and so the natural nitrogen cycle between plants and animals is lost. Also, much of the farmland in countries such as the UK is not suited to horticulture and is far more suitable as grassland for raising livestock. Ideology-driven dietary proposals raise the hackles of farming organisations sympathetic to agroecology, such as the UK's Sustainable Food Trust. Some of these diets are seen as unrealistic proposals

---

[379] The Food Foundation. Farming for 5-A-Day
[380] https://sustainablefoodtrust.org/articles/the-coronavirus-pandemic-and-future-food-security/

written by desk-based researchers with little knowledge of the practicalities of farming. Even the flexitarian diet-based EAT-Lancet Commission report has been accused by the Sustainable Food Trust of "a fundamental lack of agricultural understanding" because "if fully implemented, the recommendations would make it impossible to introduce sustainable and restorative farming systems in countries like the UK, where a high proportion of farmland is only suitable for growing grass." [381] As the Trust went on, "a key weakness in the report is the failure to fully differentiate between livestock that are part of the problem and those that are an essential component of sustainable agricultural systems." [382]

## Farmers

A healthy diet is inextricably linked to a healthy farming system and yet the needs of farmers are often forgotten in the debate about sustainable food production. Farmers must be able to produce economically competitive products, and if meat production is to decrease this should be linked to producing higher quality meat. The issue of meat is much discussed by farmers, such as in the pages of the UK's Farmer's Weekly. [383] Farmers can adapt but they need financial incentives if they are to produce food in a more sustainable way. [384] Subsidies that currently favour intensive farming need to be redirected to enable the necessary structural changes to farming that follow agroecological principles. It is equally important that farmers don't receive subsidies that simply allow them to export meat if home demand decreases. This will do nothing for GHG emissions. [385] Irish farmers are currently seeing major opportunities in exporting beef to China, a business that was worth

---

[381] https://sustainablefoodtrust.org/articles/eat-lancet-reports-recommendations-are-at-odds-with-sustainable-food-production/

[382] https://sustainablefoodtrust.org/articles/eat-reports-recommendations-are-at-odds-with-sustainable-food-production/?utm_source=SFT+Newsletter&utm_campaign=12138ade40-Newsletter_26_10_2017_COPY_01&utm_medium=email&utm_term=0_bf20bccf24-12138ade40-105160197

[383] https://www.fwi.co.uk/livestock/health-welfare/meat-eaters-or-vegetarians-who-has-the-better-arguments

[384] https://sustainablefoodtrust.org/articles/if-we-want-sustainable-food-systems-its-all-about-the-money

[385] https://www.theguardian.com/environment/2019/sep/10/no-need-to-cut-beef-to-tackle-climate-crisis-say-farmers

€9m in 2018 and is expected to grow to €120m in a few years time. [386] In the UK, the National Farmers Union has also demonstrated signs of resistance to change because of the lure of export markets. [387] As the NFU president Minette Batters has said: "We don't plan to make any cuts. We think we can do it without changing levels of production. Everybody's diet is up to individuals to choose, but there are other parts of the world that are hungry for high-quality meat." This comes against the significant concerns from organisations such as the Committee on Climate Change that beef production needs to decrease.

We need a farming system where the players genuinely act for the common good and are able to do this within a fair, economically viable and productive system. One that restores doing public good to the heart of its actions. Studies have found that organic farming is at least as profitable for the farmer as intensive farming [702]. Agroecology also provides the opportunity for farmers to diversify their business into nature activities on the farm and by exploiting their agro-ecological infrastructures such as ponds, paths, hedges and woods. The desire of people to reconnect with nature is enormous.

Farmers will need to be protected financially during a transition to this new way of farming since retaining economic stability is of far greater concern to most farmers than preventing climate change. [388] Government farming subsidies will be of paramount importance for helping farmers make an agroecological shift. Consumers are not without influence though since consumer decisions about what they want to buy influence government policy and so the subsidies that governments are willing to provide to farmers.

Agribusinesses fearful of drastically reduced sales of fertilisers, pesticides and animal feed will inevitably intensely lobby governments to maintain the status quo. The story of metaldehyde - the active ingredient in slug pellets - illustrates how these dynamics can play out, and why it is so important to provide incentives and support to farmers. Following expert advice, slug pellets containing metaldehyde were due to be banned in the UK in 2020. As

---

[386] https://www.irishexaminer.com/breakingnews/business/columnists/irish-food-taps-chinas-appetite-for-beef-964880.html
[387] https://www.theguardian.com/environment/2019/sep/10/no-need-to-cut-beef-to-tackle-climate-crisis-say-farmers
[388] survey cited in RSA Food, Farming and Countryside Commission (2019) Our Future in the Land

the UK Expert Committee on Pesticides and the Health and Safety Executive said "metaldehyde poses an unacceptable risk to birds and mammals." [389] This was endorsed by the then Environment Secretary Michael Gove who declared "the advice is clear that the risks to wildlife are simply too great – and we must all play our part in helping to protect the environment." Metaldehyde has also been found in drinking water. [390] Farmers use metaldehyde to protect crops such as rapeseed oil, winter beans, sugar beet and brassicas. There is an alternative (ferric phosphate) but it is more expensive and no mechanism was put in place to ensure farmers were not out of pocket when switching. So unsurprisingly the ban was challenged. A metaldehyde manufacturer took legal action to bring Mr Gove's decision before the High Court. And won. [391] A decision supported by the Scottish NFU. [392] This was a sad day for our thrushes and hedgehogs and indeed anyone drinking metaldehyde-contaminated water. [393] The (unsurprising) moral of this story is that farmers may be prepared to change to help protect the environment but not if they are out of pocket as a consequence.

In their 2018 report, the UK government advisory body the Committee on Climate Control identified that UK agriculture had been far less successful at reducing GHG emissions than transport and power generation [(674)]. In response to the CCC report, the president of the NFU issued a robust statement: "The NFU has been clear with its position on British farming's role in tackling climate change. Reducing livestock numbers in the UK is not a part of that policy. We are disappointed to see the Committee on Climate Change include that recommendation in its report. The report simply does not recognise the environmental benefits grass-fed beef and sheep production brings to the UK." She went on to say: "Despite our concerns over parts of the report, British farmers are committed to playing their part to reach government targets. We are committed to doing so in a way that fulfills

[389] https://www.gov.uk/government/news/restrictions-on-the-use-of-metaldehyde-to-protect-wildlife

[390] https://www.theguardian.com/environment/blog/2013/jul/10/slug-pesticides-metaldehyde-drinking-water

[391] https://www.farminguk.com/news/metaldehyde-slug-pellet-ban-overturned_53580.html

[392] https://www.nfus.org.uk/news/news/high-court-ruling-on-metaldehyde-must-see-science-based-decision-process-adopted

[393] https://www.telegraph.co.uk/gardening/problem-solving/slug-pellets-ban-lifted-legal-challenge-manufacturer/

farmers' responsibility to the public in providing domestic food and delivering food security for the nation." [394]

According to the CCC, half of farmers consider GHGs important when making decisions about their farming practices, but - worryingly - the other half "placed little or no importance on considering emissions when making decisions and/or thought their farm did not produce GHG emissions" [674]. For those farmers not undertaking any actions to reduce GHG emissions, 47% did not believe any action was necessary. At present, efforts to change farming practice are through voluntary agreements and so it is not really surprising that, according to the CCC, emission savings are unlikely to be achieved. Whereas most of the sectors with significant GHG emissions, such as energy and transport, are achieving reductions, this is not the case with agriculture which has remained fairly constant over the last decade [678].

Many EU farmers feel increasingly angry at what they perceive as attacks on their livelihoods and are digging in rather than engaging in a dialogue about transitioning to a more environmentally friendly way of farming. [395] This intransigence can be because farmers feel locked in to their current farming practices for economic or social reasons. Reducing current methods of livestock production in the UK is particularly important since it accounts for 70% of agricultural emissions. But decommissioning a dairy unit and buying a combine harvester is an expensive undertaking and the switch might not suit the land and climate. Some farmers are diversifying into areas outside traditional farming such as tourism, hospitality, retail and renewable energy. [396] Changing farming practices to agroecology also offer huge opportunities without the need to abandon the principles of farming itself. In Normandy, France an engineer turned farmer is selling carbon neutral beef at the same price as conventional beef. He achieves his carbon neutrality by only grass

[394] https://www.bbc.com/news/science-environment-46214864
https://www.nfuonline.com/news/latest-news/nfu-response-to-committee-on-climate-change-report/
[395] https://www.nytimes.com/aponline/2019/11/27/business/ap-eu-france-farmers-protests.html
[396] https://www.fwi.co.uk/business/diversification/subsidy-shake-up-triggers-boom-in-farm-diversification

feeding, by heating the barns with wood and by having solar panels on the barn roofs. Who would not want to choose his beef over its rivals? [397]

## Are there viable alternative farming strategies?

When drawing up their definition of a sustainable diet, the WHO/FAO had the insight to realise that a sustainable diet should not only have a low environmental impact whilst promoting health and wellbeing, but also be accessible, affordable, safe, equitable and culturally acceptable [704]. Agroecology encompasses all of these broad societal values. But what about the alternatives? A subject as multifaceted as food that does not take all aspects identified by the WHO into account can have unintended consequences. I will illustrate this with a few suggested alternatives to the agroecological model.

Some argue that we should intensively produce food in small areas (so-called sustainable intensification) as this will free up more countryside. By intensifying food production in a smaller area, the land spared from agriculture can be rewilded, afforested or used to grow bioenergy crops. An extreme version of rewilding is the idea of preserving half the planet for nature. However, it has recently been estimated that this "half planet" proposal would adversely affect over a billion people - hardly a realistic proposal [705].

Sustainable intensification is predicated on the assumption that crop and animal yields can further increase. But this is contrary to a lot of the evidence which is finding that yields of maize, rice, wheat and soybean have now plateaued, and there are also concerns about increasing the productivity in livestock by more intensive practices because this would confine more and more animals indoors [685]. This idea of land *sparing* contrasts with agroecology, which is based on land *sharing* - where farming activities intermingle more with nature.

Rather than sustainable intensification, we need more animals living outdoors in natural extended environments: We need sustainable *exten*sification for animals. And for crops, rather than simply growing more and focusing on yield, we also need to improve nutritional value by growing them organically.

---

[397] The Connexion journal Nov, 2019.

So for crops we need *nutritional* intensification. So rather than sustainable intensification we need *sustainable extensification* for animals and *nutritional intensification* for crops.

There is no doubt that well-chosen vegetarian and vegan diets are good for the environment, and more and more people are switching to them [706]. But poor choices can cause significant environmental harm. [398] Switching to a meat-free diet may cut out the GHG emissions from beef and lamb but there may be few environmental gains by going vegetarian if the meat is simply replaced with a higher consumption of dairy [707]. Since taste is many peoples' top reason for choosing what to eat, the reduced taste palette of a meat-free diet may be compensated for with more imported "exotic" plant foods. Many of these, such as avocadoes and almonds, have high water requirements, which can imperil local supplies, and some of these imported produce require high levels of pesticide and fertiliser use.[399] There are also the environmental impacts from importing tropical fruit and veg, much of which is airfreighted. [400]

Many vegan foods replace meat and dairy with soy and palm products. But this puts ever more demand on land and is devastating the rain forests in SE Asia and the Amazon. Unless the palm oil is fully certified there is a real danger it has come from plantations grown on deforested land, which further diminishes the habitat of already endangered species. The UK supermarket chain Iceland is to be applauded for introducing a ban on all palm oil in its own brand products. [401] Not importing environmental damage from other countries is in the DNA of agroecological farming, but it is not a prerequisite for becoming vegan or vegetarian.

Advocating veganism as the solution to sustainable eating has become fashionable in some academic circles and with food writers. But it is out of touch with the vast majority of people in Europe and the US where eating

[398] https://fcrn.org.uk/fcrn-blogs/helen-breewood/are-modern-plant-based-diets-and-foods-actually-sustainable

[399] https://www.bbc.com/future/article/20200211-why-the-vegan-diet-is-not-always-green

[400] https://www.independent.co.uk/life-style/food-and-drink/veganism-environment-veganuary-friendly-food-diet-damage-hodmedods-protein-crops-jack-monroe-a8177541.html

[401] http://www.bbc.co.uk/news/business-43696948

https://www.theguardian.com/environment/2018/apr/10/iceland-to-be-first-uk-supermarket-to-cut-palm-oil-from-own-brand-products

https://www.bbc.com/future/article/20200109-what-are-the-alternatives-to-palm-oil

animal products is an integral part of the pleasures of daily life and part of the national culture. The French living without cheeses or the Germans without salamis is hard to imagine. Insisting on veganism is like saying everyone should give up cars and use bikes and public transport. Most people agree that we should be switching to electric cars but would be strongly opposed to completely banning all cars. (And as I mentioned earlier, many farmers who raise animals would switch to the export market if their own domestic market declined.)

Vegetarianism (unlike veganism) brings with it the not insignificant animal welfare issue of what to do with male animals. As they do not providing milk, dairy or eggs, they are surplus to requirements. Even in our omnivore-dominated world where male chickens and livestock are reared for their meat, there are still billions of surplus male animals born every year. Most are quickly dispatched: chickens are minced alive or gassed and calves may be left to die after a few days, shot, or - if they are really unlucky - transported in often appalling conditions to countries where they are raised for veal. [402] There are a few glimmers of light in these appalling conditions. France has announced that it will ban the culling of chickens from the end of 2021. [403] A French company called Poulehouse has pre-empted this by producing eggs that does not involve killing the male chicks (by identifying males early in incubation) and also that allows the hens to grow old gracefully. [404]

Some, with a far more radical vision than mere veganism, advocate replacing farm animals with industrially-raised insects [708] and meat cells grown in large vats. [405] Some of these visionaries predict that by 2030 the number of cows in the U.S. will have halved and will lead to the cattle farming industry going bankrupt [709]. The path to agroecology also leads to a drop in the number of cows but this path would end with a sustainable cattle population not one where they have been completely ousted by vats of cultured cells. Abandoning nature as our source of sustenance and having it displaced by a technocratic future may seem science fiction, but it could rapidly become a reality if the vision of some think tanks is realised.

---

[402] https://www.theguardian.com/environment/2020/jan/20/it-would-be-kinder-to-shoot-them-irelands-calves-set-for-live-export.
[403] https://www.bbc.com/news/world-europe-51301915
[404] https://fr.wikipedia.org/wiki/Poulehouse
[405] Can these products be called meat? see MeatAnaloguesChatham.pdf Or more recent info??

Eating insects is likely to remain objectionable for most people in the west and using them ground up as meal as an ingredient in processed foods is simply creating another generation of UPFs. But using insects as (ideally live) animal feed, especially for pigs and chickens, is highly compatible with agroecology. After all, eating insects is part of the diet and foraging instinct of wild chickens and pigs. Insects are also very nutritious. Some such as maggots can be raised on manure or fed on food waste and so can be part of a natural agroecological cycle, and they can be grown locally. They are a promising area for the future of animal feed. [406]

Of far greater commercial interest at the moment is cultured meat. There is little doubt that compared to livestock, culturing cellular meat reduces land use and methane emissions. But reductions in GHG emissions are less clear. Whilst it is true that cultured cells don't produce methane, they do need to be kept warm, mixed and aerated and this will require enormous amounts of energy. One estimate is that replacing meat with cultured meat would use almost one quarter of all the world's energy [710]! Producing energy is currently one of the main contributors to GHG emissions (in the form of $CO_2$), and cultured meat will only substantially reduce GHG emissions if the energy for growing cultured meat comes from decarbonised/renewable sources. It is worth remembering that the cultured meat industry is competing with a very efficient processing unit called a cow. Cattle consume grass, a product that is inedible for humans and that uses the sun as a free and non-polluting source of energy; and cattle provide a wide range of end products, not only meat and milk but also leather and many others. [407] In agroecology, cattle and other farm animals provide manure-fertiliser and are a key part in the circular farming economy. Without farm animals, the regenerative farming system of agroecology is broken and this would have severe knock on effects for how the rest of our food is produced since it will require an even higher reliance on chemical fertilisers for crop production and even greater dangers of soil degradation - both major generators of GHGs. These knock-on effects of environmental damage are not usually factored in when comparing the environmental impacts of animal-derived versus cell culture-derived meat.

---

[406] http://www.poultrynews.co.uk/news/the-benefits-of-insect-based-poultry-feed.html
https://www.sciencemag.org/news/2015/10/feature-why-insects-could-be-ideal-animal-feed
[407] https://theconversation.com/why-cows-are-getting-a-bad-rap-in-lab-grown-meat-debate-103716

It remains to be seen whether or not cultured meat becomes acceptable to vegans and vegetarians since there is the problem that most cultured cells are grown in solutions that include blood products from cattle foetuses (known as foetal calf serum). This is needed to provide essential growth stimulants, and alternatives would need to be used to grow a product acceptable for vegans. Cultured cells must be produced under sterile conditions and this commonly involves using antibiotics. [408] The current use of antibiotics in farm animals is a concern because of its implication in the spread of multi-drug resistant strains of bacteria.

These issues are potentially solvable, but will require the right actions by the cultured meat industries. This is far from assured since the food industry is motivated to minimise costs and maximise profits. Unless there is regulation, it seems quite possible that, as with many other food products, cultured meat will be produced to various standards: a more expensive/upmarket product that avoids antibiotics and foetal calf serum, and uses decarbonised energy sources, and other products that do not make these commitments and can be sold more cheaply. Because of legitimate industry concerns for commercial secrecy, there could be an issue with regulation. This concern for commercial secrecy is a portent that cultured meat production will create similar issues to other sectors of the industrial food industry. One of these is domination by a small number of corporations; and indeed there are already signs this is starting to happen. [409] Some experts, such as agricultural ecologist Michel Pimbert and food systems expert Colin Anderson, at Coventry University, have concerns that this type of food production will bring it under the control of financial markets where what we eat is traded as a commodity - rather than as the single most important item for human health. [410]

At the beginning of this chapter, I referred to the idea that producing food for the common good is now as important as the good of the individual. This conclusion comes from a Group of Chief Scientific Advisors to the EU in

---

[408] Although the industry claims it will not need antibiotics this remains to be seen. https://www.foodnavigator-usa.com/Article/2018/10/25/Cell-based-meat-cos-Please-stop-calling-us-lab-grown-meat-and-we-don-t-use-antibiotics-in-full-scale-production
[409] Such as the World Economic Forum's "Transformative Twelve"
[410] https://theconversation.com/the-battle-for-the-future-of-farming-what-you-need-to-know-106805

their report Towards a Sustainable Food System published in 2020. [411] In their report they stated that "Food must be viewed more as a common good rather than as a consumer good" and that to achieve a sustainable food system" the central goal of all relevant policy development and assessment must be to ensure food sustainability in all its aspects: environmental, social and economic." Removing financial gain as the single motivation of food production is central to the future of sustainable food production.

Of course, farmers must turn a profit, just as other players in the food chain must. But this should be balanced with social responsibility. We happily pay for the service of GPs, police, teachers and others since we recognise that the vast majority act in our best interests, motivated by a sense of duty to society. In the cultural arts, musicians, actors and others express and act primarily through a humanitarian drive and we happily pay for this. In agri-culture too, most farmers are in the profession because they want to provide nutritious food at a fair price for which they can rightly expect reasonable payment. Cooking a family meal is a scaled-down act for the common good.

All these acts help make human society work. When the motivation of acting for the common good has disappeared and the over-arching motivation is financial gain we don't feel so good: a health sector manipulating our worries to sell us an unnecessary medicine or procedure; a security sector overselling insurance policies; the factory farmer minimising animal welfare standards in order to maximise profit and then hiding this from customers. Quite rightly we feel ripped off, and there may be a deeper sense of unease that because the common good has been undermined the stability of society is also being undermined.

Over the last few decades, the undermining of the common good has accelerated, and no more so than between people producing industrial foods and their customers. Advertising campaigns by food manufacturers are guilty of deceiving customers with illusory ideas about how their food is produced. The dominant profit motive often undermines the common good and this has come at a very high cost to our health, to animal welfare, to farmers' ability to earn a living and to the environment. Already many consumers living in urban areas are disengaged from food systems and have little knowledge of farms

---

[411] Towards a Sustainable Food System (2020) Group of Chief Scientific Advisors. European Commission

and how their food is produced. This disconnect is reinforced by retailers who manipulate prices so that they bear little relationship to the true cost to the farmer.

The disconnect would rapidly increase with techno foods, where the only reason to maintain standards is to increase profits. Creating profit through Intellectual Property Rights is the raison d'être for many of the players in this new market. [412] By completely supplanting the farmer from food production with its long tradition of food quality control and replacing this tried and tested system with the financial-industrial sector is of great concern.

Techno foods also threaten our connection with the natural world. If we turn to techno foods and no longer feel the need for the natural world to provide our food, we may lose the ability to feel the need to preserve nature as well. The American biologist E.O. Wilson in his book *Biophilia* hypothesised that we have an innate tendency to seek connections with nature and other forms of life. He postulated that one reason why this trait evolved was to appreciate and acknowledge the importance of plants and animals for our sustenance and hence the need to sustain the natural environment. Feeling part of the natural world is also embedded in James Lovelock's Gaia theory, as the idea of the Earth as a self-regulatory organism. If we see ourselves as part of the community of Gaia then, it could be argued, we are far less likely to inflict harm, since it would be *self*-harm. The hubristic belief that we can dominate and control Gaia is a dangerous path. George Orwell wrote his own bleak vision of the future in his book *1984*, and coincidentally, E.O. Wilson's *Biophilia* was published in 1984. Less of a coincidence is that both Big Brother and the food industry risk uncoupling our close dependent relationship with nature.

There may be a place for consuming small amounts of techno products where these provide particular nutrients. However, until the technology is very advanced it seems likely that the product will be used more as an ingredient in a UPF, much as the meat substitute Quorn is today, and this will come with all the problems with UPFs discussed in chapter 7. [413] Our current physiological health relies on a supply of natural foods, a partnership between

---

[412] https://lachefnet.wordpress.com/2018/06/10/lab-meat-more-hype-than-substance/
[413] https://www.theguardian.com/lifeandstyle/2018/feb/12/quorn-revolution-rise-ultra-processed-fake-meat

Nature and our bodies that has evolved over millennia. If we switch to techno foods we may well need an arsenal of medical technologies to cope with the chronic diseases that result from this new generation of UPFs: manufactured props for a manufactured diet.

## The agroecological Med diet

The Med diet is possibly both the healthiest diet in the world and *for* the world. Producing the foods for a Med diet by agroecological farming would be a great partnership. A plant-based and planet-based diet. In the past this was a marriage of necessity since the limited economic means of many Mediterranean peasant farmers meant that purchasing fertilisers and other expensive inputs for their farms was not an option. So an agroecological Med diet is both a vision for the future, and one that harks back to the past.

The French think tank IDDRI has developed a detailed model for an environmentally sustainable European agroecology food system, and this could form the basis for developing a Med diet agroecology system. The IDDRI model, called TYFA - GHG (Ten Years for Agroecology in Europe - Green House Gases), is designed to achieve net zero carbon by 2050 (the date set by the Intergovernmental Panel on Climate Change in their 2018 report). It incorporates key agroecological farming practices. These include managing permanent grassland by livestock according to agroecological principles and using grass and animal manure for biogas generation. Properly managed grassland and arable land would sequester large amounts of carbon from the atmosphere. [414] In accordance with the principles of agroecology, the TYFA GHG model is organic and uses no imported animal feed. The IDDRI team have demonstrated that their agroecological farming system could feed the entire EU population and reach zero net carbon by 2050 whilst still retaining some meat consumption [690]. The EU has welcomed the IDDRI report as a viable path towards improving food production. [415]

It is highly likely that an agroecological system along the lines of the IDDRI model would be able to produce sufficient food for a Med diet to feed the EU whilst still reaching carbon neutrality by 2050. Meat production is the main

---

[414] Carbon sequestration is a controversial issue and the feasibility of this is fully discussed in the IDDRI report.

[415] https://www.ifoam-eu.org/en/news/2019/04/16/press-release-ifoam-eu-welcomes-new-iddri-study-agroecology-and-carbon-neutrality

contributor to agricultural GHGs and the TYFA GHG model is based on a daily meat consumption of 88 grams. The amount of meat eaten as part of a traditional Med diet is far lower than this. Investigators from the Seven Countries study (see ch. 9) estimated that for the traditional Cretan diet, average meat consumption (red meat and chicken) was 35 grams per day [554]. This suggests that modifying the TYFA GHG model for the Med diet could achieve substantially lower GHG emissions since the livestock herd would be substantially reduced. Maintaining the same area of grassland with a far lower number of livestock would also increase the amount of grass available for hay and silage, and any surplus could be used for biogas generation.

Even based on existing non-agroecological farming systems, GHG emissions from a Med diet compare favourably with other dietary patterns. Estimates generally show that producing foods for a Med diet have a far lower environmental impact than for a standard western diet. In one study, producing foods for a Med diet reduced GHGs by almost three quarters, halved land and energy use, and reduced water use by a third compared with a typical Spanish diet [711]. A lot of this is down to the lower amounts of meat and dairy in the Med diet. Not surprisingly, GHGs and land use for a vegan diet are even lower than for a Med diet [712]. But for the health benefits and social acceptability reasons discussed earlier, I do not believe this means we should switch to a vegan diet. A great benefit of agroecology is that much of the land doubles as a biodiverse and carbon-sequestering habitat, especially because of the extensive grassland. The IDDRI agroecological model is not compatible with a vegan diet since livestock are an essential component of the nutrient cycling needed for the IDDRI agroecological model to work.

Meat from chickens is generally considered to be healthier and so the greater emphasis on meat from ruminants (because they feed on local grassland) in an agroecological Med diet might seem at odds with achieving the healthiest Med diet. However there are many factors that influence meat's health. There is no strong evidence that the small amount of red meat cooked the Mediterranean way and then eaten as part of a Med diet is harmful, and meat is an excellent source of many nutrients. Just as there is good evidence that the benefits of small amounts of alcohol - rather than none or too much - may be optimal for health, so too it is possible that this is the case with red meat eaten as part of a Med diet. For alcohol, this has been demonstrated in various epidemiological studies by assessing people's health when they follow a "Mediterranean drinking pattern". At the moment, no one has evaluated a comparable "Mediterranean meat-eating pattern" (see ch. 12).

## Our responsibilities as food citizens

Poor quality food produced to low environmental standards is often cheaper, but its true cost is simply being externalised to other sectors: to the extra costs to health services, and to the extra costs to the environment, which are already estimated to be costing 3% of global GDP. As the RSA said in their report "Farm gate prices are low; and whilst food in the supermarkets is getting cheaper, the true cost of that policy is simply passed off elsewhere in society – in a degraded environment, spiraling ill-health and impoverished high streets" [713].

At the moment, we have little way of knowing the carbon footprint and other environmental costs of the foods we buy. Agroecology is a very environmentally favourable food system, but identifying products that meet agroecology standards is difficult. "Organic" encompasses some of the values of agroecology. For instance, the Soil Association in the UK requires meat accredited as "organic" to also comply with broader issues of animal welfare and sustainability. France has a designation system called the *Haute Valeur Environnementale*. [416] But "organic" does not always represent broader ethical concerns. Agribusinesses sees "organic" as a niche market to be exploited whilst still continuing with other conventional - including industrial - ways of food production [685]. The region around the Southern Spanish city of Almeria produces a significant part of the fruit and vegetables eaten in North European countries such as Germany and the UK. Much of the organic produce, as with the conventionally grown produce, is produced under plastic in the infamous plastic cities. This has created an area of considerable ecological damage and not one associated with the ecological benefits of agroecology. The working conditions of the migrant workers are similar to those of those working on conventional grown produce - poor wages and workers rights, and often-extreme heat. [417] However, at least the workers are

---

[416] Although this has been accused of greenwashing by the Green Party because of allowing GM foods https://fr.wikipedia.org/wiki/Haute_Valeur_Environnementale
[417] https://www.theguardian.com/global-development/2020/may/01/no-food-water-masks-or-gloves-migrant-farm-workers-in-spain-at-crisis-point
https://www.theguardian.com/business/2011/feb/07/spain-salad-growers-slaves-charities

not being exposed to the pesticides and other chemicals of conventional farming (714).

Foods produced to higher ecological standards do cost more, but this is money being investing for the good of society and for future generations. In the UK, we are used to paying some of the lowest food prices in Europe. For the less well off, a coupon system could help subsidise the costs of better quality foods. [418] There are currently many proposals for costing foods according to their true costs to society such as by using carbon and meat taxes, with the idea that the polluter pays. In the meantime, many in society do see supporting local farmers a price worth paying for. We need to shift from a low cost to a true cost agricultural system.

The economic model of supply and demand predicts that if there is the demand for a food product the market will adjust to supply it. As food citizens our choices can convince supermarkets, food firms and ultimately farmers and governments of the type of food we want. The groundswell of dissatisfaction with our food system is growing as more people swap being passive food consumers to becoming active food citizens. One example of this is with the giant US meat company Tyson, which has responded to consumer demand by announcing that it is investing in plant proteins such as quinoa and lentils and other non-meat protein sources. [419] Some of the most powerful movements for change have been citizen-led: bottom-up from the people and not top-down from government. Citizen-led change is a powerful way to create the food system best suited for person and planet.

Being a food citizen starts with our own buying choices. While a UK food consumer expects fresh veg out of season in the UK flown to be flown in from distant places, the UK food citizen will wait for local seasonal veg. Food citizens are not prepared to disregard the razing of Indonesian rainforest and so avoid palm oil products. Food citizens accept that chicken and pork should be produced sustainably, and are prepared to pay a premium to avoid chicken

---

[418] This would be along the lines of other schemes such as healthy start food vouchers in England https://www.theguardian.com/society/2018/may/25/poorer-families-england-healthy-start-free-food-vouchers
[419] Tyson produces a fifth of all meat consumed in the US, https://www.bloomberg.com/news/features/2018-08-15/tyson-s-quest-to-be-your-one-stop-protein-shop

and pigs that have been fed on soya beans from land that was once an Amazonian rainforest.

Being a food citizen goes beyond personal choices and can give a greater sense of empowerment. Insisting on local, seasonal produce helps create a virtuous circle between food citizens and suppliers. Eventually this will lead to funding bodies and governments providing the finance needed for farmers to transition to agroecological farming. As a very helpful food citizen report from the New Citizenship Project put it, "it is our deeper nature to be Citizens, at our happiest when acting for a purpose that takes us beyond ourselves, and at our fullest when we are shaping what the options are, not just choosing between them" (715).

By interconnecting with nature and respecting nature's cycles, an agroecological Med diet is in harmony with our body and in harmony with nature. Describing how systems interconnect to regulate the climate, the author and climate activist Rebecca Solnit describes how "climate change is based on science. But if you delve into it deeply enough it is a kind is a kind of mysticism without mystification, a recognition of the beautiful interconnection of all life and the systems – weather, water, soil, seasons, ocean pH – on which that life depends." [420] Interconnectedness, whether it is with the climate or with food, has consequences. As Ms Solnit went on: "To acknowledge that everything is connected is to acknowledge that our actions have consequences and therefore responsibilities."

It is these responsibilities that we, the present generation, must take on board to ensure that our food is produced in a sustainable way for future generations. Sustainable development was first defined in a 1987 report *Our Common Future* by Gro Harlem Brundtland, the head of the UN Commission set up to define sustainability. In her definition she emphasised our responsibilities by saying that sustainable development should meet "the needs of the present without compromising the ability of future generations to meet their own needs". There is no better contemporary example to illustrate how a dietary choice can have dire consequences than considering a certain food market in Wuhan, China.

---

[420] https://www.theguardian.com/commentisfree/2019/mar/19/why-youll-never-meet-a-white-supremacist-who-cares-about-climate-change

Agroecology acknowledges that because dietary choices have consequences, these choices come with responsibilities. This is why, like other ecologically-minded agriculture systems, agroecology has a social element [716]. This includes social justice and is why agroecology prefers agriculture to be local and on an appropriate scale. As the FAO notes, industrial-scale livestock production threatens social justice by diminishing the market opportunities and competitiveness of small rural producers. [421]

Social justice also underpins the custom of villagers sharing common land to graze livestock. Each villager uses his or her fair share of this common resource. This system has been a successful part of local farming for hundreds of years because it works for the benefit of all. The opposite - the "tragedy of the commons" - occurs when resources are no longer shared. Instead, individuals act independently in their own self-interest. This is contrary to the common good and ends by depleting the resource for all. [422] The negative impact of self-interest in industrialised food production acting against the common good is now playing out on a global scale. And as we are seeing with the climate crisis, this further industrialisation of food production is risking a "tragedy of the planet".

Ultimately, the approach to how we eat comes down to how we view the world. It was the French gastronome Jean Anthelme Brillat-Savarin who coined the famous phrase "Tell me what you eat, and I will tell you what you are." This can be read in either direction and the inverse is equally true: Tell me what you are and I will tell you what you eat. This perspective it backed up by surveys in the US that found that the political leanings of an individual are a strong predictor of that individual's dietary choice. In one survey, liberals were 28% more likely to eat fresh fruit daily than conservatives and 10% of liberals said they were vegetarian compared to 3% of conservatives. [423] Michael Pollan said "eating is a political act". It seems that our politics act on our eating choices too.

One example of how agroecology expresses societal concerns is by the desire to shorten the food supply chain by reducing the number of intermediaries.

---

[421] FAO, 2003. World Agriculture : towards 2015/2030. see CIWF-Report-SDG-Goals.pdf
[422] https://en.wikipedia.org/wiki/Tragedy_of_the_commons
[423] https://www.livescience.com/14302-political-ideology-liberal-conservative-food-choices.html

Buying directly from the producer achieves this, but this can be difficult in countries such as the UK where even "farmer's markets" often do not involve much selling directly by the farmer. This contrasts with some other European countries where a producer selling directly to the public is still a common sight. One consequence of the Covid-19 crisis has been a surge in online food purchases direct from producers. Faced with the prospect of rotting pineapple and jackfruit during Covid-19 restrictions, farmers in the North East Indian town of Meghalaya started direct selling online with great success and far higher profitability. [424] Many similar producers have found that direct selling is far more profitable than going through a middleman and are trying to develop this new business model.

Various organisations already exist to promote community-supported agriculture. In France there is AMAP - the *Association pour le Maintien d'une Agriculture Paysanne* (Association for the Maintenance of a Peasant Agriculture) where members of the public guarantee to buy produce each week. Another example to bring farmers and the public closer together is Farmwel which envisages treating farming more like a public service, and, like schools and hospitals, to have a panel of citizens, helping make decisions such as in farm management. [425] This elevates farmers who produce healthful food to their rightful place as guardians of our health, much like a doctor working in preventative medicine.

The shortest food chain of all is to grow your own. A simple agroecological cycle is to compost your food waste and use this to fertilise your land to grow a few veg. In the UK, councils provide subsidised compost bins.[426]

This discussion can be summed in the eloquent words of the RSA report that described agroecological food production as existing in "A world where farming is largely chemical free thanks to precision farming. Livestock is fed on pasture or leftovers. Chickens thrive in agroforestry systems; outdoor pigs consume the little waste that's left in the food system. One where everyone can afford healthy food and can grow it themselves if they want to and where

[424] https://www.theguardian.com/global-development/2020/jul/06/farmers-markets-go-hi-tech-how-online-sales-are-saving-indian-farmers
[425] http://farmwel.blogspot.com
[426] https://getcomposting.com/en-gb/composters/

we focus our collective ingenuity on the health and wellbeing of the planet and of all the life." (713)

# 15. Postscript - Inflamed bodies on an inflamed planet

A body inflamed by chronic disease and a planet enflamed by burning forests. We are witnessing the rise of both personal and planetary fever. And there is ample evidence that our food choices are a major reason for both of these dangerous states. We need to cook food that doesn't cook the planet.

In his eco-psychology book Person/Planet, Theodore Roszak said "I believe there is a connection, one that becomes visible when we realise that both person and planet are threatened by the same enemy." The common enemy, he believed, was "the bigness of things". This bigness comes from multi-national companies, and one of these, the agri-food industry, is currently a major contributor to both personal and planetary fever.

Even if we cannot all be a Greta Thunberg or a David Attenborough, grassroot actions by ordinary people can nurture societal change. [427] As Prof Lorraine Whitmarsh from Cardiff University has said, "policymakers don't feel they have the mandate to take ambitious action unless there is grassroots demand for it." Just as grass roots nurture pastureland so too our grass-root actions can nurture change to a more ecologically friendly way of farming and eating. The theme of big versus small is hardly new - Roszak wrote his book over 40 years ago. But this does not make it any less relevant today and the stakes are now higher than ever for both person and for planet.[428]

A second theme running through this book has been how, through co-evolution, healthy foods harmonize with our body's needs. This contrasts with Charles Darwin's view of evolution as being driven by "survival of the fittest". Striving for domination is unlikely to be the best way for us to survive as a species in the future. It has been suggested that cooperation not competition

---

[427] https://www.bbc.com/news/science-environment-49756280
[428] Some choose to act as citizen scientists by volunteering in projects that contribute to our scientific understanding of biodiversity by recording wildlife numbers see p. 69 in REDF: state-of-nature-uk-report-2016.pdf

was crucial to the evolution of all forms of human cultural cognition, including language [717]. Cooperation is everywhere in nature from flowers providing nectar for insects in exchange for pollination services, to the relationship between mycorrhizal fungi and trees, to the relationship between us and our gut microbiome. These symbiotic relationships have led to survival of the friendliest rather than the fittest.

Perhaps only by revisiting this will we survive as a species.

# Appendices

## Abbreviations

| AICR | American Institute for Cancer Research |
|------|----------------------------------------|
| ALA | Alpha linolenic acid |
| Am. | American |
| BAC | Blood alcohol concentration |
| BHF | British Heart Foundation |
| CCC | Committee on Climate Change |
| CHD | Coronary heart disease |
| COPD | Chronic obstructive pulmonary disease |
| CVD | Cardiovascular disease |
| DALY | Disability-adjusted life year (the number of years lost due to ill-health, disability or early death) |
| DHA | Docosahexaenoic acid |
| EPA | Eicosapentaenoic acid |
| EPIC | European Prospective Investigation into Cancer (a multi-centre prospective cohort study) |
| EVOO | Extra virgin olive oil |
| GHG | Greenhouse gas |
| MCFA | Medium chain fatty acid |
| Med diet | Mediterranean diet |
| MUFA | Monounsaturated fatty acid |
| NDNS | National Diet and Nutrition Survey (UK organisation) |
| NHANES | National Health and Nutrition Examination Survey (US organisation) |
| NIH | National Institutes of Health |

| OAC | Oesophageal adenocarcinoma |
|-----|---------------------------|
| PUFA | Polyunsaturated fatty acid |
| RCT | Randomised control trial |
| RDA | Recommended daily allowance |
| RNI | Reference nutrient intake |
| ROS | Reactive oxygen species |
| SSB | Sugar-sweetened beverage |
| SFA | Saturated fatty acid |
| UPF | Ultra-processed food |
| WCRF | World Cancer Research Fund |
| YLD | Years Lived with Disability (ie a measure of poor health or morbidity) |

## Definitions

| All-cause death | Death from any cause |
|-----------------|---------------------|
| Enzymes | A type of protein that helps change one chemical into another eg if you eat too much sugar, enzymes change some of the sugar into fat. Often, a lot of enzymes work together as a team |
| Incidence | The number of people who develop a specific disease or experience a specific health-related event during a particular time period (such as a month or year) |
| Industrially processed food | Food produced by refining and adding chemicals |
| Macronutrient | Carbohydrates, fats or proteins |
| Micronutrient | Vitamins or minerals |
| Morbidity | Disease in a population |

| | |
|---|---|
| Mortality rate | Number of deaths in a given time |
| Naturally processed food | Food produced by natural, biological processing methods |
| Polysaccharide | A type of carbohydrate consisting of many sugar molecules joined together |
| Premature death | Death that occurs before the average age of death in a given country (eg in UK and US this equates to death before 75) |
| Prevalence | The number of people in a population who are currently living with the disease |

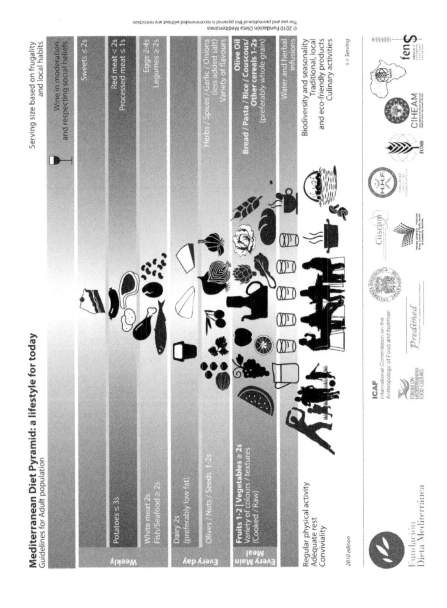

# Mediterranean Diet Pyramid: a lifestyle for today
Guidelines for Adult population

Serving size based on frugality and respecting social beliefs

Wine in moderation and respecting social beliefs

Sweets ≤ 2s

Red meat < 2s
Processed meat ≤ 1s

Eggs 2-4s
Legumes ≥ 2s

**Weekly**

Potatoes ≤ 3s

White meat 2s
Fish/Seafood ≥ 2s

Herbs / Spices / Garlic / Onions
(less added salt)
Variety of flavours

Olive Oil
Bread / Pasta / Rice / Couscous /
Other cereals 1-2s
(preferably whole grain)

**Every day**

Dairy 2s
(preferably low fat)

Olives / Nuts / Seeds 1-2s

Water and Herbal infusions

**Every Main Meal**

Fruits 1-2 | Vegetables ≥ 2s
Variety of colours / textures
(Cooked / Raw)

Biodiversity and seasonality
Traditional, local
and eco-friendly products
Culinary activities

Regular physical activity
Adequate rest
Conviviality

2010 edition

s = Serving

Fundación
Dieta Mediterránea

ICAF
International Commission on the
Anthropology of Food and Nutrition

Predimed

CIHEAM

fen S

# References

1. Marsh DR, Schroeder DG, Dearden KA *et al.* (2004) The power of positive deviance. *BMJ* **329**, 1177-1179.
2. Hill AB (1965) The Environment and Disease: Association or Causation? *Proc R Soc Med* **58**, 295-300.
3. Hoffman R, Gerber M (2011) *The Mediterranean diet : health & science.* Oxford: Wiley-Blackwell.
4. Katz DL, Meller S (2014) Can we say what diet is best for health? *Annu Rev Public Health* **35**, 83-103.
5. Scheelbeek P, Green R, Papier K *et al.* (2020) Health impacts and environmental footprints of diets that meet the Eatwell Guide recommendations: analyses of multiple UK studies. *BMJ Open* **10**, e037554.
6. Lee J, Pase M, Pipingas A *et al.* (2015) Switching to a 10-day Mediterranean-style diet improves mood and cardiovascular function in a controlled crossover study. *Nutrition* **31**, 647-652.
7. Radd-Vagenas S, Duffy SL, Naismith SL *et al.* (2018) Effect of the Mediterranean diet on cognition and brain morphology and function: a systematic review of randomized controlled trials. *Am J Clin Nutr* **107**, 389-404.
8. CNN (2018) US life expectancy drops for second year in a row. https://edition.cnn.com/2017/12/21/health/us-life-expectancy-study/index.html
9. BBC (2018) Life expectancy progress in UK 'stops for first time'. https://www.bbc.co.uk/news/health-45638646
10. Hiam L, Harrison D, McKee M *et al.* (2018) Why is life expectancy in England and Wales 'stalling'? *J Epidemiol Community Health* **72**, 404-408.
11. Iacobucci G (2019) A third of premature deaths in England are linked to social inequality, study finds. *BMJ* **367**, l6883.
12. Mahase E (2019) A decade on from Marmot, why are health inequalities widening? *BMJ* **365**, l4251.
13. Expert Scientific and Clinical Advisory Panel (2018) *Emerging evidence on the NHS Health Check: findings and recommendations.*
14. Kaeberlein M (2018) How healthy is the healthspan concept? *Geroscience* **40**, 361-364.
15. Bray GA, Kim KK, Wilding JPH *et al.* (2017) Obesity: a chronic relapsing progressive disease process. A position statement of the World Obesity Federation. *Obes Rev* **18**, 715-723.
16. Schnurr TM, Jakupovic H, Carrasquilla GD *et al.* (2020) Obesity, unfavourable lifestyle and genetic risk of type 2 diabetes: a case-cohort study. *Diabetologia* 10.1007/s00125-020-05140-5.
17. Barnes AS (2011) The epidemic of obesity and diabetes: trends and treatments. *Tex Heart Inst J* **38**, 142-144.
18. Kelly T, Yang W, Chen CS *et al.* (2008) Global burden of obesity in 2005 and projections to 2030. *Int J Obes (Lond)* **32**, 1431-1437.
19. Snook KR, Hansen AR, Duke CH *et al.* (2018) Notice of Retraction and Replacement. Snook et al. Change in percentages of adults with overweight or obesity trying to lose weight, 1988-2014. JAMA. 2017;317(9):971-973. *JAMA* **320**, 2485-2486.
20. Davies SC (2018) Annual Report of the Chief Medical Officer, 2018 Health 2040 – Better Health Within Reach.
21. Mahase E (2019) Prevention green paper lacks ambition, say critics. *BMJ* **366**, l4829.
22. Braveman P, Gottlieb L (2014) The social determinants of health: it's time to consider the causes of the causes. *Public Health Rep* **129 Suppl 2**, 19-31.
23. Anon (Vol 393 May 25, 2019)      Confronting heart disease and health inequality in the

UK. *The Lancet* **393**, 2100.

24. Loopstra R, McKee M, Katikireddi SV *et al.* (2016) Austerity and old-age mortality in England: a longitudinal cross-local area analysis, 2007-2013. *J R Soc Med* **109**, 109-116.

25. Lancet (2018) UK life science research: time to burst the biomedical bubble. *The Lancet* **392**.

26. All Party Parliamentary Group for Longevity (2020) *The Health of the Nation A Strategy for Healthier Longer Lives*.

27. Harland JI (2009) An assessment of the economic and heart health benefits of replacing saturated fat in the diet with monounsaturates in the form of rapeseed (canola) oilnbu_1756. *Nutrition Bulletin* **34**, 174–184.

28. Alageel S, Gulliford MC (2019) Health checks and cardiovascular risk factor values over six years' follow-up: Matched cohort study using electronic health records in England. *PLoS Med* **16**, e1002863.

29. Huffman MD, Xavier D, Perel P (2017) Uses of polypills for cardiovascular disease and evidence to date. *Lancet* **389**, 1055-1065.

30. Webster R, Grobbee D, Rodgers A (2019) The 2016 Joint European Prevention Guidelines and the uses of polypills: Time to update the evidence. *Eur J Prev Cardiol* 10.1177/2047487319872660, 2047487319872660.

31. Carlos S, de Irala J, Hanley M *et al.* (2014) The use of expensive technologies instead of simple, sound and effective lifestyle interventions: a perpetual delusion. *J Epidemiol Community Health* **68**, 897-904.

32. Thorpe KE, Philyaw M (2012) The medicalization of chronic disease and costs. *Annu Rev Public Health* **33**, 409-423.

33. Li Y, Schoufour J, Wang DD *et al.* (2020) Healthy lifestyle and life expectancy free of cancer, cardiovascular disease, and type 2 diabetes: prospective cohort study. *BMJ* **368**, l6669.

34. Salen P, de Lorgeril M (2011) The Okinawan diet: a modern view of an ancestral healthy lifestyle. *World Rev Nutr Diet* **102**, 114-123.

35. Pes GM, Tolu F, Dore MP *et al.* (2015) Male longevity in Sardinia, a review of historical sources supporting a causal link with dietary factors. *Eur J Clin Nutr* **69**, 411-418.

36. Islami F, Goding Sauer A, Miller KD *et al.* (2018) Proportion and number of cancer cases and deaths attributable to potentially modifiable risk factors in the United States. *CA Cancer J Clin* **68**, 31-54.

37. Lourida I, Hannon E, Littlejohns TJ *et al.* (2019) Association of Lifestyle and Genetic Risk With Incidence of Dementia. *JAMA* 10.1001/jama.2019.9879.

38. Akbaraly T, Sabia S, Hagger-Johnson G *et al.* (2013) Does overall diet in midlife predict future aging phenotypes? A cohort study. *Am J Med* **126**, 411-419 e413.

39. Newton JN, Briggs AD, Murray CJ *et al.* (2015) Changes in health in England, with analysis by English regions and areas of deprivation, 1990-2013: a systematic analysis for the Global Burden of Disease Study 2013. *Lancet* **386**, 2257-2274.

40. Halpern D, Harper H (2020) *Making it easier to live well: addressing the behavioural and environmental drivers of ill health. The Health of the Nation A Strategy for Healthier Longer Lives.* All Party Parliamentary Group for Longevity.

41. Corfe S (2018) *What are the barriers to eating healthily in the UK?* : Social Market Foundation.

42. Ludwig J, Sanbonmatsu L, Gennetian L *et al.* (2011) Neighborhoods, obesity, and diabetes-- a randomized social experiment. *N Engl J Med* **365**, 1509-1519.

43. Lasko-Skinner R (2020) *Turning the Tables. Making Healthier Choices Easier for Consumers.* Demos.

44. Browne S, Minozzi S, Bellisario C *et al.* (2018) Effectiveness of interventions aimed at improving dietary behaviours among people at higher risk of or with chronic non-communicable diseases: an overview of systematic reviews. *Eur J Clin Nutr* 10.1038/s41430-018-0327-3.

45. Mikkelsen BE (2011) Images of foodscapes: introduction to foodscape studies and their application in the study of healthy eating out-of-home environments. *Perspect Public Health* **131**,

209-216.

46. Mozaffarian D, Angell SY, Lang T *et al.* (2018) Role of government policy in nutrition-barriers to and opportunities for healthier eating. *BMJ* **361**, k2426.

47. Willett W, Rockstrom J, Loken B *et al.* (2019) Food in the Anthropocene: the EAT-Lancet Commission on healthy diets from sustainable food systems. *Lancet* **393**, 447-492.

48. McGill R, Anwar E, Orton L *et al.* (2015) Are interventions to promote healthy eating equally effective for all? Systematic review of socioeconomic inequalities in impact. *BMC Public Health* **15**, 457.

49. Hunt (In press) How food companies use social media to influence policy debates: a framework of Australian ultra-processed food industry Twitter data. *Public Health Nutrition.*

50. Bes-Rastrollo M, Schulze MB, Ruiz-Canela M *et al.* (2013) Financial conflicts of interest and reporting bias regarding the association between sugar-sweetened beverages and weight gain: a systematic review of systematic reviews. *PLoS Med* **10**, e1001578; discussion e1001578.

51. Dyer O (2019) International Life Sciences Institute is advocate for food and drink industry, say researchers. *BMJ* **365**, l4037.

52. MacGregor GA, He FJ, Pombo-Rodrigues S (2015) Food and the responsibility deal: how the salt reduction strategy was derailed. *BMJ* **350**, h1936.

53. Laverty AA, Kypridemos C, Seferidi P *et al.* (2019) Quantifying the impact of the Public Health Responsibility Deal on salt intake, cardiovascular disease and gastric cancer burdens: interrupted time series and microsimulation study. *J Epidemiol Community Health* 10.1136/jech-2018-211749.

54. Knai C, James L, Petticrew M *et al.* (2017) An evaluation of a public-private partnership to reduce artificial trans fatty acids in England, 2011-16. *Eur J Public Health* **27**, 605-608.

55. Panjwani C, Caraher M (2014) The Public Health Responsibility Deal: brokering a deal for public health, but on whose terms? *Health Policy* **114**, 163-173.

56. Scrinis G, Monteiro CA (2018) Ultra-processed foods and the limits of product reformulation. *Public Health Nutr* **21**, 247-252.

57. Ronit K, Jensen JD (2014) Obesity and industry self-regulation of food and beverage marketing: a literature review. *Eur J Clin Nutr* **68**, 753-759.

58. Moodie R, Stuckler D, Monteiro C *et al.* (2013) Profits and pandemics: prevention of harmful effects of tobacco, alcohol, and ultra-processed food and drink industries. *Lancet* **381**, 670-679.

59. Brownell KD (2012) Thinking forward: the quicksand of appeasing the food industry. *PLoS Med* **9**, e1001254.

60. Capewell S, Lloyd-Williams F (2018) The role of the food industry in health: lessons from tobacco? *Br Med Bull* **125**, 131-143.

61. Mialon M, Mialon J, Andrade GC *et al.* (2019) 'We must have a sufficient level of profitability': food industry submissions to the French parliamentary inquiry on industrial food. *Crit Pub Health.*

62. The Lancet (2017) The UK's inadequate plan for reducing childhood obesity. *Lancet* **390**, 822.

63. Dalglish SL (2020) COVID-19 gives the lie to global health expertise. *Lancet* **395**, 1189.

64. Mozaffarian D, Forouhi NG (2018) Dietary guidelines and health-is nutrition science up to the task? *BMJ* **360**, k822.

65. Capewell S, Cairney P, Clarke A (2018) Should action take priority over further research on public health? *BMJ* **360**, k292.

66. Swinburn B, Moore M (2014) Urgently needed: voices for integrity in public policy making. *Aust N Z J Public Health* **38**, 505.

67. Cooper BE, Lee WE, Goldacre BM *et al.* (2012) The quality of the evidence for dietary advice given in UK national newspapers. *Public Underst Sci* **21**, 664-673.

68. Chowdhury R, Warnakula S, Kunutsor S *et al.* (2014) Association of Dietary, Circulating, and Supplement Fatty Acids With Coronary Risk: A Systematic Review and Meta-analysis. *Ann*

*Intern Med* **160**.
69. Schoenfeld JD, Ioannidis JP (2013) Is everything we eat associated with cancer? A systematic cookbook review. *Am J Clin Nutr* **97**, 127-134.
70. Castell S (2014) *Public Attitudes to Science 2014*. Ipsos MORI.
71. O'Key V, Hugh-Jones S (2010) I don't need anybody to tell me what I should be doing'. A discursive analysis of maternal accounts of (mis)trust of healthy eating information. *Appetite* **54**, 524-532.
72. Alonso-Alonso M, Woods SC, Pelchat M *et al.* (2015) Food reward system: current perspectives and future research needs. *Nutr Rev* **73**, 296-307.
73. Hoffman SJ, Tan C (2015) Biological, psychological and social processes that explain celebrities' influence on patients' health-related behaviors. *Arch Public Health* **73**, 3.
74. Diamandis EP, Bouras N (2018) Hubris and Sciences. *F1000Res* **7**, 133.
75. Sies H (1988) A new parameter for sex education. *Nature* **332**, 495.
76. Cofield SS, Corona RV, Allison DB (2010) Use of Causal Language in Observational Studies of Obesity and Nutrition. *Obes Facts* **3**, 353–356.
77. Field AE, Coakley EH, Must A *et al.* (2001) Impact of overweight on the risk of developing common chronic diseases during a 10-year period. *Arch Intern Med* **161**, 1581-1586.
78. Wakeford R (2015) Association and causation in epidemiology - half a century since the publication of Bradford Hill's interpretational guidance. *J R Soc Med* **108**, 4-6.
79. Martinez-Gonzalez MA, Gea A, Ruiz-Canela M (2019) The Mediterranean Diet and Cardiovascular Health. *Circ Res* **124**, 779-798.
80. Willett WC, Stampfer MJ (2013) Current evidence on healthy eating. *Annu Rev Public Health* **34**, 77-95.
81. Spiegelhalter D (2016) How old are you, really? Communicating chronic risk through 'effective age' of your body and organs. *BMC Med Inform Decis Mak* **16**, 104.
82. Kim R, Lee DH, Subramanian SV (2019) Understanding the obesity epidemic. *BMJ* **366**, l4409.
83. Ronksley PE, Brien SE, Turner BJ *et al.* (2011) Association of alcohol consumption with selected cardiovascular disease outcomes: a systematic review and meta-analysis. *BMJ* **342**, d671.
84. Realdon S, Antonello A, Arcidiacono D *et al.* (2016) Adherence to WCRF/AICR lifestyle recommendations for cancer prevention and the risk of Barrett's esophagus onset and evolution to esophageal adenocarcinoma: results from a pilot study in a high-risk population. *Eur J Nutr* **55**, 1563-1571.
85. Yip CSC, Lam W, Fielding R (2018) A summary of meat intakes and health burdens. *Eur J Clin Nutr* **72**, 18-29.
86. Arcidiacono D, Antonello A, Fassan M *et al.* (2017) Insulin promotes HER2 signaling activation during Barrett's Esophagus carcinogenesis. *Dig Liver Dis* **49**, 630-638.
87. Kim YI (2018) Folate and cancer: a tale of Dr. Jekyll and Mr. Hyde? *Am J Clin Nutr* **107**, 139-142.
88. Allen NE, Beral V, Casabonne D *et al.* (2009) Moderate alcohol intake and cancer incidence in women. *J Natl Cancer Inst* **101**, 296-305.
89. Liu S, Willett WC, Stampfer MJ *et al.* (2000) A prospective study of dietary glycemic load, carbohydrate intake, and risk of coronary heart disease in US women. *Am J Clin Nutr* **71**, 1455-1461.
90. Lairon D, Defoort C, Martin JC *et al.* (2009) Nutrigenetics: links between genetic background and response to Mediterranean-type diets. *Public Health Nutr* **12**, 1601-1606.
91. Schulze MB, Martinez-Gonzalez MA, Fung TT *et al.* (2018) Food based dietary patterns and chronic disease prevention. *BMJ* **361**, k2396.
92. Ludwig DS, Willett WC, Volek JS *et al.* (2018) Dietary fat: From foe to friend? *Science* **362**, 764-770.
93. Gardner CD, Trepanowski JF, Del Gobbo LC *et al.* (2018) Effect of Low-Fat vs Low-

Carbohydrate Diet on 12-Month Weight Loss in Overweight Adults and the Association With Genotype Pattern or Insulin Secretion: The DIETFITS Randomized Clinical Trial. *JAMA* **319**, 667-679.

94. Huntriss R, Campbell M, Bedwell C (2018) The interpretation and effect of a low-carbohydrate diet in the management of type 2 diabetes: a systematic review and meta-analysis of randomised controlled trials. *Eur J Clin Nutr* **72**, 311-325.

95. Forouhi NG, Misra A, Mohan V *et al.* (2018) Dietary and nutritional approaches for prevention and management of type 2 diabetes. *BMJ* **361**, k2234.

96. Seidelmann SB, Claggett B, Cheng S *et al.* (2018) Dietary carbohydrate intake and mortality: a prospective cohort study and meta-analysis. *Lancet Public Health* **3**, e419-e428.

97. Mann T (2018) Why do dieters regain weight? *Psychological Science Agenda.*

98. Hoffman R (2017) Micronutrient deficiencies in the elderly - could ready meals be part of the solution? *J Nutr Sci* **6**, e2.

99. Astrup A, Bugel S (2018) Overfed but undernourished: recognizing nutritional inadequacies/deficiencies in patients with overweight or obesity. *Int J Obes (Lond)* 10.1038/s41366-018-0143-9.

100. Shao A, Drewnowski A, Willcox DC *et al.* (2017) Optimal nutrition and the ever-changing dietary landscape: a conference report. *Eur J Nutr* **56**, 1-21.

101. Mocchegiani E, Costarelli L, Giacconi R *et al.* (2014) Micronutrient-gene interactions related to inflammatory/immune response and antioxidant activity in ageing and inflammation. A systematic review. *Mech Ageing Dev* **136-137**, 29-49.

102. Chen P, Li C, Li X *et al.* (2014) Higher dietary folate intake reduces the breast cancer risk: a systematic review and meta-analysis. *Br J Cancer* **110**, 2327-2338.

103. Ames BN (2006) Low micronutrient intake may accelerate the degenerative diseases of aging through allocation of scarce micronutrients by triage. *Proc Natl Acad Sci U S A* **103**, 17589-17594.

104. McKay DL, Perrone G, Rasmussen H *et al.* (2000) The effects of a multivitamin/mineral supplement on micronutrient status, antioxidant capacity and cytokine production in healthy older adults consuming a fortified diet. *J Am Coll Nutr* **19**, 613-621.

105. Fenech MF (2010) Dietary reference values of individual micronutrients and nutriomes for genome damage prevention: current status and a road map to the future. *Am J Clin Nutr* **91**, 1438S-1454S.

106. Scarborough P, Rayner M (2014) When nutrient profiling can (and cannot) be useful. *Public Health Nutr* **17**, 2637-2640.

107. Tseng M, Hodge A (2014) Profiling foods and diets. *Public Health Nutr* **17**, 2625.

108. Bates B, Lennox A, Prentice A *et al.* (2014) National Diet and Nutrition Survey: Results from Years 1 to 4 (combined) of the Rolling Programme for 2008 and 2009 to 2011 and 2012. Appendicies and Tables. https://www.gov.uk/government/statistics/national-diet-and-nutrition-survey-results-from-years-1-to-4-combined-of-the-rolling-programme-for-2008-and-2009-to-2011-and-2012 (accessed July 2016)

109. Veronese N, Solmi M, Caruso MG *et al.* (2018) Dietary fiber and health outcomes: an umbrella review of systematic reviews and meta-analyses. *Am J Clin Nutr* **107**, 436-444.

110. Lunn J, Buttriss JL (2007) Carbohydrates and dietary fibre. *Nutrition Bulletin* **32**, 21-64.

111. Nyambe-Silavwe H, Williamson G (2016) Polyphenol- and fibre-rich dried fruits with green tea attenuate starch-derived postprandial blood glucose and insulin: a randomised, controlled, single-blind, cross-over intervention. *Br J Nutr* **116**, 443-450.

112. Muller M, Canfora EE, Blaak EE (2018) Gastrointestinal Transit Time, Glucose Homeostasis and Metabolic Health: Modulation by Dietary Fibers. *Nutrients* **10**.

113. Desai MS, Seekatz AM, Koropatkin NM *et al.* (2016) A Dietary Fiber-Deprived Gut Microbiota Degrades the Colonic Mucus Barrier and Enhances Pathogen Susceptibility. *Cell* **167**, 1339-1353 e1321.

114. Valdes AM, Walter J, Segal E *et al.* (2018) Role of the gut microbiota in nutrition and

health. *BMJ* **361**, k2179.

115. Gentile CL, Weir TL (2018) The gut microbiota at the intersection of diet and human health. *Science* **362**, 776-780.

116. Lockyer S, Nugent AP (2017) Health effects of resistant starch. *Nutrition Bulletin* **42**, 10-41.

117. Read NW, Welch IM, Austen CJ *et al.* (1986) Swallowing food without chewing; a simple way to reduce postprandial glycaemia. *Br J Nutr* **55**, 43-47.

118. Rose C, Parker A, Jefferson B *et al.* (2015) The Characterization of Feces and Urine: A Review of the Literature to Inform Advanced Treatment Technology. *Crit Rev Environ Sci Technol* **45**, 1827-1879.

119. Tresserra-Rimbau A, Rimm EB, Medina-Remon A *et al.* (2014) Polyphenol intake and mortality risk: a re-analysis of the PREDIMED trial. *BMC Med* **12**, 77-88.

120. Seibold P, Vrieling A, Johnson TS *et al.* (2014) Enterolactone concentrations and prognosis after postmenopausal breast cancer: assessment of effect modification and meta-analysis. *Int J Cancer* **135**, 923-933.

121. Akuffo KO, Beatty S, Peto T *et al.* (2017) The Impact of Supplemental Antioxidants on Visual Function in Nonadvanced Age-Related Macular Degeneration: A Head-to-Head Randomized Clinical Trial. *Invest Ophthalmol Vis Sci* **58**, 5347-5360.

122. Evans JR, Lawrenson JG (2017) Antioxidant vitamin and mineral supplements for slowing the progression of age-related macular degeneration. *Cochrane Database Syst Rev* **7**, CD000254.

123. Lindbergh CA, Renzi-Hammond LM, Hammond BR *et al.* (2018) Lutein and Zeaxanthin Influence Brain Function in Older Adults: A Randomized Controlled Trial. *J Int Neuropsychol Soc* **24**, 77-90.

124. Chapman NA, Jacobs RJ, Braakhuis AJ (2018) Role of diet and food intake in age-related macular degeneration: a systematic review. *Clin Exp Ophthalmol* 10.1111/ceo.13343.

125. Knobbe CA, Stojanoska M (2017) The 'Displacing Foods of Modern Commerce' Are the Primary and Proximate Cause of Age-Related Macular Degeneration: A Unifying Singular Hypothesis. *Med Hypotheses* **109**, 184-198.

126. Zakynthinos G, Varzakas T (2016) Carotenoids: From Plants to Food Industry. *Current Research in Nutrition and Food Science* **4**, 38-51.

127. Yang L, Ling W, Du Z *et al.* (2017) Effects of Anthocyanins on Cardiometabolic Health: A Systematic Review and Meta-Analysis of Randomized Controlled Trials. *Adv Nutr* **8**, 684-693.

128. Miller JA, Pappan K, Thompson PA *et al.* (2015) Plasma metabolomic profiles of breast cancer patients after short-term limonene intervention. *Cancer Prev Res (Phila)* **8**, 86-93.

129. Manios Y, Antonopoulou S, Kaliora AC *et al.* (2005) Dietary intake and biochemical risk factors for cardiovascular disease in two rural regions of Crete. *J Physiol Pharmacol* **56 Suppl 1**, 171-181.

130. Menendez JA, Joven J, Aragones G *et al.* (2013) Xenohormetic and anti-aging activity of secoiridoid polyphenols present in extra virgin olive oil: a new family of gerosuppressant agents. *Cell Cycle* **12**, 555-578.

131. Devillier P, Naline E, Grassin-Delyle S (2015) The pharmacology of bitter taste receptors and their role in human airways. *Pharmacol Ther* **155**, 11-21.

132. Kim JH, Ellwood PE, Asher MI (2009) Diet and asthma: looking back, moving forward. *Respir Res* **10**, 49.

133. Hawley SA, Fullerton MD, Ross FA *et al.* (2012) The ancient drug salicylate directly activates AMP-activated protein kinase. *Science* **336**, 918-922.

134. Hardie DG (2014) AMP-activated protein kinase: maintaining energy homeostasis at the cellular and whole-body levels. *Annu Rev Nutr* **34**, 31-55.

135. Orsinia F, Maggio A, Rouphael Y *et al.* (2016) "Physiological quality" of organically grown vegetables. *Scientia Horticulturae* **208**, 131-139.

136. Saiko P, Szakmary A, Jaeger W *et al.* (2008) Resveratrol and its analogs: defense against cancer, coronary disease and neurodegenerative maladies or just a fad? *Mutat Res* **658**, 68-94.

137. Ramirez-Garza SL, Laveriano-Santos EP, Marhuenda-Munoz M *et al.* (2018) Health

Effects of Resveratrol: Results from Human Intervention Trials. *Nutrients* **10**.

138. Mie A, Andersen HR, Gunnarsson S *et al.* (2017) Human health implications of organic food and organic agriculture: a comprehensive review. *Environ Health* **16**, 111.

139. Kesarwani K, Gupta R, Mukerjee A (2013) Bioavailability enhancers of herbal origin: an overview. *Asian Pac J Trop Biomed* **3**, 253-266.

140. Pannu N, Bhatnagar A (2019) Resveratrol: from enhanced biosynthesis and bioavailability to multitargeting chronic diseases. *Biomed Pharmacother* **109**, 2237-2251.

141. Tresserra-Rimbau A, Medina-Remon A, Perez-Jimenez J *et al.* (2013) Dietary intake and major food sources of polyphenols in a Spanish population at high cardiovascular risk: the PREDIMED study. *Nutr Metab Cardiovasc Dis* **23**, 953-959.

142. Monteiro CA, Cannon G, Levy RB *et al.* (2019) Ultra-processed foods: what they are and how to identify them. *Public Health Nutr* **22**, 936-941.

143. Rico-Campa A, Martinez-Gonzalez MA, Alvarez-Alvarez I *et al.* (2019) Association between consumption of ultra-processed foods and all cause mortality: SUN prospective cohort study. *BMJ* **365**, l1949.

144. Monteiro CA, Moubarac JC, Levy RB *et al.* (2018) Household availability of ultra-processed foods and obesity in nineteen European countries. *Public Health Nutr* **21**, 18-26.

145. Rauber F, da Costa Louzada ML, Steele EM *et al.* (2018) Ultra-Processed Food Consumption and Chronic Non-Communicable Diseases-Related Dietary Nutrient Profile in the UK (2008(-)2014). *Nutrients* **10**.

146. Adams J, White M (2015) Characterisation of UK diets according to degree of food processing and associations with socio-demographics and obesity: cross-sectional analysis of UK National Diet and Nutrition Survey (2008-12). *Int J Behav Nutr Phys Act* **12**, 160.

147. Lustig RH (2017) Processed Food-An Experiment That Failed. *JAMA Pediatr* **171**, 212-214.

148. Mendonca RD, Pimenta AM, Gea A *et al.* (2016) Ultraprocessed food consumption and risk of overweight and obesity: the University of Navarra Follow-Up (SUN) cohort study. *Am J Clin Nutr* **104**, 1433-1440.

149. Rauber F, Steele EM, Louzada M *et al.* (2020) Ultra-processed food consumption and indicators of obesity in the United Kingdom population (2008-2016). *PLoS One* **15**, e0232676.

150. Nardocci M, Leclerc BS, Louzada ML *et al.* (2018) Consumption of ultra-processed foods and obesity in Canada. *Can J Public Health* 10.17269/s41997-018-0130-x.

151. Hall KD, Ayuketah A, Brychta R *et al.* (2019) Ultra-Processed Diets Cause Excess Calorie Intake and Weight Gain: An Inpatient Randomized Controlled Trial of Ad Libitum Food Intake. *Cell Metab* 10.1016/j.cmet.2019.05.008.

152. Fiolet T, Srour B, Sellem L *et al.* (2018) Consumption of ultra-processed foods and cancer risk: results from NutriNet-Sante prospective cohort. *BMJ* **360**, k322.

153. Schnabel L, Kesse-Guyot E, Alles B *et al.* (2019) Association Between Ultraprocessed Food Consumption and Risk of Mortality Among Middle-aged Adults in France. *JAMA Intern Med* 10.1001/jamainternmed.2018.7289.

154. Kim H, Hu EA, Rebholz CM (2019) Ultra-processed food intake and mortality in the USA: results from the Third National Health and Nutrition Examination Survey (NHANES III, 1988-1994). *Public Health Nutr* 10.1017/S1368980018003890, 1-9.

155. Adjibade M, Julia C, Alles B *et al.* (2019) Prospective association between ultra-processed food consumption and incident depressive symptoms in the French NutriNet-Sante cohort. *BMC Med* **17**, 78.

156. Haut Conseil de la Santé Publique (2017) Avis relatif à la révision des repères alimentaires pour les adultes du futur Programme National Nutrition Santé 2017-2021. http://www.hcsp.fr/Explore.cgi/Telecharger?NomFichier=hcspa20170216_reperesalimentaire sactua2017.pdf

157. Ministry of Health of Brazil. Dietary Guidelines for the Brazilian population (2014) Dietary Guidelines for the Brazilian population.

http://189.28.128.100/dab/docs/portaldab/publicacoes/guia_alimentar_populacao_ingles.pdf

158. Mialona M, Sêrodio P, Scagliusia FB (2018) Criticism of the NOVA classification: who are the protagonists? *World Nutrition* **9**, 176-240.

159. Hebebrand J, Albayrak O, Adan R *et al.* (2014) "Eating addiction", rather than "food addiction", better captures addictive-like eating behavior. *Neurosci Biobehav Rev* **47**, 295-306.

160. Fardet A, Rock E (2020) How to protect both health and food system sustainability? A holistic 'global health'-based approach via the 3V rule proposal. *Public Health Nutr* 10.1017/S136898002000227X, 1-17.

161. Jun S, Cowan AE, Bhadra A *et al.* (2020) Older adults with obesity have higher risks of some micronutrient inadequacies and lower overall dietary quality compared to peers with a healthy weight, National Health and Nutrition Examination Surveys (NHANES), 2011-2014. *Public Health Nutr* **23**, 2268-2279.

162. Louzada ML, Martins AP, Canella DS *et al.* (2015) Impact of ultra-processed foods on micronutrient content in the Brazilian diet. *Rev Saude Publica* **49**, 45.

163. Louzada M, Ricardo CZ, Steele EM *et al.* (2018) The share of ultra-processed foods determines the overall nutritional quality of diets in Brazil. *Public Health Nutr* **21**, 94-102.

164. Martinez Steele E, Popkin BM, Swinburn B *et al.* (2017) The share of ultra-processed foods and the overall nutritional quality of diets in the US: evidence from a nationally representative cross-sectional study. *Popul Health Metr* **15**, 6.

165. Calton JB (2010) Prevalence of micronutrient deficiency in popular diet plans. *J Int Soc Sports Nutr* **7**, 24.

166. Aslam MF, Ellis PR, Berry SE *et al.* (2018) Enhancing mineral bioavailability from cereals: Current strategies and future perspectives. *Nutrition Bulletin* **43**, 184-188.

167. Gibson GE, Hirsch JA, Fonzetti P *et al.* (2016) Vitamin B1 (thiamine) and dementia. *Ann N Y Acad Sci* 10.1111/nyas.13031 [Epub ahead of print].

168. Hoffman R (2016) Thiamine deficiency in the Western diet and dementia risk. *Br J Nutr* **116**, 188-189.

169. Verrill L, Wood D, Cates S *et al.* (2017) Vitamin-Fortified Snack Food May Lead Consumers to Make Poor Dietary Decisions. *J Acad Nutr Diet* **117**, 376-385.

170. Baltacıoğl C (2017) Effect of Different Frying Methods on the Total trans Fatty Acid Content and Oxidative Stability of Oils. *JAOCS*.

171. Davies IG, Blackham T, Jaworowska A *et al.* (2016) Saturated and trans-fatty acids in UK takeaway food. *Int J Food Sci Nutr* **67**, 217-224.

172. Mozaffarian D, Aro A, Willett WC (2009) Health effects of trans-fatty acids: experimental and observational evidence. *Eur J Clin Nutr* **63 Suppl 2**, S5-21.

173. Allen K, Pearson-Stuttard J, Hooton W *et al.* (2015) Potential of trans fats policies to reduce socioeconomic inequalities in mortality from coronary heart disease in England: cost effectiveness modelling study. *BMJ* **351**, h4583.

174. Zinocker MK, Lindseth IA (2018) The Western Diet-Microbiome-Host Interaction and Its Role in Metabolic Disease. *Nutrients* **10**.

175. Imamura F, O'Connor L, Ye Z *et al.* (2015) Consumption of sugar sweetened beverages, artificially sweetened beverages, and fruit juice and incidence of type 2 diabetes: systematic review, meta-analysis, and estimation of population attributable fraction. *BMJ* **351**, h3576.

176. Chazelas E, Srour B, Desmetz E *et al.* (2019) Sugary drink consumption and risk of cancer: results from NutriNet-Sante prospective cohort. *BMJ* **366**, l2408.

177. Suez J, Korem T, Zeevi D *et al.* (2014) Artificial sweeteners induce glucose intolerance by altering the gut microbiota. *Nature* **514**, 181-186.

178. Singh RK, Chang HW, Yan D *et al.* (2017) Influence of diet on the gut microbiome and implications for human health. *J Transl Med* **15**, 73.

179. Ritz E, Hahn K, Ketteler M *et al.* (2012) Phosphate additives in food--a health risk. *Dtsch Arztebl Int* **109**, 49-55.

180. Weide A, Riehl S, Zeidi M *et al.* (2018) A systematic review of wild grass exploitation in

relation to emerging cereal cultivation throughout the Epipalaeolithic and aceramic Neolithic of the Fertile Crescent. *PLOS One* **13**.

181. Parada J, Aguilera JM (2007) Food microstructure affects the bioavailability of several nutrients. *J Food Sci* **72**, R21-32.

182. Johnston KL, Clifford MN, Morgan LM (2002) Possible role for apple juice phenolic compounds in the acute modification of glucose tolerance and gastrointestinal hormone secretion in humans. *J Sci Food Agric* **82**, 1800-1805.

183. de Graaf C, Kok FJ (2010) Slow food, fast food and the control of food intake. *Nat Rev Endocrinol* **6**, 290-293.

184. Bolhuis DP, Forde CG, Cheng Y *et al.* (2014) Slow food: sustained impact of harder foods on the reduction in energy intake over the course of the day. *PLoS One* **9**, e93370.

185. Astrup A, Bertram HC, Bonjour JP *et al.* (2019) WHO draft guidelines on dietary saturated and trans fatty acids: time for a new approach? *BMJ* **366**, l4137.

186. Virtamo J, Pietinen P, Huttunen JK *et al.* (2003) Incidence of cancer and mortality following alpha-tocopherol and beta-carotene supplementation: a postintervention follow-up. *JAMA* **290**, 476-485.

187. Bjelakovic G, Nikolova D, Gluud C (2014) Antioxidant supplements and mortality. *Curr Opin Clin Nutr Metab Care* **17**, 40-44.

188. Jenkins DJA, Spence JD, Giovannucci EL *et al.* (2018) Supplemental Vitamins and Minerals for CVD Prevention and Treatment. *J Am Coll Cardiol* **71**, 2570-2584.

189. Malcolm ADB (2019) Folate: Deja vu – all over again. *Nutrition Bulletin* **44**, 2-3.

190. Abbasi J (2018) Another Nail in the Coffin for Fish Oil Supplements. *JAMA* **319**, 1851-1852.

191. Abdelhamid AS, Brown TJ, Brainard JS *et al.* (2018) Omega-3 fatty acids for the primary and secondary prevention of cardiovascular disease. *Cochrane Database Syst Rev* **7**, CD003177.

192. Manson JE, Cook NR, Lee IM *et al.* (2019) Marine n-3 Fatty Acids and Prevention of Cardiovascular Disease and Cancer. *N Engl J Med* **380**, 23-32.

193. Wang W, Yang H, Johnson D *et al.* (2017) Chemistry and biology of omega-3 PUFA peroxidation-derived compounds. *Prostaglandins Other Lipid Mediat* **132**, 84-91.

194. Seeram NP, Schulman RN, Heber D (2006) *Pomegranates : ancient roots to modern medicine, Medicinal and aromatic plants--industrial profiles ; v 43.* Boca Raton: CRC/Taylor & Francis.

195. Nelson KM, Dahlin JL, Bisson J *et al.* (2017) The Essential Medicinal Chemistry of Curcumin. *J Med Chem* **60**, 1620-1637.

196. Nelson KM, Dahlin JL, Bisson J *et al.* (2017) Curcumin May (Not) Defy Science. *ACS Med Chem Lett* **8**, 467-470.

197. Patanwala I, King MJ, Barrett DA *et al.* (2014) Folic acid handling by the human gut: implications for food fortification and supplementation. *Am J Clin Nutr* **100**, 593-599.

198. Berr C, Akbaraly T, Arnaud J *et al.* (2009) Increased selenium intake in elderly high fish consumers may account for health benefits previously ascribed to omega-3 fatty acids. *J Nutr Health Aging* **13**, 14-18.

199. de Kok TM, van Breda SG, Manson MM (2008) Mechanisms of combined action of different chemopreventive dietary compounds: a review. *Eur J Nutr* **47 Suppl 2**, 51-59.

200. Parker TL, Miller SA, Myers LE *et al.* (2010) Evaluation of synergistic antioxidant potential of complex mixtures using oxygen radical absorbance capacity (ORAC) and electron paramagnetic resonance (EPR). *J Agric Food Chem* **58**, 209-217.

201. Micha R, Penalvo JL, Cudhea F *et al.* (2017) Association Between Dietary Factors and Mortality From Heart Disease, Stroke, and Type 2 Diabetes in the United States. *JAMA* **317**, 912-924.

202. Schwingshackl L, Schwedhelm C, Hoffmann G *et al.* (2017) Food groups and risk of all-cause mortality: a systematic review and meta-analysis of prospective studies. *Am J Clin Nutr* **105**, 1462-1473.

203. Hoffman R, Ranjbar G, Madden AM (2016) Inhibition of the glycaemic response by

onion: a comparison between lactose-tolerant and lactose-intolerant adults. *Eur J Clin Nutr* **70**, 1089-1091.

204. Sun L, Goh HJ, Govindharajulu P *et al.* (2020) Postprandial glucose, insulin and incretin responses differ by test meal macronutrient ingestion sequence (PATTERN study). *Clin Nutr* **39**, 950-957.

205. Fardet A, Rock E (2018) Perspective: Reductionist Nutrition Research Has Meaning Only within the Framework of Holistic and Ethical Thinking. *Adv Nutr* **9**, 655-670.

206. da Silva R, Bach-Faig A, Raido Quintana B *et al.* (2009) Worldwide variation of adherence to the Mediterranean diet, in 1961-1965 and 2000-2003. *Public Health Nutr* **12**, 1676-1684.

207. Bach-Faig A, Berry EM, Lairon D *et al.* (2011) Mediterranean diet pyramid today. Science and cultural updates. *Public Health Nutr* **14**, 2274-2284.

208. Maillot M, Issa C, Vieux F *et al.* (2011) The shortest way to reach nutritional goals is to adopt Mediterranean food choices: evidence from computer-generated personalized diets. *Am J Clin Nutr* **94**, 1127-1137.

209. Conde C, Delrot S, Geros H (2008) Physiological, biochemical and molecular changes occurring during olive development and ripening. *J Plant Physiol* **165**, 1545-1562.

210. Estruch R, Ros E, Salas-Salvado J *et al.* (2013) Primary prevention of cardiovascular disease with a Mediterranean diet. *N Engl J Med* **368**, 1279-1290.

211. Estruch R, Ros E, Salas-Salvado J *et al.* (2018) Primary Prevention of Cardiovascular Disease with a Mediterranean Diet Supplemented with Extra-Virgin Olive Oil or Nuts. *N Engl J Med* **378**, e34.

212. De Lorgeril M, Salen P, Martin JL *et al.* (1996) Effect of a mediterranean type of diet on the rate of cardiovascular complications in patients with coronary artery disease. Insights into the cardioprotective effect of certain nutriments. *J Am Coll Cardiol* **28**, 1103-1108.

213. Martinez-Gonzalez MA, Buil-Cosiales P, Corella D *et al.* (2019) Cohort Profile: Design and methods of the PREDIMED-Plus randomized trial. *Int J Epidemiol* **48**, 387-388o.

214. Salas-Salvado J, Diaz-Lopez A, Ruiz-Canela M *et al.* (2019) Effect of a Lifestyle Intervention Program With Energy-Restricted Mediterranean Diet and Exercise on Weight Loss and Cardiovascular Risk Factors: One-Year Results of the PREDIMED-Plus Trial. *Diabetes Care* **42**, 777-788.

215. Koloverou E, Esposito K, Giugliano D *et al.* (2014) The effect of Mediterranean diet on the development of type 2 diabetes mellitus: a meta-analysis of 10 prospective studies and 136,846 participants. *Metabolism* **63**, 903-911.

216. Neuenschwander M, Ballon A, Weber KS *et al.* (2019) Role of diet in type 2 diabetes incidence: umbrella review of meta-analyses of prospective observational studies. *BMJ* **366**, l2368.

217. Dinu M, Pagliai G, Casini A *et al.* (2018) Mediterranean diet and multiple health outcomes: an umbrella review of meta-analyses of observational studies and randomised trials. *Eur J Clin Nutr* **72**, 30-43.

218. Lourida I, Soni M, Thompson-Coon J *et al.* (2013) Mediterranean diet, cognitive function, and dementia: a systematic review. *Epidemiology* **24**, 479-489.

219. Solfrizzi V, Agosti P, Lozupone M *et al.* (2018) Nutritional Intervention as a Preventive Approach for Cognitive-Related Outcomes in Cognitively Healthy Older Adults: A Systematic Review. *J Alzheimers Dis* **64**, S229-S254.

220. Bundy R, Minihane AM (2018) Diet, exercise and dementia: The potential impact of a Mediterranean diet pattern and physical activity on cognitive health in a UK population. *Nutrition Bulletin* **43**, 284–289.

221. Cardenas D (2013) Let not thy food be confused with thy medicine: The Hippocratic misquotation. *e-SPEN Journal* **8**, e260-e262.

222. Morley JE, Morris JC, Berg-Weger M *et al.* (2015) Brain health: the importance of recognizing cognitive impairment: an IAGG consensus conference. *J Am Med Dir Assoc* **16**, 731-739.

223. World Cancer Research Fund/American Institute for Cancer Research (2018) *Continuous Update Project Expert Report: Diet, Nutrition, Physical Activity and Breast Cancer Survivors.*

224. Weigl J, Hauner H, Hauner D (2018) Can Nutrition Lower the Risk of Recurrence in Breast Cancer? *Breast Care (Basel)* **13**, 86-91.

225. Vadiveloo M, Lichtenstein AH, Anderson C *et al.* (2020) Rapid Diet Assessment Screening Tools for Cardiovascular Disease Risk Reduction Across Healthcare Settings: A Scientific Statement From the American Heart Association. *Circ Cardiovasc Qual Outcomes* 10.1161/HCQ.0000000000000094,

226. Megson IL, Whitfield PD, Zabetakis I (2016) Lipids and cardiovascular disease: where does dietary intervention sit alongside statin therapy? *Food Funct* **7**, 2603-2614.

227. Newman D (2013) Mediterranean Diet for 5 Years for Heart Disease Prevention (Without Known Heart Disease) http://www.thennt.com/nnt/mediterranean-diet-for-heart-disease-prevention-without-known-heart-disease/

228. Bonaccio M, Di Castelnuovo A, Costanzo S *et al.* (2019) Impact of combined healthy lifestyle factors on survival in an adult general population and in high-risk groups: prospective results from the Moli-sani Study. *J Intern Med* **286**, 207-220.

229. Perreault S, Blais L, Lamarre D *et al.* (2005) Persistence and determinants of statin therapy among middle-aged patients for primary and secondary prevention. *Br J Clin Pharmacol* **59**, 564-573.

230. Marventano S, Vetrani C, Vitale M *et al.* (2017) Whole Grain Intake and Glycaemic Control in Healthy Subjects: A Systematic Review and Meta-Analysis of Randomized Controlled Trials. *Nutrients* **9**.

231. Feinman RD, Pogozelski WK, Astrup A *et al.* (2015) Dietary carbohydrate restriction as the first approach in diabetes management: Critical review and evidence base. *Nutrition* **31**, 1-13.

232. Lockyer S, Stanner S (2016) Coconut oil – a nutty idea? *Nutrition Bulletin* **41**, 42-54.

233. Rosato V, Temple NJ, La Vecchia C *et al.* (2019) Mediterranean diet and cardiovascular disease: a systematic review and meta-analysis of observational studies. *Eur J Nutr* **58**, 173-191.

234. Toledo E, Salas-Salvado J, Donat-Vargas C *et al.* (2015) Mediterranean Diet and Invasive Breast Cancer Risk Among Women at High Cardiovascular Risk in the PREDIMED Trial: A Randomized Clinical Trial. *JAMA Intern Med* **175**, 1752-1760.

235. van den Brandt PA, Schulpen M (2017) Mediterranean diet adherence and risk of postmenopausal breast cancer: results of a cohort study and meta-analysis. *Int J Cancer* **140**, 2220-2231.

236. Couto E, Sandin S, Lof M *et al.* (2013) Mediterranean dietary pattern and risk of breast cancer. *PLoS One* **8**, e55374.

237. Cade JE, Taylor EF, Burley VJ *et al.* (2011) Does the Mediterranean dietary pattern or the Healthy Diet Index influence the risk of breast cancer in a large British cohort of women? *Eur J Clin Nutr* **65**, 920-928.

238. Turati F, Carioli G, Bravi F *et al.* (2018) Mediterranean Diet and Breast Cancer Risk. *Nutrients* **10**.

239. Kafatos A, Verhagen H, Moschandreas J *et al.* (2000) Mediterranean diet of Crete: foods and nutrient content. *J Am Diet Assoc* **100**, 1487-1493.

240. Esmarck B, Andersen JL, Olsen S *et al.* (2001) Timing of postexercise protein intake is important for muscle hypertrophy with resistance training in elderly humans. *J Physiol* **535**, 301-311.

241. Van Cauter E, Polonsky KS, Scheen AJ (1997) Roles of circadian rhythmicity and sleep in human glucose regulation. *Endocr Rev* **18**, 716-738.

242. Jakubowicz D, Barnea M, Wainstein J *et al.* (2013) High caloric intake at breakfast vs. dinner differentially influences weight loss of overweight and obese women. *Obesity (Silver Spring)* **21**, 2504-2512.

243. Fardet A (2010) New hypotheses for the health-protective mechanisms of whole-grain cereals: what is beyond fibre? *Nutr Res Rev* **23**, 65-134.

244. Ruddick-Collins LC, Johnston JD, Morgan PJ *et al.* (2018) The Big Breakfast Study: Chrono-nutrition influence on energy expenditure and bodyweight. *Nutr Bull* **43**, 174-183.

245. Si Hassen W, Castetbon K, Tichit C *et al.* (2018) Energy, nutrient and food content of snacks in French adults. *Nutr J* **17**, 33.

246. Harris (2015) *Binge BritainA look at the UK's snacking habits in conjunction with The Grocer.*

247. O'Connor L, Brage S, Griffin SJ *et al.* (2015) The cross-sectional association between snacking behaviour and measures of adiposity: the Fenland Study, UK. *Br J Nutr* **114**, 1286-1293.

248. Hull S, Re R, Chambers L *et al.* (2015) A mid-morning snack of almonds generates satiety and appropriate adjustment of subsequent food intake in healthy women. *Eur J Nutr* **54**, 803-810.

249. Miller R, Benelam B, Stanner SA *et al.* (2013) Is snacking good or bad for health: An overview. *Nutrition Bulletin* **38**, 302–322.

250. Boyland EJ, Harrold JA, Dovey TM *et al.* (2013) Food choice and overconsumption: effect of a premium sports celebrity endorser. *J Pediatr* **163**, 339-343.

251. Vinson JA, Zubik L, Bose P *et al.* (2005) Dried fruits: excellent in vitro and in vivo antioxidants. *J Am Coll Nutr* **24**, 44-50.

252. Sayon-Orea C, Bes-Rastrollo M, Carlos S *et al.* (2013) Association between sleeping hours and siesta and the risk of obesity: the SUN Mediterranean Cohort. *Obes Facts* **6**, 337-347.

253. Naska A, Oikonomou E, Trichopoulou A *et al.* (2007) Siesta in healthy adults and coronary mortality in the general population. *Arch Intern Med* **167**, 296-301.

254. Aune D, Giovannucci E, Boffetta P *et al.* (2017) Fruit and vegetable intake and the risk of cardiovascular disease, total cancer and all-cause mortality-a systematic review and dose-response meta-analysis of prospective studies. *Int J Epidemiol* **46**, 1029-1056.

255. White RR, Hall MB (2017) Nutritional and greenhouse gas impacts of removing animals from US agriculture. *Proc Natl Acad Sci U S A* **114**, E10301-E10308.

256. Satija A, Bhupathiraju SN, Spiegelman D *et al.* (2017) Healthful and Unhealthful Plant-Based Diets and the Risk of Coronary Heart Disease in U.S. Adults. *J Am Coll Cardiol* **70**, 411-422.

257. Hoffman R (2017) Can the paleolithic diet meet the nutritional needs of older people? *Maturitas* **95**, 63-64.

258. Manousou S, Stal M, Larsson C *et al.* (2018) A Paleolithic-type diet results in iodine deficiency: a 2-year randomized trial in postmenopausal obese women. *Eur J Clin Nutr* **72**, 124-129.

259. World Economic Forum (2019) *Meat: the Future series. Alternative Proteins.*

260. Ministry of Health of Brazil SoHC, Primary Health Care Department, (2014) *Dietary Guidelines for the Brazilian population.*

261. Papadaki A, Johnson L, Toumpakari Z *et al.* (2018) Validation of the English Version of the 14-Item Mediterranean Diet Adherence Screener of the PREDIMED Study, in People at High Cardiovascular Risk in the UK. *Nutrients* **10**.

262. Eyre H, Kahn R, Robertson RM *et al.* (2004) Preventing cancer, cardiovascular disease, and diabetes: a common agenda for the American Cancer Society, the American Diabetes Association, and the American Heart Association. *Stroke* **35**, 1999-2010.

263. Valavanidis A, Vlachogianni T, Fiotakis K (2009) Tobacco smoke: involvement of reactive oxygen species and stable free radicals in mechanisms of oxidative damage, carcinogenesis and synergistic effects with other respirable particles. *Int J Environ Res Public Health* **6**, 445-462.

264. Zhou LX, Sun CL, Wei LJ *et al.* (2016) Lower cognitive function in patients with age-related macular degeneration: a meta-analysis. *Clin Interv Aging* **11**, 215-223.

265. Johnson EJ, McDonald K, Caldarella SM *et al.* (2008) Cognitive findings of an exploratory trial of docosahexaenoic acid and lutein supplementation in older women. *Nutr Neurosci* **11**, 75-83.

266. Age-Related Eye Disease Study 2 Research G, Chew EY, Clemons TE *et al.* (2014)

Secondary analyses of the effects of lutein/zeaxanthin on age-related macular degeneration progression: AREDS2 report No. 3. *JAMA Ophthalmol* **132**, 142-149.

267. Cevenini E, Monti D, Franceschi C (2013) Inflamm-ageing. *Curr Opin Clin Nutr Metab Care* **16**, 14-20.

268. Ferrucci L, Fabbri E (2018) Inflammageing: chronic inflammation in ageing, cardiovascular disease, and frailty. *Nat Rev Cardiol* **15**, 505-522.

269. Hunt KJ, Walsh BM, Voegeli D *et al.* (2010) Inflammation in aging part 2: implications for the health of older people and recommendations for nursing practice. *Biol Res Nurs* **11**, 253-260.

270. Malafarina V, Uriz-Otano F, Iniesta R *et al.* (2012) Sarcopenia in the elderly: diagnosis, physiopathology and treatment. *Maturitas* **71**, 109-114.

271. Ridker PM, Everett BM, Thuren T *et al.* (2017) Antiinflammatory Therapy with Canakinumab for Atherosclerotic Disease. *N Engl J Med* **377**, 1119-1131.

272. Stone NJ, Robinson JG, Lichtenstein AH *et al.* (2014) 2013 ACC/AHA guideline on the treatment of blood cholesterol to reduce atherosclerotic cardiovascular risk in adults: a report of the American College of Cardiology/American Heart Association Task Force on Practice Guidelines. *J Am Coll Cardiol* **63**, 2889-2934.

273. Mainous AG, 3rd, Tanner RJ, Baker R *et al.* (2014) Prevalence of prediabetes in England from 2003 to 2011: population-based, cross-sectional study. *BMJ Open* **4**, e005002.

274. Huang Y, Cai X, Qiu M *et al.* (2014) Prediabetes and the risk of cancer: a meta-analysis. *Diabetologia* **57**, 2261-2269.

275. Riccardi G, Rivellese AA, Giacco R (2008) Role of glycemic index and glycemic load in the healthy state, in prediabetes, and in diabetes. *Am J Clin Nutr* **87**, 269S-274S.

276. Augustin LS, Kendall CW, Jenkins DJ *et al.* (2015) Glycemic index, glycemic load and glycemic response: An International Scientific Consensus Summit from the International Carbohydrate Quality Consortium (ICQC). *Nutr Metab Cardiovasc Dis* **25**, 795-815.

277. Cai X, Zhang Y, Li M *et al.* (2020) Association between prediabetes and risk of all cause mortality and cardiovascular disease: updated meta-analysis. *BMJ* **370**, m2297.

278. Reaven GM (1988) Banting lecture 1988. Role of insulin resistance in human disease. *Diabetes* **37**, 1595-1607.

279. Haslam DW, James WP (2005) Obesity. *Lancet* **366**, 1197-1209.

280. van Vliet-Ostaptchouk JV, Nuotio ML, Slagter SN *et al.* (2014) The prevalence of metabolic syndrome and metabolically healthy obesity in Europe: a collaborative analysis of ten large cohort studies. *BMC Endocr Disord* **14**, 9.

281. Bray GA, Heisel WE, Afshin A *et al.* (2018) The Science of Obesity Management: An Endocrine Society Scientific Statement. *Endocr Rev* **39**, 79-132.

282. Bell JA, Kivimaki M, Hamer M (2014) Metabolically healthy obesity and risk of incident type 2 diabetes: a meta-analysis of prospective cohort studies. *Obes Rev* **15**, 504-515.

283. Mongraw-Chaffin M, Foster MC, Anderson CAM *et al.* (2018) Metabolically Healthy Obesity, Transition to Metabolic Syndrome, and Cardiovascular Risk. *J Am Coll Cardiol* **71**, 1857-1865.

284. Matta J, Nasreddine L, Jomaa L *et al.* (2016) Metabolically Healthy Overweight and Obesity Is Associated with Higher Adherence to a Traditional Dietary Pattern: A Cross-Sectional Study among Adults in Lebanon. *Nutrients* **8**.

285. Eguaras S, Toledo E, Buil-Cosiales P *et al.* (2015) Does the Mediterranean diet counteract the adverse effects of abdominal adiposity? *Nutr Metab Cardiovasc Dis* **25**, 569-574.

286. Trinchieri G (2012) Cancer and inflammation: an old intuition with rapidly evolving new concepts. *Annu Rev Immunol* **30**, 677-706.

287. Morrison L, Laukkanen JA, Ronkainen K *et al.* (2016) Inflammatory biomarker score and cancer: A population-based prospective cohort study. *BMC Cancer* **16**, 80.

288. Ligibel JA, Alfano CM, Courneya KS *et al.* (2014) American Society of Clinical Oncology position statement on obesity and cancer. *J Clin Oncol* **32**, 3568-3574.

289. Akinyemiju T, Moore JX, Pisu M *et al.* (2018) A Prospective Study of Obesity, Metabolic

Health, and Cancer Mortality. *Obesity (Silver Spring)* **26**, 193-201.

290. Gunter MJ, Xie X, Xue X *et al.* (2015) Breast cancer risk in metabolically healthy but overweight postmenopausal women. *Cancer Res* **75**, 270-274.

291. Rose DP, Gracheck PJ, Vona-Davis L (2015) The Interactions of Obesity, Inflammation and Insulin Resistance in Breast Cancer. *Cancers (Basel)* **7**, 2147-2168.

292. Kabat GC, Kim MY, Lee JS *et al.* (2017) Metabolic Obesity Phenotypes and Risk of Breast Cancer in Postmenopausal Women. *Cancer Epidemiol Biomarkers Prev* **26**, 1730-1735.

293. Gunter MJ, Hoover DR, Yu H *et al.* (2009) Insulin, insulin-like growth factor-I, and risk of breast cancer in postmenopausal women. *J Natl Cancer Inst* **101**, 48-60.

294. World Cancer Research Fund/American Institute for Cancer Research (2017) *Continuous Update Project Report: Diet, Nutrition, Physical Activity and Breast Cancer.*

295. World Cancer Research Fund/American Institute for Cancer Research (2018) *Continuous Update Project Expert Report. Diet, nutrition, physical activity and breast cancer survivors.*

296. Friedenreich CM, Neilson HK, Farris MS *et al.* (2016) Physical Activity and Cancer Outcomes: A Precision Medicine Approach. *Clin Cancer Res* **22**, 4766-4775.

297. Martinez JA, Chalasani P, Thomson CA *et al.* (2016) Phase II study of metformin for reduction of obesity-associated breast cancer risk: a randomized controlled trial protocol. *BMC Cancer* **16**, 500.

298. Zahedi H, Djalalinia S, Sadeghi O *et al.* (2018) Dietary Inflammatory Potential Score and Risk of Breast Cancer: Systematic Review and Meta-analysis. *Clin Breast Cancer* **18**, e561-e570.

299. Masclee GM, Coloma PM, de Wilde M *et al.* (2014) The incidence of Barrett's oesophagus and oesophageal adenocarcinoma in the United Kingdom and The Netherlands is levelling off. *Aliment Pharmacol Ther* **39**, 1321-1330.

300. Kapoor H, Agrawal DK, Mittal SK (2015) Barrett's esophagus: recent insights into pathogenesis and cellular ontogeny. *Transl Res* **166**, 28-40.

301. Arnold M, Soerjomataram I, Ferlay J *et al.* (2015) Global incidence of oesophageal cancer by histological subtype in 2012. *Gut* **64**, 381-387.

302. Edgren G, Adami HO, Weiderpass E *et al.* (2013) A global assessment of the oesophageal adenocarcinoma epidemic. *Gut* **62**, 1406-1414.

303. Spechler SJ (2014) Does Barrett's esophagus regress after surgery (or proton pump inhibitors)? *Dig Dis* **32**, 156-163.

304. Kavanagh ME, O'Sullivan KE, O'Hanlon C *et al.* (2014) The esophagitis to adenocarcinoma sequence; the role of inflammation. *Cancer Lett* **345**, 182-189.

305. Jankowski JAZ, de Caestecker J, Love SB *et al.* (2018) Esomeprazole and aspirin in Barrett's oesophagus (AspECT): a randomised factorial trial. *Lancet* **392**, 400-408.

306. Doyle SL, Donohoe CL, Finn SP *et al.* (2012) IGF-1 and its receptor in esophageal cancer: association with adenocarcinoma and visceral obesity. *Am J Gastroenterol* **107**, 196-204.

307. Salvayre R, Negre-Salvayre A, Camare C (2016) Oxidative theory of atherosclerosis and antioxidants. *Biochimie* **125**, 281-296.

308. Wang A, Yang Y, Su Z *et al.* (2017) Association of Oxidized Low-Density Lipoprotein With Prognosis of Stroke and Stroke Subtypes. *Stroke* **48**, 91-97.

309. DiSabato DJ, Quan N, Godbout JP (2016) Neuroinflammation: the devil is in the details. *J Neurochem* **139 Suppl 2**, 136-153.

310. Arnold SE, Arvanitakis Z, Macauley-Rambach SL *et al.* (2018) Brain insulin resistance in type 2 diabetes and Alzheimer disease: concepts and conundrums. *Nat Rev Neurol* **14**, 168-181.

311. Ferreira ST, Clarke JR, Bomfim TR *et al.* (2014) Inflammation, defective insulin signaling, and neuronal dysfunction in Alzheimer's disease. *Alzheimers Dement* **10**, S76-S83.

312. Arvanitakis Z, Wilson RS, Bienias JL *et al.* (2004) Diabetes mellitus and risk of Alzheimer disease and decline in cognitive function. *Arch Neurol* **61**, 661-666.

313. Liu CH, Abrams ND, Carrick DM *et al.* (2017) Biomarkers of chronic inflammation in disease development and prevention: challenges and opportunities. *Nat Immunol* **18**, 1175-1180.

314. Van Hecke T, J. VC, De Smet S (2017) Oxidation During Digestion of Meat: Interactions

with the Diet and Helicobacter pylori Gastritis, and Implications on Human Health. *Comprehensive Reviews in Food Science and Food Safety* **16**, 214-233.

315. Yuhara H, Steinmaus C, Cohen SE *et al.* (2011) Is diabetes mellitus an independent risk factor for colon cancer and rectal cancer? *Am J Gastroenterol* **106**, 1911-1921; quiz 1922.

316. Masters RC, Liese AD, Haffner SM *et al.* (2010) Whole and refined grain intakes are related to inflammatory protein concentrations in human plasma. *J Nutr* **140**, 587-594.

317. Montonen J, Boeing H, Fritsche A *et al.* (2013) Consumption of red meat and whole-grain bread in relation to biomarkers of obesity, inflammation, glucose metabolism and oxidative stress. *Eur J Nutr* **52**, 337-345.

318. Shivappa N, Steck SE, Hurley TG *et al.* (2014) Designing and developing a literature-derived, population-based dietary inflammatory index. *Public Health Nutr* **17**, 1689-1696.

319. Ruiz-Canela M, Bes-Rastrollo M, Martinez-Gonzalez MA (2016) The Role of Dietary Inflammatory Index in Cardiovascular Disease, Metabolic Syndrome and Mortality. *Int J Mol Sci* **17**.

320. Zhong X, Guo L, Zhang L *et al.* (2017) Inflammatory potential of diet and risk of cardiovascular disease or mortality: A meta-analysis. *Sci Rep* **7**, 6367.

321. Tyrovolas S, Haro JM, Foscolou A *et al.* (2018) Anti-Inflammatory Nutrition and Successful Ageing in Elderly Individuals: The Multinational MEDIS Study. *Gerontology* **64**, 3-10.

322. Li D, Hao X, Li J *et al.* (2018) Dose-response relation between dietary inflammatory index and human cancer risk: evidence from 44 epidemiologic studies involving 1,082,092 participants. *Am J Clin Nutr* **107**, 371-388.

323. Lu Y, Shivappa N, Lin Y *et al.* (2016) Diet-related inflammation and oesophageal cancer by histological type: a nationwide case-control study in Sweden. *Eur J Nutr* **55**, 1683-1694.

324. Shivappa N, Hebert JR, Anderson LA *et al.* (2017) Dietary inflammatory index and risk of reflux oesophagitis, Barrett's oesophagus and oesophageal adenocarcinoma: a population-based case-control study. *Br J Nutr* **117**, 1323-1331.

325. Turati F, Tramacere I, La Vecchia C *et al.* (2013) A meta-analysis of body mass index and esophageal and gastric cardia adenocarcinoma. *Ann Oncol* **24**, 609-617.

326. World Cancer Research Fund / American Institute for Cancer Research (2018) *Continuous Update Porject Expert Report 2018. Diet, nutrition, physical activity and oesophageal cancer.*

327. Maret-Ouda J, El-Serag HB, Lagergren J (2016) Opportunities for Preventing Esophageal Adenocarcinoma. *Cancer Prev Res (Phila)* **9**, 828-834.

328. Kwiecien S, Magierowski M, Majka J *et al.* (2019) Curcumin: A Potent Protectant against Esophageal and Gastric Disorders. *Int J Mol Sci* **20**.

329. Rawat N, Alhamdani A, McAdam E *et al.* (2012) Curcumin abrogates bile-induced NF-kappaB activity and DNA damage in vitro and suppresses NF-kappaB activity whilst promoting apoptosis in vivo, suggesting chemopreventative potential in Barrett's oesophagus. *Clin Transl Oncol* **14**, 302-311.

330. Subramaniam D, Ponnurangam S, Ramamoorthy P *et al.* (2012) Curcumin induces cell death in esophageal cancer cells through modulating Notch signaling. *PLoS One* **7**, e30590.

331. Pophali PA, Sharma AN, Kossack S *et al.* (2016) Modulation of Esophageal Inflammation in Obese Barrett's Esophagus Subjects by Omega-3 Free Fatty Acids: A Potential Strategy for Prevention of Esophageal Adenocarcinoma . *Gastroenterology* **150**, S9.

332. Schulpen M, Peeters PH, van den Brandt PA (2019) Mediterranean diet adherence and risk of esophageal and gastric cancer subtypes in the Netherlands Cohort Study. *Gastric Cancer* **22**, 663-674.

333. Li WQ, Park Y, Wu JW *et al.* (2013) Index-based dietary patterns and risk of esophageal and gastric cancer in a large cohort study. *Clin Gastroenterol Hepatol* **11**, 1130-1136 e1132.

334. Urpi-Sarda M, Casas R, Chiva-Blanch G *et al.* (2012) Virgin olive oil and nuts as key foods of the Mediterranean diet effects on inflammatory biomakers related to atherosclerosis. *Pharmacol Res* **65**, 577-583.

335. Barbaresko J, Koch M, Schulze MB *et al.* (2013) Dietary pattern analysis and biomarkers of low-grade inflammation: a systematic literature review. *Nutr Rev* **71**, 511-527.

336. Ostan R, Lanzarini C, Pini E *et al.* (2015) Inflammaging and cancer: a challenge for the Mediterranean diet. *Nutrients* **7**, 2589-2621.

337. Alkerwi A, Vernier C, Crichton GE *et al.* (2014) Cross-comparison of diet quality indices for predicting chronic disease risk: findings from the Observation of Cardiovascular Risk Factors in Luxembourg (ORISCAV-LUX) study. *Br J Nutr* 10.1017/S0007114514003456, 1-11.

338. Garcia-Arellano A, Ramallal R, Ruiz-Canela M *et al.* (2015) Dietary Inflammatory Index and Incidence of Cardiovascular Disease in the PREDIMED Study. *Nutrients* **7**, 4124-4138.

339. Bonaccio M, Di Castelnuovo A, Costanzo S *et al.* (2019) Interaction between Mediterranean diet and statins on mortality risk in patients with cardiovascular disease: Findings from the Moli-sani Study. *Int J Cardiol* **276**, 248-254.

340. Steck SE, Shivappa N, Tabung FK *et al.* (2014) The Dietary Inflammatory Index: A New Tool for Assessing Diet Quality Based on Inflammatory Potential. *The Digest* **49**, 1-9.

341. Myles IA (2014) Fast food fever: reviewing the impacts of the Western diet on immunity. *Nutr J* **13**, 61.

342. Ruiz-Nunez B, Dijck-Brouwer DA, Muskiet FA (2016) The relation of saturated fatty acids with low-grade inflammation and cardiovascular disease. *J Nutr Biochem* **36**, 1-20.

343. Iwata NG, Pham M, Rizzo NO *et al.* (2011) Trans fatty acids induce vascular inflammation and reduce vascular nitric oxide production in endothelial cells. *PLoS One* **6**, e29600.

344. Tall AR, Yvan-Charvet L (2015) Cholesterol, inflammation and innate immunity. *Nat Rev Immunol* **15**, 104-116.

345. Galli C, Calder PC (2009) Effects of fat and fatty acid intake on inflammatory and immune responses: a critical review. *Ann Nutr Metab* **55**, 123-139.

346. Calder PC (2015) Functional Roles of Fatty Acids and Their Effects on Human Health. *JPEN J Parenter Enteral Nutr* **39**, 18S-32S.

347. Gayet-Boyer C, Tenenhaus-Aziza F, Prunet C *et al.* (2014) Is there a linear relationship between the dose of ruminant trans-fatty acids and cardiovascular risk markers in healthy subjects: results from a systematic review and meta-regression of randomised clinical trials. *Br J Nutr* **112**, 1914-1922.

348. Rudkowska I (2016) Talking about trans fatty acids. *Maturitas* **84**, 1-2.

349. Carrigan MA, Uryasev O, Frye CB *et al.* (2015) Hominids adapted to metabolize ethanol long before human-directed fermentation. *Proc Natl Acad Sci U S A* **112**, 458-463.

350. Rodrigo R, Miranda A, Vergara L (2011) Modulation of endogenous antioxidant system by wine polyphenols in human disease. *Clin Chim Acta* **412**, 410-424.

351. Franco R, Navarro G, Martinez-Pinilla E (2019) Antioxidants versus Food Antioxidant Additives and Food Preservatives. *Antioxidants (Basel)* **8**.

352. Kerr BJ, Kellner TA, Shurson GC (2015) Characteristics of lipids and their feeding value in swine diets. *J Anim Sci Biotechnol* **6**, 30.

353. Blaak EE, Antoine JM, Benton D *et al.* (2012) Impact of postprandial glycaemia on health and prevention of disease. *Obes Rev* **13**, 923-984.

354. Minihane AM, Vinoy S, Russell WR *et al.* (2015) Low-grade inflammation, diet composition and health: current research evidence and its translation. *Br J Nutr* **114**, 999-1012.

355. Calder PC, Ahluwalia N, Brouns F *et al.* (2011) Dietary factors and low-grade inflammation in relation to overweight and obesity. *Br J Nutr* **106 Suppl 3**, S5-78.

356. Camargo A, Delgado-Lista J, Garcia-Rios A *et al.* (2012) Expression of proinflammatory, proatherogenic genes is reduced by the Mediterranean diet in elderly people. *Br J Nutr* **108**, 500-508.

357. Bogani P, Galli C, Villa M *et al.* (2007) Postprandial anti-inflammatory and antioxidant effects of extra virgin olive oil. *Atherosclerosis* **190**, 181-186.

358. Thazhath SS, Wu T, Bound MJ *et al.* (2014) Changes in meal composition and duration

affect postprandial endothelial function in healthy humans. *Am J Physiol Gastrointest Liver Physiol* **307**, G1191-1197.

359. Karaaslan C, Suzen S (2015) Antioxidant properties of melatonin and its potential action in diseases. *Curr Top Med Chem* **15**, 894-903.

360. Favero G, Rodella LF, Reiter RJ *et al.* (2014) Melatonin and its atheroprotective effects: a review. *Mol Cell Endocrinol* **382**, 926-937.

361. Dehghan M, Mente A, Zhang X *et al.* (2017) Associations of fats and carbohydrate intake with cardiovascular disease and mortality in 18 countries from five continents (PURE): a prospective cohort study. *Lancet* **390**, 2050-2062.

362. Ludwig DS, Hu FB, Tappy L *et al.* (2018) Dietary carbohydrates: role of quality and quantity in chronic disease. *BMJ* **361**, k2340.

363. Bhupathiraju SN, Tobias DK, Malik VS *et al.* (2014) Glycemic index, glycemic load, and risk of type 2 diabetes: results from 3 large US cohorts and an updated meta-analysis. *Am J Clin Nutr* **100**, 218-232.

364. Cowie DM, Parsons JP, Raphael T (1924) INSULIN AND MENTAL DEPRESSION. *Arch NeurPsych* **12**, 522-533.

365. Lee SH, Zabolotny JM, Huang H *et al.* (2016) Insulin in the nervous system and the mind: Functions in metabolism, memory, and mood. *Mol Metab* **5**, 589-601.

366. Berger A (2016) Insulin resistance and reduced brain glucose metabolism in the aetiology of Alzheimer's disease. *Journal of Insulin Resistance* **1**.

367. Cherbuin N, Sachdev P, Anstey KJ (2012) Higher normal fasting plasma glucose is associated with hippocampal atrophy: The PATH Study. *Neurology* **79**, 1019-1026.

368. Floud S, Simpson RF, Balkwill A *et al.* (2020) Body mass index, diet, physical inactivity, and the incidence of dementia in 1 million UK women. *Neurology* **94**, e123-e132.

369. Ozawa M, Shipley M, Kivimaki M *et al.* (2017) Dietary pattern, inflammation and cognitive decline: The Whitehall II prospective cohort study. *Clin Nutr* **36**, 506-512.

370. Jacka FN, Cherbuin N, Anstey KJ *et al.* (2015) Western diet is associated with a smaller hippocampus: a longitudinal investigation. *BMC Med* **13**, 215.

371. Bredesen DE (2014) Reversal of cognitive decline: a novel therapeutic program. *Aging (Albany NY)* **6**, 707-717.

372. Lehtisalo J, Levalahti E, Lindstrom J *et al.* (2019) Dietary changes and cognition over 2 years within a multidomain intervention trial-The Finnish Geriatric Intervention Study to Prevent Cognitive Impairment and Disability (FINGER). *Alzheimers Dement* **15**, 410-417.

373. Ngandu T, Lehtisalo J, Solomon A *et al.* (2015) A 2 year multidomain intervention of diet, exercise, cognitive training, and vascular risk monitoring versus control to prevent cognitive decline in at-risk elderly people (FINGER): a randomised controlled trial. *Lancet* **385**, 2255-2263.

374. Frith E, Shivappa N, Mann JR *et al.* (2018) Dietary inflammatory index and memory function: population-based national sample of elderly Americans. *Br J Nutr* **119**, 552-558.

375. Chen X, Maguire B, Brodaty H *et al.* (2019) Dietary Patterns and Cognitive Health in Older Adults: A Systematic Review. *J Alzheimers Dis* **67**, 583-619.

376. McGrattan AM, McGuinness B, McKinley MC *et al.* (2019) Diet and Inflammation in Cognitive Ageing and Alzheimer's Disease. *Curr Nutr Rep* **8**, 53-65.

377. Shakersain B, Santoni G, Larsson SC *et al.* (2016) Prudent diet may attenuate the adverse effects of Western diet on cognitive decline. *Alzheimers Dement* **12**, 100-109.

378. Knight A, Bryan J, Murphy K (2016) Is the Mediterranean diet a feasible approach to preserving cognitive function and reducing risk of dementia for older adults in Western countries? New insights and future directions. *Ageing Res Rev* **25**, 85-101.

379. Power R, Prado-Cabrero A, Mulcahy R *et al.* (2019) The Role of Nutrition for the Aging Population: Implications for Cognition and Alzheimer's Disease. *Annu Rev Food Sci Technol* **10**, 619-639.

380. Cunnane SC, Courchesne-Loyer A, Vandenberghe C *et al.* (2016) Can Ketones Help

Rescue Brain Fuel Supply in Later Life? Implications for Cognitive Health during Aging and the Treatment of Alzheimer's Disease. *Front Mol Neurosci* **9**, 53.

381. Fortier M, Castellano CA, Croteau E *et al.* (2019) A ketogenic drink improves brain energy and some measures of cognition in mild cognitive impairment. *Alzheimers Dement* **15**, 625-634.

382. Vandenberghe C, St-Pierre V, Pierotti T *et al.* (2017) Tricaprylin Alone Increases Plasma Ketone Response More Than Coconut Oil or Other Medium-Chain Triglycerides: An Acute Crossover Study in Healthy Adults. *Curr Dev Nutr* **1**, e000257.

383. Hellín P, Lopez M-B, Jordan M-J *et al.* (1998) Fatty acids in Murciano-Granadina goats' milk. *Lait* **78**, 363-369.

384. Fernando WM, Martins IJ, Goozee KG *et al.* (2015) The role of dietary coconut for the prevention and treatment of Alzheimer's disease: potential mechanisms of action. *Br J Nutr* **114**, 1-14.

385. Offermanns S, Schwaninger M (2015) Nutritional or pharmacological activation of HCA(2) ameliorates neuroinflammation. *Trends Mol Med* **21**, 245-255.

386. Cherbuin N, Anstey KJ (2012) The Mediterranean diet is not related to cognitive change in a large prospective investigation: the PATH Through Life study. *Am J Geriatr Psychiatry* **20**, 635-639.

387. Hornedo-Ortega R, Cerezo AB, de Pablos RM *et al.* (2018) Phenolic Compounds Characteristic of the Mediterranean Diet in Mitigating Microglia-Mediated Neuroinflammation. *Front Cell Neurosci* **12**, 373.

388. de Pablos RM, Espinosa-Oliva AM, Hornedo-Ortega R *et al.* (2019) Hydroxytyrosol protects from aging process via AMPK and autophagy; a review of its effects on cancer, metabolic syndrome, osteoporosis, immune-mediated and neurodegenerative diseases. *Pharmacol Res* **143**, 58-72.

389. Bakhta K, Cecillon E, Lacombe E *et al.* (2019) Alzheimer's disease and neurodegenerative diseases in France. *Lancet* **394**, 466-467.

390. Jacka FN, O'Neil A, Opie R *et al.* (2017) A randomised controlled trial of dietary improvement for adults with major depression (the 'SMILES' trial). *BMC Med* **15**, 23.

391. Parletta N, Zarnowiecki D, Cho J *et al.* (2019) A Mediterranean-style dietary intervention supplemented with fish oil improves diet quality and mental health in people with depression: A randomized controlled trial (HELFIMED). *Nutr Neurosci* **22**, 474-487.

392. Bot M, Brouwer IA, Roca M *et al.* (2019) Effect of Multinutrient Supplementation and Food-Related Behavioral Activation Therapy on Prevention of Major Depressive Disorder Among Overweight or Obese Adults With Subsyndromal Depressive Symptoms: The MooDFOOD Randomized Clinical Trial. *JAMA* **321**, 858-868.

393. Firth J, Gangwisch JE, Borisini A *et al.* (2020) Food and mood: how do diet and nutrition affect mental wellbeing? *BMJ* **369**, m2382.

394. Schlesinger S, Chan DSM, Vingeliene S *et al.* (2017) Carbohydrates, glycemic index, glycemic load, and breast cancer risk: a systematic review and dose-response meta-analysis of prospective studies. *Nutr Rev* **75**, 420-441.

395. Sieri S, Krogh V (2017) Dietary glycemic index, glycemic load and cancer: An overview of the literature. *Nutr Metab Cardiovasc Dis* **27**, 18-31.

396. Maiorino MI, Bellastella G, Giugliano D *et al.* (2017) Can diet prevent diabetes? *J Diabetes Complications* **31**, 288-290.

397. Esposito K, Maiorino MI, Bellastella G *et al.* (2015) A journey into a Mediterranean diet and type 2 diabetes: a systematic review with meta-analyses. *BMJ Open* **5**, e008222.

398. Ley SH, Hamdy O, Mohan V *et al.* (2014) Prevention and management of type 2 diabetes: dietary components and nutritional strategies. *Lancet* **383**, 1999-2007.

399. Giovannucci E, Harlan DM, Archer MC *et al.* (2010) Diabetes and cancer: a consensus report. *Diabetes Care* **33**, 1674-1685.

400. Nohmi T (2018) Thresholds of Genotoxic and Non-Genotoxic Carcinogens. *Toxicol Res* **34**, 281-290.

401. Friedenreich CM, Shaw E, Neilson HK *et al.* (2017) Epidemiology and biology of physical activity and cancer recurrence. *J Mol Med (Berl)* **95**, 1029-1041.

402. Kyu HH, Bachman VF, Alexander LT *et al.* (2016) Physical activity and risk of breast cancer, colon cancer, diabetes, ischemic heart disease, and ischemic stroke events: systematic review and dose-response meta-analysis for the Global Burden of Disease Study 2013. *BMJ* **354**, i3857.

403. Lahart IM, Metsios GS, Nevill AM *et al.* (2015) Physical activity, risk of death and recurrence in breast cancer survivors: A systematic review and meta-analysis of epidemiological studies. *Acta Oncol* **54**, 635-654.

404. Friedenreich CM (2011) Physical activity and breast cancer: review of the epidemiologic evidence and biologic mechanisms. *Recent Results Cancer Res* **188**, 125-139.

405. Friedenreich CM, Neilson HK, Lynch BM (2010) State of the epidemiological evidence on physical activity and cancer prevention. *Eur J Cancer* **46**, 2593-2604.

406. Burkewitz K, Zhang Y, Mair WB (2014) AMPK at the nexus of energetics and aging. *Cell Metab* **20**, 10-25.

407. McCarty MF (2014) AMPK activation--protean potential for boosting healthspan. *Age (Dordr)* **36**, 641-663.

408. Martucci M, Ostan R, Biondi F *et al.* (2017) Mediterranean diet and inflammaging within the hormesis paradigm. *Nutr Rev* **75**, 442-455.

409. Salminen A, Kaarniranta K (2012) AMP-activated protein kinase (AMPK) controls the aging process via an integrated signaling network. *Ageing Res Rev* **11**, 230-241.

410. Leonov A, Arlia-Ciommo A, Piano A *et al.* (2015) Longevity extension by phytochemicals. *Molecules* **20**, 6544-6572.

411. Burkewitz K, Weir HJ, Mair WB (2016) AMPK as a Pro-longevity Target. *EXS* **107**, 227-256.

412. Halikas A, Gibas KJ (2018) AMPK induced memory improvements in the diabetic population: A case study. *Diabetes Metab Syndr* **12**, 1141-1146.

413. Witkamp RF, van Norren K (2018) Let thy food be thy medicine....when possible. *Eur J Pharmacol* **836**, 102-114.

414. EUFIC (2012) *Fruit and vegetable consumption in Europe - do Europeans get enough?* .

415. Maguire ER, Monsivais P (2015) Socio-economic dietary inequalities in UK adults: an updated picture of key food groups and nutrients from national surveillance data. *Br J Nutr* **113**, 181-189.

416. Hiam L, Dorling D (2018) Government's misplaced prevention agenda. *BMJ* **363**, k5134.

417. Boeing H, Bechthold A, Bub A *et al.* (2012) Critical review: vegetables and fruit in the prevention of chronic diseases. *Eur J Nutr* **51**, 637-663.

418. World Cancer Research Fund/American Institute for Cancer Research (2018) *Continuous Update Project Expert Report. Wholegrains, vegetables and fruit and the risk of cancer.*

419. Zheng JS, Sharp SJ, Imamura F *et al.* (2020) Association of plasma biomarkers of fruit and vegetable intake with incident type 2 diabetes: EPIC-InterAct case-cohort study in eight European countries. *BMJ* **370**, m2194.

420. Wang X, Ouyang Y, Liu J *et al.* (2014) Fruit and vegetable consumption and mortality from all causes, cardiovascular disease, and cancer: systematic review and dose-response meta-analysis of prospective cohort studies. *BMJ* **349**, g4490.

421. Leenders M, Boshuizen HC, Ferrari P *et al.* (2014) Fruit and vegetable intake and cause-specific mortality in the EPIC study. *Eur J Epidemiol* **29**, 639-652.

422. Akash MS, Rehman K, Chen S (2014) Spice plant Allium cepa: dietary supplement for treatment of type 2 diabetes mellitus. *Nutrition* **30**, 1128-1137.

423. Liu F, Prabhakar M, Ju J *et al.* (2017) Effect of inulin-type fructans on blood lipid profile and glucose level: a systematic review and meta-analysis of randomized controlled trials. *Eur J Clin Nutr* **71**, 9-20.

424. Coe S, Ryan L (2016) Impact of polyphenol-rich sources on acute postprandial glycaemia:

a systematic review. *J Nut Sci* **5**, 1-11.

425. Hord NG, Tang Y, Bryan NS (2009) Food sources of nitrates and nitrites: the physiologic context for potential health benefits. *Am J Clin Nutr* **90**, 1-10.

426. Hodge AM, English DR, O'Dea K *et al.* (2004) Glycemic index and dietary fiber and the risk of type 2 diabetes. *Diabetes Care* **27**, 2701-2706.

427. Buchner FL, Bueno-de-Mesquita HB, Ros MM *et al.* (2010) Variety in fruit and vegetable consumption and the risk of lung cancer in the European prospective investigation into cancer and nutrition. *Cancer Epidemiol Biomarkers Prev* **19**, 2278-2286.

428. DuPont MS, Mondin Z, Williamson G *et al.* (2000) Effect of variety, processing, and storage on the flavonoid glycoside content and composition of lettuce and endive. *J Agric Food Chem* **48**, 3957-3964.

429. McCarty MF, DiNicolantonio JJ (2014) Are organically grown foods safer and more healthful than conventionally grown foods? *Br J Nutr* **112**, 1589-1591.

430. Baudry J (2018) Association of Frequency of Organic Food Consumption With Cancer Risk Findings From the NutriNet-Santé Prospective Cohort Study.

431. Bradbury KE, Balkwill A, Spencer EA *et al.* (2014) Organic food consumption and the incidence of cancer in a large prospective study of women in the United Kingdom. *Br J Cancer* **110**, 2321-2326.

432. Reiss R, Johnston J, Tucker K *et al.* (2012) Estimation of cancer risks and benefits associated with a potential increased consumption of fruits and vegetables. *Food Chem Toxicol* **50**, 4421-4427.

433. Baranski M, Srednicka-Tober D, Volakakis N *et al.* (2014) Higher antioxidant and lower cadmium concentrations and lower incidence of pesticide residues in organically grown crops: a systematic literature review and meta-analyses. *Br J Nutr* **112**, 794-811.

434. The Expert Committee on Pesticide Residues in Food (2018) *Report on the pesticide residues monitoring programme: Quarter 1 2018.*

435. Zhang L, Rana I, Shaffer RM *et al.* (2019) Exposure to glyphosate-based herbicides and risk for non-Hodgkin lymphoma: A meta-analysis and supporting evidence. *Mutat Res* **781**, 186-206.

436. Benbrook CM (2016) Trends in glyphosate herbicide use in the United States and globally. *Environ Sci Eur* **28**, 3.

437. Kamel F, Hoppin JA (2004) Association of pesticide exposure with neurologic dysfunction and disease. *Environ Health Perspect* **112**, 950-958.

438. Lukowicz C, Ellero-Simatos S, Regnier M *et al.* (2018) Metabolic Effects of a Chronic Dietary Exposure to a Low-Dose Pesticide Cocktail in Mice: Sexual Dimorphism and Role of the Constitutive Androstane Receptor. *Environ Health Perspect* **126**, 067007.

439. Vian MA, Tomao V, Coulomb PO *et al.* (2006) Comparison of the anthocyanin composition during ripening of Syrah grapes grown using organic or conventional agricultural practices. *J Agric Food Chem* **54**, 5230-5235.

440. Birch LL, Fisher JO (1998) Development of eating behaviors among children and adolescents. *Pediatrics* **101**, 539-549.

441. Turnwald BP, Boles DZ, Crum AJ (2017) Association Between Indulgent Descriptions and Vegetable Consumption: Twisted Carrots and Dynamite Beets. *JAMA Intern Med* **177**, 1216-1218.

442. Hoffman R, Gerber M (2015) Food Processing and the Mediterranean Diet. *Nutrients* **7**, 7925-7964.

443. Cavagnaro PF, Camargo A, Galmarini CR *et al.* (2007) Effect of cooking on garlic (Allium sativum L.) antiplatelet activity and thiosulfinates content. *J Agric Food Chem* **55**, 1280-1288.

444. Song K, Milner JA (1999) Heating garlic inhibits its ability to suppress 7, 12-dimethylbenz(a)anthracene-induced DNA adduct formation in rat mammary tissue. *J Nutr* **129**, 657-661.

445. Song K, Milner JA (2001) The influence of heating on the anticancer properties of garlic. *J*

*Nutr* **131**, 1054S-1057S.

446. Jin ZY, Wu M, Han RQ *et al.* (2013) Raw garlic consumption as a protective factor for lung cancer, a population-based case-control study in a Chinese population. *Cancer Prev Res (Phila)* **6**, 711-718.

447. Bosetti C, Tzonou A, Lagiou P *et al.* (2000) Fraction of prostate cancer incidence attributed to diet in Athens, Greece. *Eur J Cancer Prev* **9**, 119-123.

448. Rinaldi de Alvarenga JF, Quifer-Rada P, Francetto Juliano F *et al.* (2019) Using Extra Virgin Olive Oil to Cook Vegetables Enhances Polyphenol and Carotenoid Extractability: A Study Applying the sofrito Technique. *Molecules* **24**.

449. Gillick S, Quested T (2018) *Household food waste: restated data for 2007-2015.* WRAP.

450. Collaborators GBDD (2019) Health effects of dietary risks in 195 countries, 1990-2017: a systematic analysis for the Global Burden of Disease Study 2017. *Lancet* **393**, 1958-1972.

451. Benisi-Kohansal S, Saneei P, Salehi-Marzijarani M *et al.* (2016) Whole-Grain Intake and Mortality from All Causes, Cardiovascular Disease, and Cancer: A Systematic Review and Dose-Response Meta-Analysis of Prospective Cohort Studies. *Adv Nutr* **7**, 1052-1065.

452. Reynolds A, Mann J, Cummings J *et al.* (2019) Carbohydrate quality and human health: a series of systematic reviews and meta-analyses. *Lancet* 10.1016/S0140-6736(18)31809-9.

453. Jarvi AE, Karlstrom BE, Granfeldt YE *et al.* (1999) Improved glycemic control and lipid profile and normalized fibrinolytic activity on a low-glycemic index diet in type 2 diabetic patients. *Diabetes Care* **22**, 10-18.

454. Runchey SS, Valsta LM, Schwarz Y *et al.* (2013) Effect of low- and high-glycemic load on circulating incretins in a randomized clinical trial. *Metabolism* **62**, 188-195.

455. Scientific Advisory Committee on Nutrition (2015) *Carbohydrates and Health.*

456. Vitaglione P, Mennella I, Ferracane R *et al.* (2015) Whole-grain wheat consumption reduces inflammation in a randomized controlled trial on overweight and obese subjects with unhealthy dietary and lifestyle behaviors: role of polyphenols bound to cereal dietary fiber. *Am J Clin Nutr* **101**, 251-261.

457. Boz H (2015) Ferulic Acid in Cereals – a Review. *Czech J Food Sci* **33**, 107.

458. Belobrajdic DP, Bird AR (2013) The potential role of phytochemicals in wholegrain cereals for the prevention of type-2 diabetes. *Nutr J* **12**, 62.

459. Yu L, Nanguet AL, Beta T (2013) Comparison of Antioxidant Properties of Refined and Whole Wheat Flour and Bread. *Antioxidants (Basel)* **2**, 370-383.

460. Chen Y, Ross AB, Aman P *et al.* (2004) Alkylresorcinols as markers of whole grain wheat and rye in cereal products. *J Agric Food Chem* **52**, 8242-8246.

461. Jonnalagadda SS, Harnack L, Liu RH *et al.* (2011) Putting the whole grain puzzle together: health benefits associated with whole grains--summary of American Society for Nutrition 2010 Satellite Symposium. *J Nutr* **141**, 1011S-1022S.

462. Roberts C, Steer T, Maplethorpe N *et al.* (2018) National diet and nutrition survey results from years 7 and 8 (combined) of the rolling programme (2014/2015–2015/2016).

463. Shepherd SJ, Gibson PR (2013) Nutritional inadequacies of the gluten-free diet in both recently-diagnosed and long-term patients with coeliac disease. *J Hum Nutr Diet* **26**, 349-358.

464. Korsmo-Haugen HK, Brurberg KG, Mann J *et al.* (2019) Carbohydrate quantity in the dietary management of type 2 diabetes: A systematic review and meta-analysis. *Diabetes Obes Metab* **21**, 15-27.

465. Stamataki NS, Yanni AE, Karathanos VT (2017) Bread making technology influences postprandial glucose response: a review of the clinical evidence. *Br J Nutr* **117**, 1001-1012.

466. Gobbetti M, Rizzello CG, Di Cagno R *et al.* (2014) How the sourdough may affect the functional features of leavened baked goods. *Food Microbiol* **37**, 30-40.

467. Lopez HW, Krespine V, Guy C *et al.* (2001) Prolonged fermentation of whole wheat sourdough reduces phytate level and increases soluble magnesium. *J Agric Food Chem* **49**, 2657-2662.

468. Rodriguez-Ramiro I, Brearley CA, Bruggraber SF *et al.* (2017) Assessment of iron

bioavailability from different bread making processes using an in vitro intestinal cell model. *Food Chem* **228**, 91-98.

469. L.K. K, L.D. V, Amnuaycheewa P *et al.* (2015) A Grounded Guide to Gluten: How Modern Genotypes and Processing Impact Wheat Sensitivity. *Comprehensive Reviews in Food Science and Food Safety* **14**, 285-302.

470. Greco L, Gobbetti M, Auricchio R *et al.* (2011) Safety for patients with celiac disease of baked goods made of wheat flour hydrolyzed during food processing. *Clin Gastroenterol Hepatol* **9**, 24-29.

471. Robinson E, Chambers K (2018) The challenge of increasing wholegrain intake in the UK. *Nutrition Bulletin* **43** 135–146.

472. Mann KD, Pearce MS, McKevith B *et al.* (2015) Low whole grain intake in the UK: results from the National Diet and Nutrition Survey rolling programme 2008-11. *Br J Nutr* **113**, 1643-1651.

473. Gardner CD, Hartle JC, Garrett RD *et al.* (2019) Maximizing the intersection of human health and the health of the environment with regard to the amount and type of protein produced and consumed in the United States. *Nutr Rev* **77**, 197-215.

474. Messina V (2014) Nutritional and health benefits of dried beans. *Am J Clin Nutr* **100 Suppl 1**, 437S-442S.

475. Henry CJ, Heppell N (2002) Nutritional losses and gains during processing: future problems and issues. *Proc Nutr Soc* **61**, 145-148.

476. Goni I, Valentin-Gamazo C (2003) Chickpea flour ingredient slows glycemic response to pasta in healthy volunteers. *Food Chemistry* **81**, 511-515.

477. Schlormann W, Birringer M, Bohm V *et al.* (2015) Influence of roasting conditions on health-related compounds in different nuts. *Food Chem* **180**, 77-85.

478. Sabate J, Oda K, Ros E (2010) Nut consumption and blood lipid levels: a pooled analysis of 25 intervention trials. *Arch Intern Med* **170**, 821-827.

479. Ortega RM, Palencia A, Lopez-Sobaler AM (2006) Improvement of cholesterol levels and reduction of cardiovascular risk via the consumption of phytosterols. *Br J Nutr* **96 Suppl 1**, S89-93.

480. Luu HN, Blot WJ, Xiang YB *et al.* (2015) Prospective evaluation of the association of nut/peanut consumption with total and cause-specific mortality. *JAMA Intern Med* **175**, 755-766.

481. Ros E (2015) Nuts and CVD. *Br J Nutr* **113 Suppl 2**, S111-120.

482. Peterson J, Dwyer J, Adlercreutz H *et al.* (2010) Dietary lignans: physiology and potential for cardiovascular disease risk reduction. *Nutr Rev* **68**, 571-603.

483. Mason JK, Thompson LU (2014) Flaxseed and its lignan and oil components: can they play a role in reducing the risk of and improving the treatment of breast cancer? *Appl Physiol Nutr Metab* **39**, 663-678.

484. Smeds AI, Eklund PC, Sjoholm RE *et al.* (2007) Quantification of a broad spectrum of lignans in cereals, oilseeds, and nuts. *J Agric Food Chem* **55**, 1337-1346.

485. Boucher BA, Wanigaratne S, Harris SA *et al.* (2018) Postdiagnosis Isoflavone and Lignan Intake in Newly Diagnosed Breast Cancer Patients: Cross-Sectional Survey Shows Considerable Intake from Previously Unassessed High-Lignan Foods. *Curr Dev Nutr* **2**, nzx009.

486. Krigasa N, Lazarib D, Maloupac E *et al.* (2015) Introducing Dittany of Crete (Origanum dictamnus L.) to gastronomy: A new culinary concept for a traditionally used medicinal plant. *International Journal of Gastronomy and Food Science*, 112-118.

487. Trichopoulou A (2012) Diversity v. globalization: traditional foods at the epicentre. *Public Health Nutr* **15**, 951-954.

488. Vasilopoulou E, Georga K, Bjoerkov Joergensen M *et al.* (2005) The antioxidant properties of Greek foods and the flavonoid content of the Mediterranean menu. *Curr Med Chem* **5**, 1-13??

489. Mueller M, Hobiger S, Jungbauer A (2010) Anti-inflammatory activity of extracts from fruits, herbs and spices. *Food Chemistry* **122**, 987-996.

490. Dragland S, Senoo H, Wake K *et al.* (2003) Several culinary and medicinal herbs are important sources of dietary antioxidants. *J Nutr* **133**, 1286-1290.

491. Deyno S, Eneyew K, Seyfe S *et al.* (2019) Efficacy and safety of cinnamon in type 2 diabetes mellitus and pre-diabetes patients: A meta-analysis and meta-regression. *Diabetes Res Clin Pract* **156**, 107815.

492. Medagama AB (2015) The glycaemic outcomes of Cinnamon, a review of the experimental evidence and clinical trials. *Nutr J* **14**, 108.

493. Opara EI (2019) Culinary herbs and spices: what can human studies tell us about their role in the prevention of chronic non-communicable diseases? *J Sci Food Agric* **99**, 4511-4517.

494. Visioli F, Franco M, Toledo E *et al.* (2018) Olive oil and prevention of chronic diseases: Summary of an International conference. *Nutr Metab Cardiovasc Dis* **28**, 649-656.

495. Schwingshackl L, Hoffmann G (2014) Monounsaturated fatty acids, olive oil and health status: a systematic review and meta-analysis of cohort studies. *Lipids Health Dis* **13**, 154.

496. Covas MI, Nyyssonen K, Poulsen HE *et al.* (2006) The effect of polyphenols in olive oil on heart disease risk factors: a randomized trial. *Ann Intern Med* **145**, 333-341.

497. Henderson L, Gregory J, Irving K *et al.* (2003) *The National Diet and Nutrition Survey: adults aged 19 to 64 years. Volume 2: Energy, protein, carbohydrate, fat and alcohol intake.* London: TSO.

498. Gaforio JJ, Visioli F, Alarcon-de-la-Lastra C *et al.* (2019) Virgin Olive Oil and Health: Summary of the III International Conference on Virgin Olive Oil and Health Consensus Report, JAEN (Spain) 2018. *Nutrients* **11**.

499. St-Laurent-Thibault C, Arseneault M, Longpre F *et al.* (2011) Tyrosol and hydroxytyrosol, two main components of olive oil, protect N2a cells against amyloid-beta-induced toxicity. Involvement of the NF-kappaB signaling. *Curr Alzheimer Res* **8**, 543-551.

500. Zamora-Zamoraa F, Martínez-Galiano JM, Gaforioc JJ *et al.* (2018) Effects of olive oil on blood pressure: A systematic review and meta-analysis. *GRASAS Y ACEITES 69 (4)* **69**, 1-9.

501. Buckland G, Mayen AL, Agudo A *et al.* (2012) Olive oil intake and mortality within the Spanish population (EPIC-Spain). *Am J Clin Nutr* **96**, 142-149.

502. Estruch R, Martinez-Gonzalez MA, Corella D *et al.* (2016) Effect of a high-fat Mediterranean diet on bodyweight and waist circumference: a prespecified secondary outcomes analysis of the PREDIMED randomised controlled trial. *Lancet Diabetes Endocrinol* **4**, 666-676.

503. Mancini JG, Filion KB, Atallah R *et al.* (2016) Systematic Review of the Mediterranean Diet for Long-Term Weight Loss. *Am J Med* **129**, 407-415 e404.

504. (2020) Dietary patterns associated with obesity outcomes in adults: an umbrella review. *Public Health Nutrition.*

505. Hall KD, Kahan S (2018) Maintenance of lost weight and long-term management of obesity. *Med Clin North Am* **102**, 183–197.

506. Sihag J, Jones PJH (2018) Oleoylethanolamide: The role of a bioactive lipid amide in modulating eating behaviour. *Obes Rev* **19**, 178-197.

507. Wang S, Li X, Rodrigues R *et al.* (2014) *Packaging influences on olive oil quality: A review of the literature.* UC Davis Olive Center.

508. Gargouri B, Zribi A, Bouaziz M (2015) Effect of containers on the quality of Chemlali olive oil during storage. *J Food Sci Technol* **52**, 1948-1959.

509. Leitzmann MF, Kurth T (2012) Fried foods and the risk of coronary heart disease. *BMJ* **344**, d8274.

510. Dobarganes C, Marquez-Ruiz G (2015) Possible adverse effects of frying with vegetable oils. *Br J Nutr* **113 Suppl 2**, S49-57.

511. Hoffman R, Gerber M (2014) Can rapeseed oil replace olive oil as part of a Mediterranean-style diet? *Br J Nutr* **112**, 1882-1895.

.512. Silva L, Pinto J, Carrola J *et al.* (2010) Oxidative stability of olive oil after food processing and comparison with other vegetable oils. *Food Chemistry* **121** 1177–1187.

513. Kummerow FA (2013) Interaction between sphingomyelin and oxysterols contributes to atherosclerosis and sudden death. *Am J Cardiovasc Dis* **3**, 17-26.

514. Medina I, Sacchi R, Aubourg S (1995) A C-NMR study of lipid alteration during fish canning: effect of filling medium. *J Sci Food Agric* **69**, 445-450.

515. Pedersen A, Baumstark MW, Marckmann P *et al.* (2000) An olive oil-rich diet results in higher concentrations of LDL cholesterol and a higher number of LDL subfraction particles than rapeseed oil and sunflower oil diets. *J Lipid Res* **41**, 1901-1911.

516. Ghazani SM, García-Llatas G, Marangoni AG (2013) Minor constituents in canola oil processed by traditional and minimal refining methods. *Journal of the American Oil Chemists' Society* **90**, 743-756.

517. de Lorgeril M, Salen P, Martin JL *et al.* (1999) Mediterranean diet, traditional risk factors, and the rate of cardiovascular complications after myocardial infarction: final report of the Lyon Diet Heart Study. *Circulation* **99**, 779-785.

518. de Lorgeril M, Salen P (2006) The Mediterranean-style diet for the prevention of cardiovascular diseases. *Public Health Nutr* **9**, 118-123.

519. Lauretti E, Pratico D (2017) Effect of canola oil consumption on memory, synapse and neuropathology in the triple transgenic mouse model of Alzheimer's disease. *Sci Rep* **7**, 17134.

520. Neelakantan N, Seah JYH, van Dam RM (2020) The Effect of Coconut Oil Consumption on Cardiovascular Risk Factors: A Systematic Review and Meta-Analysis of Clinical Trials. *Circulation* 10.1161/CIRCULATIONAHA.119.043052.

521. Zong G, Li Y, Wanders AJ *et al.* (2016) Intake of individual saturated fatty acids and risk of coronary heart disease in US men and women: two prospective longitudinal cohort studies. *BMJ* **355**, i5796.

522. Love HJ, Sulikowski D (2018) Of Meat and Men: Sex Differences in Implicit and Explicit Attitudes Toward Meat. *Front Psychol* **9**, 559.

523. Beardsworth A, Bryman A, Keil T (2002) Women, men and food: the significance of gender for nutritional attitudes and choices. . *Br Food J* **104**, 470–491.

524. Ponzio E, Mazzarini G, Gasperi G *et al.* (2015) The Vegetarian Habit in Italy: Prevalence and Characteristics of Consumers. *Ecol Food Nutr* **54**, 370–379.

525. Torjesen I (2019) WHO pulls support from initiative promoting global move to plant based foods. *BMJ* **365**, l1700.

526. Macdiarmid JI, Whybrow S (2019) Nutrition from a climate change perspective. *Proc Nutr Soc* 10.1017/S0029665118002896, 1-8.

527. von Keyserlingk MAG, Cestari AA, Franks B *et al.* (2017) Dairy cows value access to pasture as highly as fresh feed. *Scientific Reports* **7**.

528. Scherer L, Tomasik B, Rueda O *et al.* (2018) Framework for integrating animal welfare into life cycle sustainability assessment. *Int J Life Cycle Assess* **23**, 1476-1490.

529. Buckwell A, Nadeu E (2018) *What is the Safe Operating Space for EU Livestock?* : RISE Foundation, Brussels.

530. Clark B, Stewart GB, Panzone LA *et al.* (2017) Citizens, consumers and farm animal welfare: A meta-analysis of willingness-to-pay studies. *Food Policy* **68**, 112–127.

531. Zheng Y, Li Y, Satija A *et al.* (2019) Association of changes in red meat consumption with total and cause specific mortality among US women and men: two prospective cohort studies. *BMJ* **365**, l2110.

532. Wolk A (2017) Potential health hazards of eating red meat. *J Intern Med* **281**, 106-122.

533. World Cancer Research Fund / American Institute for Cancer Research (2018) Continuous Update Project Expert Report. Meat, fish and dairy products and the risk of cancer.

534. Hara A, Sasazuki S, Inoue M *et al.* (2012) Zinc and heme iron intakes and risk of colorectal cancer: a population-based prospective cohort study in Japan. *Am J Clin Nutr* **96**, 864-873.

535. Demeyer D, Mertens B, De Smet S *et al.* (2016) Mechanisms Linking Colorectal Cancer to the Consumption of (Processed) Red Meat: A Review. *Crit Rev Food Sci Nutr* **56**, 2747-2766.

536. de Vogel J, Jonker-Termont DS, van Lieshout EM *et al.* (2005) Green vegetables, red meat and colon cancer: chlorophyll prevents the cytotoxic and hyperproliferative effects of haem in

rat colon. *Carcinogenesis* **26**, 387-393.

537. Balder HF, Vogel J, Jansen MC *et al.* (2006) Heme and chlorophyll intake and risk of colorectal cancer in the Netherlands cohort study. *Cancer Epidemiol Biomarkers Prev* **15**, 717-725.

538. Kruger C, Zhou Y (2018) Red meat and colon cancer: A review of mechanistic evidence for heme in the context of risk assessment methodology. *Food Chem Toxicol* **118**, 131-153.

539. PENSABENE JW, FIDDLER W, GATES RA *et al.* (1974) EFFECT OF FRYING AND OTHER COOKING CONDITIONS ON NITROSOPYRROLIDINE FORMATION IN BACON. *Journal of Food Science* **39**, 314-316.

540. Etemadi A, Sinha R, Ward MH *et al.* (2017) Mortality from different causes associated with meat, heme iron, nitrates, and nitrites in the NIH-AARP Diet and Health Study: population based cohort study. *BMJ* **357**, j1957.

541. Anderson JJ, Darwis NDM, Mackay DF *et al.* (2018) Red and processed meat consumption and breast cancer: UK Biobank cohort study and meta-analysis. *Eur J Cancer* **90**, 73-82.

542. Liu G, Zong G, Hu FB *et al.* (2017) Cooking Methods for Red Meats and Risk of Type 2 Diabetes: A Prospective Study of U.S. Women. *Diabetes Care* **40**, 1041-1049.

543. Sugimura T, Wakabayashi K, Nakagama H *et al.* (2004) Heterocyclic amines: Mutagens/carcinogens produced during cooking of meat and fish. *Cancer Sci* **95**, 290-299.

544. Uribarri J, Woodruff S, Goodman S *et al.* (2010) Advanced glycation end products in foods and a practical guide to their reduction in the diet. *J Am Diet Assoc* **110**, 911-916 e912.

545. Liu G, Zong G, Wu K *et al.* (2018) Meat Cooking Methods and Risk of Type 2 Diabetes: Results From Three Prospective Cohort Studies. *Diabetes Care* **41**, 1049-1060.

546. Cai W, Uribarri J, Zhu L *et al.* (2014) Oral glycotoxins are a modifiable cause of dementia and the metabolic syndrome in mice and humans. *Proc Natl Acad Sci U S A* **111**, 4940-4945.

547. Sinha R, Peters U, Cross AJ *et al.* (2005) Meat, meat cooking methods and preservation, and risk for colorectal adenoma. *Cancer Res* **65**, 8034-8041.

548. Jakszyn P, Lujan-Barroso L, Agudo A *et al.* (2013) Meat and heme iron intake and esophageal adenocarcinoma in the European Prospective Investigation into Cancer and Nutrition study. *Int J Cancer* **133**, 2744-2750.

549. Choi Y, Song S, Song Y *et al.* (2013) Consumption of red and processed meat and esophageal cancer risk: meta-analysis. *World J Gastroenterol* **19**, 1020-1029.

550. Linseisen J, Kesse E, Slimani N *et al.* (2002) Meat consumption in the European Prospective Investigation into Cancer and Nutrition (EPIC) cohorts: results from 24-hour dietary recalls. *Public Health Nutr* **5**, 1243-1258.

551. Gibis M, Kruwinnus M, Weiss J (2015) Impact of different pan-frying conditions on the formation of heterocyclic aromatic amines and sensory quality in fried bacon. *Food Chem* **168**, 383-389.

552. Tsai SJ, Jenq SN, Lee H (1996) Naturally occurring diallyl disulfide inhibits the formation of carcinogenic heterocyclic aromatic amines in boiled pork juice. *Mutagenesis* **11**, 235-240.

553. Poulsen MW, Hedegaard RV, Andersen JM *et al.* (2013) Advanced glycation endproducts in food and their effects on health. *Food Chem Toxicol* **60**, 10-37.

554. Kromhout D, Keys A, Aravanis C *et al.* (1989) Food consumption patterns in the 1960s in seven countries. *Am J Clin Nutr* **49**, 889-894.

555. Srednicka-Tober D, Baranski M, Seal C *et al.* (2016) Composition differences between organic and conventional meat: a systematic literature review and meta-analysis. *Br J Nutr* **115**, 994-1011.

556. Howe P, Meyer B, Record S *et al.* (2006) Dietary intake of long-chain omega-3 polyunsaturated fatty acids: contribution of meat sources. *Nutrition* **22**, 47-53.

557. Daley CA, Abbott A, Doyle PS *et al.* (2010) A review of fatty acid profiles and antioxidant content in grass-fed and grain-fed beef. *Nutr J* **9**, 10.

558. Nuernberg K, Dannenberger D, ., Nuernberg G (2005) Effect of a grass-based and a concentrate feeding system onmeat quality characteristics and fatty acid composition of

longissimus muscle in different cattle breeds. *Livest Prod Sci* **94**, 137–147.

559. McAfee AJ, McSorley EM, Cuskelly GJ *et al.* (2010) Red meat from animals offered a grass diet increases plasma and platelet n-3 PUFA in healthy consumers. *Br J Nutr* **105**, 80-89.

560. Simopoulos AP (2001) The Mediterranean diets: What is so special about the diet of Greece? The scientific evidence. *J Nutr* **131**, 3065S-3073S.

561. Tapsell LC (2015) Fermented dairy food and CVD risk. *Br J Nutr* **113 Suppl 2**, S131-135.

562. Crichton GE, Alkerwi A (2014) Whole-fat dairy food intake is inversely associated with obesity prevalence: findings from the Observation of Cardiovascular Risk Factors in Luxembourg study. *Nutr Res* **34**, 936-943.

563. Mozaffarian D, de Oliveira Otto MC, Lemaitre RN *et al.* (2013) trans-Palmitoleic acid, other dairy fat biomarkers, and incident diabetes: the Multi-Ethnic Study of Atherosclerosis (MESA). *Am J Clin Nutr* **97**, 854-861.

564. Griffin BA (2015) Saturated fat: guidelines to reduce coronary heart disease risk are still valid. *The Pharmaceutical Journal.*

565. Thorning TK, Bertram HC, Bonjour JP *et al.* (2017) Whole dairy matrix or single nutrients in assessment of health effects: current evidence and knowledge gaps. *Am J Clin Nutr* **105**, 1033-1045.

566. Dehghan M, Mente A, Rangarajan S *et al.* (2018) Association of dairy intake with cardiovascular disease and mortality in 21 countries from five continents (PURE): a prospective cohort study. *Lancet* 10.1016/S0140-6736(18)31812-9.

567. Sacks FM, Lichtenstein AH, Wu JHY *et al.* (2017) Dietary Fats and Cardiovascular Disease: A Presidential Advisory From the American Heart Association. *Circulation* **136**, e1-e23.

568. de Oliveira Otto MC, Mozaffarian D, Kromhout D *et al.* (2012) Dietary intake of saturated fat by food source and incident cardiovascular disease: the Multi-Ethnic Study of Atherosclerosis. *Am J Clin Nutr* **96**, 397-404.

569. Koskinen TT, Virtanen HEK, Voutilainen S *et al.* (2018) Intake of fermented and non-fermented dairy products and risk of incident CHD: the Kuopio Ischaemic Heart Disease Risk Factor Study. *Br J Nutr* **120**, 1288-1297.

570. Mozaffarian D (2016) Dietary and Policy Priorities for Cardiovascular Disease, Diabetes, and Obesity: A Comprehensive Review. *Circulation* **133**, 187-225.

571. Feeney EL, Barron R, Dible V *et al.* (2018) Dairy matrix effects: response to consumption of dairy fat differs when eaten within the cheese matrix-a randomized controlled trial. *Am J Clin Nutr* **108**, 667-674.

572. Lovegrove JA, Hobbs DA (2016) New perspectives on dairy and cardiovascular health. *Proc Nutr Soc* **75**, 247-258.

573. Collins YF, McSweeney PLH, Wilkinson MG (2003) Lipolysis and free fatty acid catabolism in cheese: a review of current knowledge. *International Dairy Journal* **13**, 841–866.

574. Harrison S, Lennon R, Holly J *et al.* (2017) Does milk intake promote prostate cancer initiation or progression via effects on insulin-like growth factors (IGFs)? A systematic review and meta-analysis. *Cancer Causes Control* **28**, 497-528.

575. Aune D, Navarro Rosenblatt DA, Chan DS *et al.* (2015) Dairy products, calcium, and prostate cancer risk: a systematic review and meta-analysis of cohort studies. *Am J Clin Nutr* **101**, 87-117.

576. Research WCRFAIfC (2018) *Diet, nutrition, physical activity ans prostate cancer.*

577. Hall WL (2017) The future for long chain n-3 PUFA in the prevention of coronary heart disease: do we need to target non-fish-eaters? *Proc Nutr Soc* **76**, 408-418.

578. Li N, Wub X, Zhuangb W (2020) Fish consumption and multiple health outcomes: Umbrella review. *Trends in Food Science & Technology 99 (2020) 273–283* **99**, 273-283.

579. Lund EK (2013) Health benefits of seafood; is it just the fatty acids? *Food Chem* **140**, 413-420.

580. Lai HT, de Oliveira Otto MC, Lemaitre RN *et al.* (2018) Serial circulating omega 3 polyunsaturated fatty acids and healthy ageing among older adults in the Cardiovascular Health

Study: prospective cohort study. *BMJ* **363**, k4067.

581. Calder PC (2017) Omega-3 fatty acids and inflammatory processes: from molecules to man. *Biochem Soc Trans* **45**, 1105-1115.

582. Manson JE, Mora S, Cook NR (2019) Marine n-3 Fatty Acids and Vitamin D Supplementation and Primary Prevention. Reply. *N Engl J Med* **380**, 1879-1880.

583. Calder PC (2014) Very long chain omega-3 (n-3) fatty acids and human health. *Eur J Lipid Sci Technol* **116**, 1280–1300.

584. Jonathan Shepherd C, Monroig O, Tocher DR (2017) Future availability of raw materials for salmon feeds and supply chain implications: The case of Scottish farmed salmon. *Aquaculture* **467**, 49–62.

585. Henriques J, Dick JR, Tocher DR *et al.* (2014) Nutritional quality of salmon products available from major retailers in the UK: content and composition of n-3 long-chain PUFA. *Br J Nutr* **112**, 964-975.

586. Fry JM (2012) *Carbon Footprint of Scottish Suspended Mussels and Intertidal Oysters; SARF078.* SARF078; Environmental Resources Management: London, UK,.

587. Venugopal V, Gopakumar K (2017) Shellfish: Nutritive Value, Health Benefits, and Consumer Safety. *Comprehensive Reviews in Food Science and Food Safety* **16**, 1219-1242.

588. Trichopoulou A, Bamia C, Trichopoulos D (2009) Anatomy of health effects of Mediterranean diet: Greek EPIC prospective cohort study. *Bmj* **338**, b2337.

589. Eleftheriou D, Benetou V, Trichopoulou A *et al.* (2018) Mediterranean diet and its components in relation to all-cause mortality: meta-analysis. *Br J Nutr* **120**, 1081-1097.

590. Moberly T (2018) Public health experts split over deal with industry funded charity. *BMJ* **362**, k3942.

591. Kypri K, McCambridge J (2018) Alcohol must be recognised as a drug. *BMJ* **362**, k3944.

592. Boban M, Stockley C, Teissedre PL *et al.* (2016) Drinking pattern of wine and effects on human health: why should we drink moderately and with meals? *Food Funct* **7**, 2937-2942.

593. Yasar S (2018) Relation between alcohol consumption in midlife and dementia in late life. *BMJ* **362**, k3164.

594. Ferrieres J (2004) The French paradox: lessons for other countries. *Heart* **90**, 107-111.

595. Bagnardi V, Rota M, Botteri E *et al.* (2013) Light alcohol drinking and cancer: a meta-analysis. *Ann Oncol* **24**, 301-308.

596. Cao Y, Willett WC, Rimm EB *et al.* (2015) Light to moderate intake of alcohol, drinking patterns, and risk of cancer: results from two prospective US cohort studies. *BMJ* **351**, h4238.

597. Trichopoulou A, Bamia C, Lagiou P *et al.* (2010) Conformity to traditional Mediterranean diet and breast cancer risk in the Greek EPIC (European Prospective Investigation into Cancer and Nutrition) cohort. *Am J Clin Nutr* **92**, 620-625.

598. Research WCRFAIfC (2018) *Diet, Nutrition, Physical Activity and Cancer A Global Perspective A Summary of the Third Expert Report.*

599. Schwingshackl L, Schwedhelm C, Galbete C *et al.* (2017) Adherence to Mediterranean Diet and Risk of Cancer: An Updated Systematic Review and Meta-Analysis. *Nutrients* **9**.

600. Kontou N, Psaltopoulou T, Soupos N *et al.* (2012) Alcohol consumption and colorectal cancer in a Mediterranean population: a case-control study. *Dis Colon Rectum* **55**, 703-710.

601. Samoli E, Lagiou A, Nikolopoulos E *et al.* (2010) Mediterranean diet and upper aerodigestive tract cancer: the Greek segment of the Alcohol-Related Cancers and Genetic Susceptibility in Europe study. *Br J Nutr* **104**, 1369-1374.

602. Owen RW, Mier W, Giacosa A *et al.* (2000) Identification of lignans as major components in the phenolic fraction of olive oil. *Clin Chem* **46**, 976-988.

603. Kyro C, Zamora-Ros R, Scalbert A *et al.* (2015) Pre-diagnostic polyphenol intake and breast cancer survival: the European Prospective Investigation into Cancer and Nutrition (EPIC) cohort. *Breast Cancer Res Treat* **154**, 389-401.

604. Davis C, Bryan J, Hodgson J *et al.* (2015) Definition of the Mediterranean Diet; a Literature Review. *Nutrients* **7**, 9139-9153.

605. Romieu I, Ferrari P, Chajes V *et al.* (2017) Fiber intake modulates the association of alcohol intake with breast cancer. *Int J Cancer* **140**, 316-321.

606. de Batlle J, Ferrari P, Chajes V *et al.* (2015) Dietary folate intake and breast cancer risk: European prospective investigation into cancer and nutrition. *J Natl Cancer Inst* **107**, 367.

607. Maciel ME, Castro GD, Castro JA (2004) Inhibition of the rat breast cytosolic bioactivation of ethanol to acetaldehyde by some plant polyphenols and folic acid. *Nutr Cancer* **49**, 94-99.

608. Maciel ME, Castro JA, Castro GD (2011) Inhibition of rat mammary microsomal oxidation of ethanol to acetaldehyde by plant polyphenols. *Hum Exp Toxicol* **30**, 656-664.

609. Wood AM, Kaptoge S, Butterworth AS *et al.* (2018) Risk thresholds for alcohol consumption: combined analysis of individual-participant data for 599 912 current drinkers in 83 prospective studies. *Lancet* **391**, 1513-1523.

610. Astrup A, Costanzo S, de Gaetano G (2018) Risk thresholds for alcohol consumption. *Lancet* **392**, 2165-2166.

611. Poli A, Marangoni F, Avogaro A *et al.* (2013) Moderate alcohol use and health: a consensus document. *Nutr Metab Cardiovasc Dis* **23**, 487-504.

612. Lundgaard I, Wang W, Eberhardt A *et al.* (2018) Beneficial effects of low alcohol exposure, but adverse effects of high alcohol intake on glymphatic function. *Sci Rep* **8**, 2246.

613. Cederbaum AI (2012) Alcohol metabolism. *Clin Liver Dis* **16**, 667-685.

614. Sanchez-Bayona R, Gea A, Gardeazabal I *et al.* (2020) Binge Drinking and Risk of Breast Cancer: Results from the SUN ('Seguimiento Universidad de Navarra') Project. *Nutrients* **12**.

615. Lachenmeier DW, Sohnius EM (2008) The role of acetaldehyde outside ethanol metabolism in the carcinogenicity of alcoholic beverages: evidence from a large chemical survey. *Food Chem Toxicol* **46**, 2903-2911.

616. Seitz HK, Becker P (2007) Alcohol metabolism and cancer risk. *Alcohol Res Health* **30**, 38-41, 44-37.

617. Gea A, Bes-Rastrollo M, Toledo E *et al.* (2014) Mediterranean alcohol-drinking pattern and mortality in the SUN (Seguimiento Universidad de Navarra) Project: a prospective cohort study. *Br J Nutr* **111**, 1871-1880.

618. Hernandez-Hernandez A, Gea A, Ruiz-Canela M *et al.* (2015) Mediterranean Alcohol-Drinking Pattern and the Incidence of Cardiovascular Disease and Cardiovascular Mortality: The SUN Project. *Nutrients* **7**, 9116-9126.

619. Haseeb S, Alexander B, Baranchuk A (2017) Wine and Cardiovascular Health: A Comprehensive Review. *Circulation* **136**, 1434-1448.

620. Bohn T (2014) Dietary factors affecting polyphenol bioavailability. *Nutr Rev* **72**, 429-452.

621. Snopek L, Mlcek J, Sochorova L *et al.* (2018) Contribution of Red Wine Consumption to Human Health Protection. *Molecules* **23**.

622. Peluso I, Manafikhi H, Reggi R *et al.* (2015) Effects of red wine on postprandial stress: potential implication in non-alcoholic fatty liver disease development. *Eur J Nutr* **54**, 497-507.

623. Lippi G, Franchini M, Guidi GC (2010) Red wine and cardiovascular health: the "French Paradox" revisited. *International Journal of Wine Research* **2**, 1-7.

624. Gorelik S, Ligumsky M, Kohen R *et al.* (2008) The stomach as a "bioreactor": when red meat meets red wine. *J Agric Food Chem* **56**, 5002-5007.

625. Kanner J, Lapidot T (2001) The stomach as a bioreactor: dietary lipid peroxidation in the gastric fluid and the effects of plant-derived antioxidants. *Free Radic Biol Med* **31**, 1388-1395.

626. Natella F, Macone A, Ramberti A *et al.* (2011) Red wine prevents the postprandial increase in plasma cholesterol oxidation products: a pilot study. *Br J Nutr* **105**, 1718-1723.

627. Renaud S, de Lorgeril M (1992) Wine, alcohol, platelets, and the French paradox for coronary heart disease. *Lancet* **339**, 1523-1526.

628. McDonald JA, Goyal A, Terry MB (2013) Alcohol Intake and Breast Cancer Risk: Weighing the Overall Evidence. *Curr Breast Cancer Rep* **5**.

629. Brooks PJ, Enoch MA, Goldman D *et al.* (2009) The alcohol flushing response: an

unrecognized risk factor for esophageal cancer from alcohol consumption. *PLoS Med* **6**, e50.

630. Kypri K, Vater T, Bowe SJ *et al.* (2014) Web-based alcohol screening and brief intervention for university students: a randomized trial. *JAMA* **311**, 1218-1224.

631. Park T (2019) *A Menu for Change*. The Behavioural Insights Team.

632. Wolfson JA, Leung CW, Richardson CR (2020) More frequent cooking at home is associated with higher Healthy Eating Index-2015 score. *Public Health Nutr* **23**, 2384-2394.

633. Flego A, Herbert J, Gibbs L *et al.* (2013) Methods for the evaluation of the Jamie Oliver Ministry of Food program, Australia. *BMC Public Health* **13**, 411.

634. Bagwell S, O'Keefe E, Doff S *et al.* (2014) *Encouraging Healthier Takeaways in Low-income Communities: Tools to support those working to encourage healthier catering amongst fast food takeaways.*

635. Jaworowska A, Blackham TM, Long R *et al.* (2014) Nutritional composition of takeaway food in the UK. *Nutrition & Food Science* **44**, 414-430.

636. Lachat C, Nago E, Verstraeten R *et al.* (2012) Eating out of home and its association with dietary intake: a systematic review of the evidence. *Obes Rev* **13**, 329-346.

637. Goffe L, Rushton S, White M *et al.* (2017) Relationship between mean daily energy intake and frequency of consumption of out-of-home meals in the UK National Diet and Nutrition Survey. *Int J Behav Nutr Phys Act* **14**, 131.

638. Roe M, Pinchen H, Church S *et al.* (2013) Trans fatty acids in a range of UK processed foods. *Food Chemistry* **140**, 427–431.

639. Thompson C, Ponsford R, Lewis D *et al.* (2018) Fast-food, everyday life and health: A qualitative study of 'chicken shops' in East London. *Appetite* **128**, 7-13.

640. Goffe L, Penn L, Adams J *et al.* (2018) The challenges of interventions to promote healthier food in independent takeaways in England: qualitative study of intervention deliverers' views. *BMC Public Health* **18**, 184.

641. Lavelle F, McGowan L, Spence M *et al.* (2016) Barriers and facilitators to cooking from 'scratch' using basic or raw ingredients: A qualitative interview study. *Appetite* **107**, 383-391.

642. Steptoe A, Deaton A, Stone AA (2015) Subjective wellbeing, health, and ageing. *Lancet* **385**, 640-648.

643. Steptoe A, Wardle J, Marmot M (2005) Positive affect and health-related neuroendocrine, cardiovascular, and inflammatory processes. *Proc Natl Acad Sci U S A* **102**, 6508-6512.

644. Hutchinson JMC (2005) Is more choice always desirable? Evidence and arguments from leks, food selection, and environmental enrichment. *Biol Rev* **80**, 73–92.

645. Pulker CE, Trapp GSA, Scott JA *et al.* (2018) Global supermarkets' corporate social responsibility commitments to public health: a content analysis. *Global Health* **14**, 121.

646. Thornton LE, Cameron AJ, McNaughton SA *et al.* (2013) Does the availability of snack foods in supermarkets vary internationally? *Int J Behav Nutr Phys Act* **10**, 56.

647. Cameron AJ, Thornton LE, McNaughton SA *et al.* (2013) Variation in supermarket exposure to energy-dense snack foods by socio-economic position. *Public Health Nutr* **16**, 1178-1185.

648. Scott C, J. S, Taylor A (2018) *Affordability of the UK's Eatwell Guide*. The Food Foundation.

649. Food Foundation (2019) The Broken Plate.

650. Snowden C (2017) *Cheap as Chips - Is a Healthy Diet Affordable? IEA Discussion Paper no. 82.* Institute of Economic Affairs.

651. Rao M, Afshin A, Singh G *et al.* (2013) Do healthier foods and diet patterns cost more than less healthy options? A systematic review and meta-analysis. *BMJ Open* **3**, e004277.

652. Afshin A, Penalvo JL, Del Gobbo L *et al.* (2017) The prospective impact of food pricing on improving dietary consumption: A systematic review and meta-analysis. *PLoS One* **12**, e0172277.

653. Bonaccio M, Bonanni AE, Di Castelnuovo A *et al.* (2012) Low income is associated with poor adherence to a Mediterranean diet and a higher prevalence of obesity: cross-sectional results from the Moli-sani study. *BMJ Open* **2**.

654. Lara J, Turbett E, McKevic A *et al.* (2015) The Mediterranean diet among British older

adults: Its understanding, acceptability and the feasibility of a randomised brief intervention with two levels of dietary advice. *Maturitas* **82**, 387-393.

655. Drewnowski A, Eichelsdoerfer P (2009) The Mediterranean diet: does it have to cost more? *Public Health Nutr* **12**, 1621-1628.

656. Marty L, Dubois C, Gaubard MS *et al.* (2015) Higher nutritional quality at no additional cost among low-income households: insights from food purchases of "positive deviants". *Am J Clin Nutr* **102**, 190-198.

657. Dubois C, Tharrey M, Darmon N (2017) Identifying foods with good nutritional quality and price for the Opticourses intervention research project. *Public Health Nutr* **20**, 3051-3059.

658. Masic U, Yeomans MR (2014) Umami flavor enhances appetite but also increases satiety. *Am J Clin Nutr* **100**, 532-538.

659. Alkerwi A, Crichton GE, Hebert JR (2015) Consumption of ready-made meals and increased risk of obesity: findings from the Observation of Cardiovascular Risk Factors in Luxembourg (ORISCAV-LUX) study. *Br J Nutr* **113**, 270-277.

660. Ohkuma T, Hirakawa Y, Nakamura U *et al.* (2015) Association between eating rate and obesity: a systematic review and meta-analysis. *Int J Obes (Lond)* **39**, 1589-1596.

661. Hurst Y, Fukuda H (2018) Effects of changes in eating speed on obesity in patients with diabetes: a secondary analysis of longitudinal health check-up data. *BMJ Open* **8**, e019589.

662. Paz-Graniel I, Babio N, Mendez I *et al.* (2019) Association between Eating Speed and Classical Cardiovascular Risk Factors: A Cross-Sectional Study. *Nutrients* **11**.

663. Shah M, Copeland J, Dart L *et al.* (2014) Slower eating speed lowers energy intake in normal-weight but not overweight/obese subjects. *J Acad Nutr Diet* **114**, 393-402.

664. Scott KA, Melhorn SJ, Sakai RR (2012) Effects of Chronic Social Stress on Obesity. *Curr Obes Rep* **1**, 16-25.

665. Ferreira Antunes JL, Toporcov TN, Biazevic MG *et al.* (2013) Joint and independent effects of alcohol drinking and tobacco smoking on oral cancer: a large case-control study. *PLoS One* **8**, e68132.

666. Schanes K, Dobernig K, Gozet B (2018) Food waste matters - A systematic review of household food waste practices and their policy implications. *Journal of Cleaner Production* **182**, 978-991.

667. Gustavsson J, Cederberg C, Sonesson U *et al.* (2011) *Global Food Losses and Food Waste.* Food and Agriculture Organization of the United Nations.

668. Schader C, Muller A, Scialabba Nel H *et al.* (2015) Impacts of feeding less food-competing feedstuffs to livestock on global food system sustainability. *J R Soc Interface* **12**, 20150891.

669. Food FaCC (2019) *Field Guide for the Future.* RSA.

670. Lenton TM, Rockstrom J, Gaffney O *et al.* (2019) Climate tipping points - too risky to bet against. *Nature* **575**, 592-595.

671. Laybourn-Langton L, Rankin L, Baxter D (2019) *This is a crisis: Facing up to the age of environmental breakdown.*

672. Sánchez-Bayoa F, Wyckhuysb KAG (2019) Worldwide decline of the entomofauna: A review of its drivers. *Biological Conservation* **232**, 8-27.

673. Mbow C, Rosenzweig C, Tubiello F *et al.* (2019) *Food security. Climate Change and Land: an IPCC special report on climate change, desertification, land degradation, sustainable land management, food security and greenhouse gas fluxes in terrestrial ecosystems.*

674. Committee on Climate Change (2018) *Reducing UK emissions 2018 Progress Report to Parliament.*

675. Clune S, Crossin E, Verghese K (2017) Systematic review of greenhouse gas emissions for different fresh food categories. *Journal of Cleaner Production* **140**, 766-783.

676. Wang T, Teague WR, Park SC *et al.* (2015) GHG Mitigation Potential of Different Grazing Strategies in the United States Southern Great Plains. *Sustainability* **7**, 13500-13521.

677. Gerber PJ, Steinfeld H, Henderson B *et al.* (2013) Tackling climate change through livestock – A global assessment of emissions and mitigation opportunities. *Food and Agriculture*

*Organization of the United Nations (FAO), Rome.*
678. Committee on Climate Change (2019) *Net Zero: The UK's contribution to stopping global warming.*
679. Wellesley L, Happer C, Froggatt A (2015) *Changing Climate, Changing Diets Pathways to Lower Meat Consumption. Chatham House Report.* Chatham House.
680. Röös E, Carlsson G, Ferawati F *et al.* (2018) Less meat, more legumes: prospects and challenges in the transition toward sustainable diets in Sweden. *Renewable Agriculture and Food Systems* https://doi.org/10.1017/S1742170518000443, 1-14.
681. Pierrehumbert RT, Eshel G (2015) Climate impact of beef: an analysis considering multiple time scales and production methods without use of global warming potentials. *Environ Res Lett* **10**.
682. Garnett T, Godde C, Muller A (2017) *Grazed and Confused.* Food Climate Research Network.
683. Lynch J (2019) Availability of disaggregated greenhouse gas emissions from beef cattle production: A systematic review. *Environmental Impact Assessment Review* **76**, 69-78.
684. Bellarby J, Tirado R, Leip A *et al.* (2013) Livestock greenhouse gas emissions and mitigation potential in Europe. *Glob Chang Biol* **19**, 3-18.
685. IPES-Food. (2016) *From uniformity to diversity: a paradigm shift from industrial agriculture to diversified agroecological systems.* . International Panel of Experts on Sustainable Food systems.
686. Kromhout D, Spaaij CJ, de Goede J *et al.* (2016) The 2015 Dutch food-based dietary guidelines. *Eur J Clin Nutr* **70**, 869-878.
687. UK Parliament Post (2020) *A resilient UK food system.*
688. Swinburn BA, Kraak VI, Allender S *et al.* (2019) The Global Syndemic of Obesity, Undernutrition, and Climate Change: The Lancet Commission report. *Lancet* **393**, 791-846.
689. Lucas T, Horton R (2019) The 21st-century great food transformation. *Lancet* **393**, 386-387.
690. Aubert P, Schwoob M, Poux X (2019) *Agroecology and carbon neutrality in Europe by 2050: what are the issues? Findings from the TYFA modelling exercise.* IDDRI.
691. The Economist Intelligence Unit (2018) *Fixing Food 2018 Best Practice Towards the Sustainability Goals.*
692. EUROPEAN COMMISSION (2020) *A Farm to Fork Strategy for a fair, healthy and environmentally-friendly food system.*
693. Piesse J, Thirtle C (2010) Agricultural R&D, technology and productivity. *Philos Trans R Soc Lond B Biol Sci* **365**, 3035-3047.
694. Altieri MA, Toledo VM (2011) The agroecological revolution in Latin America: rescuing nature, ensuring food sovereignty and empowering peasants. . *The Journal of Peasant Studies* **38**, 587–612.
695. Salazar E, Billing S, Breen M (2020) *We need to talk about chicken.* Eating Better.
696. de Boer J, Aiking H (2018) Prospects for pro-environmental protein consumption in Europe: Cultural, culinary, economic and psychological factors. *Appetite* **121**, 29-40.
697. Ryschawy J, Choisis N, Choisis JP *et al.* (2012) Mixed crop-livestock systems: an economic and environmental-friendly way of farming? *Animal* **6**, 1722-1730.
698. Commission E (2019) *THE POST-2020 COMMON AGRICULTURAL POLICY: ENVIRONMENTAL BENEFITS AND SIMPLIFICATION.*
699. Lal R (2004) Soil carbon sequestration impacts on global climate change and food security. *Science* **304**, 1623-1627.
700. Fisher MJ, Rao IM, Ayarza MA *et al.* (1994) Carbon storage by introduced deep-rooted grasses in the South American savannas. *Nature* **371**, 236-238.
701. Garnett T, Godde C, Muller A *et al.* (2017) *Grazed and confused? Ruminating on cattle, grazing systems, methane, nitrous oxide, the soil carbon sequestration question – And what it all means for greenhouse gas emissions.* Oxford, UK.: Oxford, UK: Food Climate Research Network, University of Oxford.

702. Reganold JP, Wachter JM (2016) Organic agriculture in the twenty-first century. *Nat Plants* **2**, 15221.

703. Hallmann CA, Sorg M, Jongejans E *et al.* (2017) More than 75 percent decline over 27 years in total flying insect biomass in protected areas. *PLoS One* **12**, e0185809.

704. FAO and WHO (2019) *Sustainable healthy diets – Guiding principles.* . Rome.

705. Scheliecher J, Zaehringer JG, Fastre C *et al.* (2019) Protecting half of the planet could affect over one billlion people. *Nature Sustainability* doi:10.1038/s41893-019-0423-y.

706. Aleksandrowicz L, Green R, Joy EJ *et al.* (2016) The Impacts of Dietary Change on Greenhouse Gas Emissions, Land Use, Water Use, and Health: A Systematic Review. *PLoS One* **11**, e0165797.

707. Heller MC, Keoleian GA (2015) Greenhouse gas emission estimates of U.S. dietary choices and food loss. *J Ind Ecol* **19**, 391-401.

708. van Huis A (2016) Edible insects are the future? *Proc Nutr Soc* **75**, 294-305.

709. Tubb C, Seba T (2019) *Rethinking Food and Agriculture 2020-2030*. RethinkX.

710. Lynch J, Pierrehumbert R (2019) Climate Impacts of Cultured Meat and Beef Cattle. *Front Sustain Food Syst* **3**, 1-11.

711. Saez-Almendros S, Obrador B, Bach-Faig A *et al.* (2013) Environmental footprints of Mediterranean versus Western dietary patterns: beyond the health benefits of the Mediterranean diet. *Environ Health* **12**, 118.

712. van Dooren C, Marinussen M, Blonk H *et al.* (2014) Exploring dietary guidelines based on ecological and nutritional values: A comparison of six dietary patterns. *Food Policy* **44**, 36-46.

713. Food FaCC (2019) *Our Future in the Land*. RSA.

714. Medland L (2016) Working for social sustainability: insights from a Spanish organic production enclave. *Agroecology and Sustainable Food Systems* **40**, 1133–1156.

715. New Citizenship Project (2017) *Food Citizenship*.

716. Wezel A, Bellon S, Doré T *et al.* (2009) Agroecology as a science, a movement and a practice. A review. *Agronomy for Sustainable Development* **29**, 503-515.

717. Hare B (2017) Survival of the Friendliest: Homo sapiens Evolved via Selection for Prosociality. *Annu Rev Psychol* **68**, 155-186.

444